Shocked

Shocked

Insider stories

about

Electroconvulsive therapy

Professor George Kirov

First published independently in 2020
on Amazon Kindle Direct Publishing

ISBN paperback: 9798630913944

Editor: Fiona Marshall
Interior design: Petya Tsankova
Cover design: Natalia Junqueira

To the NHS staff who have risked their lives caring for patients during the COVID-19 pandemic.

To my family who has supported and tolerated me all these years.

To my parents who would have been happy to see me write this book.

TABLE OF CONTENTS

INDEX OF ABBREVIATIONS

CBT	Cognitive Behaviour Therapy
CMT	Charcot-Marie-Tooth disease
CNV	Copy Number Variation. Deletions or duplications of large stretches of genetic material
HAM-D	Hamilton Depression Rating Scale
ECG	Electrocardiogram
ECT	Electroconvulsive Therapy
ECTAS	ECT Accreditation Service
EEG	Electroencephalogram
mC	millicoulomb, unit of electric charge. A Coulomb (1000mC) is the quantity of electricity conveyed in one second by a current of one ampere. ECT machines in the UK are set to deliver between 10mC and 1152mC. The settings increase in steps of about 11mC, so the mC settings might appear illogical.
MMSE	Mini Mental State Examination. A rating scale for global cognitive function (maximum score of 30 points)
MRI	Magnetic resonance imaging
MS	Multiple Sclerosis
NICE	National Institute for Health and Care Excellence
SHO	Senior House Officer

PREFACE

'More than half of the patients treated in our unit reach remission within 12 ECT sessions.'

Behind these dry, anonymous statistics are the personal stories of people who went through suffering and mental anguish of such severity that it resulted in this treatment of last resort. This book is about these individual stories.

I have chosen stories with more than their fair share of drama and complications, those that left stronger impressions in my memory. To protect privacy, I have changed many personal details and events, or have combined details of different patients, although never to the extent that would affect the clinical decisions that were taken in the individual cases, or their outcomes. A couple of stories are based on typical clinical scenarios, rather than on one single patient, so any similarities with real persons, except for the most unique of events, are coincidental and only reflect the fact that these presentations happen repeatedly in the clinic. These are often success stories, but I didn't spare the reader the things that can go wrong, such as the memory problems, arrhythmias and tricky decisions we have to make. The views expressed throughout the book are my own and although in my view correct, do not necessarily represent the official views of any organisation. The titles of the chapters do not imply that they contain instructions about the treatment of the respective conditions.

I AM SHOCKED

For many people, even many medical professionals, electroconvulsive therapy (ECT) is shrouded in mystery. This first story is a gentle introduction to ECT and the main concepts around it. It is about a straightforward treatment course, where everything went well, and no difficult decisions needed to be made. While the treatment was standard, the patient's story was rather more dramatic.

Catherine's husband was struggling to cope with his wife's illness. She hadn't mentioned suicide, but he had been warned to keep an eye on her. Depression was nothing new for Catherine. A few months earlier she had slipped back into another episode - her fourth in the past 10 years. The previous three episodes had all been treated successfully, responding quickly to the same antidepressant. Millions of people experience such episodes, and yet this time it seemed different. After her second bout of depression, Catherine had retired as a medical doctor but had led an active life, going to concerts, taking walks, reading books. But now, there were already signs that her depression was more serious than her previous bouts had been. It soon became evident that her usual antidepressant wasn't working. Far from it, in fact. Day after day, for nearly six months, she became gradually slower, losing interest in her usual activities, and staying at home practically all the time. She had almost stopped eating, and her weight had dropped by six kilograms. She couldn't finish anything; in fact, she was incapable of starting anything. Her answers were increasingly vague and confused, and as for questions, she had stopped asking any. Admission to hospital had been discussed, but she had refused.

Alarm bells went off for her psychiatrist who advised her husband to be vigilant. He took heed and one morning, when Catherine seemed to be spending too long in the bathroom, he went upstairs to check that she was all right. The bathroom door was locked and there was no response to his calls. A firm push on the door dislodged the flimsy latch and revealed a scene that filled him with horror: Catherine was lying in the bath, her face just above the water, as white as paper. But the bath wasn't just full of water. It appeared to be full of blood. Mr Jones rushed to pull her out. This wasn't that difficult, as she weighed even less now, having lost so much blood. On the inside of her thigh he saw a small trickle of blood. The ambulance arrived quickly. In hospital Catherine was given several litres of blood transfusion. The little cut on her thigh turned out to be quite deep. She had tried to sever her femoral artery with a pair of nail scissors. As a doctor, she knew that cutting a vein isn't a very efficient way of killing oneself, so she went for an artery, one that carries a lot of blood. She also knew that it passes close under the skin at one point and had probably felt its pulsations on several past patients while assessing the blood supply to their legs. However, Catherine wasn't a surgeon, wasn't using an adequate instrument, and probably it hurt too much in any case, so mercifully, she failed to cut it completely. Otherwise, she would have died within minutes. Doctors and farmers are very successful in completing suicides - farmers know how animals are slaughtered and also have dangerous tools to hand, sometimes even firearms. Doctors know what can kill you.

Once stabilised, Catherine was transferred to the psychiatric ward. The team didn't hesitate too much over which treatment she needed. Although her life had been saved, this patient was clearly in great danger, not just because she could kill herself suddenly and violently, but also because she could simply starve herself - she had lost another three kilograms since her admission. There was no time to wait for a second antidepressant and the added antipsychotic to work, as they could take weeks and might not prove effective anyway. Catherine was referred for ECT. She didn't consent to it but didn't object to it either. This wasn't through apathy, but through sheer incapacity. In fact, she wasn't even able to reason about her illness and the treatments at this point. Later, she told me that she had felt stupid, weak and confused, and so limited in concentration and focus that she hadn't been able to listen to the end of a song. She had been unable to think clearly for months.

When I first saw her, her speech was slow and faltering, her eyes wandering aimlessly around the room. She was unable to give clear answers even to simple questions, or to tell me what was wrong with her and when it had started. There was a vague suggestion of something shameful from her past, but her words never finished the thought that was started, her speech disintegrated into muttering, and facts remained absent. I had no doubt whatsoever that all the terrible things that she thought she had done, had happened in her mind only.

'No, no, that's wrong,' she moaned a few times, not always in response to a question. The nurses completed the picture: at times Catherine would pace along the corridor, freeze for a few seconds, and then throw herself on the floor, wringing her hands. She was suspicious of the medication offered to her and would spend minutes looking at the tablets and at the nurses offering them. On one occasion she pointed out that the staff were not real.

The Mental Capacity Act was used to treat her without her consent, as she did not object to having the treatment but had no capacity to make the decision.[1] We set up Catherine's first treatment as soon as possible. She lay down on the bed without saying anything and vacantly watched the nurses attaching wires to her body: ECG to the chest, EEG to the forehead and behind the ears, a blood pressure cuff to one arm and a pulse/oxygen meter to a finger. When everything was in place, Magdi, our consultant anaesthetist, inserted a needle into a wrist vein, and put an oxygen mask over her face. The monitor soon showed 100% oxygen saturation and Magdi injected 350mg of Thiopental into the vein. After just a few seconds, Catherine's eyes closed.

'Open your eyes,' Magdi said, to make sure she was asleep. Her eyes remained closed and there was no reaction to him stroking her eyelids. She was ready to receive Suxamethonium, a very short-acting muscle relaxant, which would prevent her from contracting her muscles during the seizure, to avoid injuries and muscle

---

[1] Patients who lack capacity to consent, but appear to adhere to the treatment, can receive ECT under the Mental Capacity Act. It is preferred as the less restrictive option, compared to sectioning under the Mental Health Act, in terms of the patient's freedom.

aches. During the next minute we kept watching out for the tiny twitches in her muscles that indicated that the muscle relaxant had found its way to the myriads of neuromuscular junctions where the nerves meet the muscles to relay the instructions for movements. After the twitches were over (the correct name is fasciculations), she was ready. Kara, our lead nurse, put a soft mouthguard between Catherine's teeth, to prevent them from being damaged, as the jaws clench strongly, even with muscle relaxation. The junior doctor placed the two electrodes over Catherine's temples. 'Impedance is fine,' pronounced Kara (the machine had performed a test of the impedance, i.e. the resistance to the electrical current caused by the skin and the skull, and a green light indicated it was within the right range). 'Happy to proceed?' she added, checking that I didn't have any objections to the precise placement of the electrodes over the patient's temples. Everything was fine, so I nodded encouragingly.

At the first treatment, we want to establish the seizure threshold, i.e. the minimum amount of electricity required to elicit a seizure, so that we don't give patients an unnecessarily high dose. Today we started with 126mC of electric charge,[2] higher than usual, as we took into account that both her use of Diazepam and her age (over 70) would make her somewhat resistant to seizures. (Diazepam is even used to stop epileptic seizures and always interferes with ECT treatment.) Kara pressed the yellow button on the ECT machine, and a warning noise

---

[2] mC = millicoulombs, a measure of electric charge. ECT machines in the UK are set to deliver between 10 and 1152mC. There will be more discussion on electric charge in this book, so you just need to keep reading.

sounded while the electric charge was delivered. Catherine's jaws clamped, and tiny muscles convulsed around the eyes, the forehead, and the cheeks, resulting in a grimace. Her fists clenched and the arms were slightly flexed at the elbows. While patients are given muscle relaxants to protect them from convulsions which are too forceful, we do want to see some muscle movement during the seizures, in order to assess the seizure quality, so we ensure the dose is not high enough to completely paralyse the patient. After 1.5 seconds the noise stopped, and Catherine's face and arms immediately relaxed. The clenching of the muscles during the delivery of the electric stimulus was not a seizure yet. In ECT, the direct effect of the repetitive electric pulses on the neurons in the brain should provoke a seizure, where the neurons start discharging spontaneously and in concert, a few seconds after the stimulation. We were watching intently for the repetitive symmetrical twitching of the muscles that should follow the electric charge. Not a muscle moved. I glanced at the EEG traces. Sometimes the patient's muscles are too well paralysed, and we can record a seizure only by the electrical activity in the brain. The trace showed a nearly flat line, with minuscule fast see-saw flickers, typically observed in a sleeping person. After about 20 seconds somebody stated, 'No fit,' and everybody nodded.

'Shall we restimulate?'

Kara asked me for approval, having already prepared the machine for another stimulation. Up to two re-stimulations can be administered according to our protocol but only if the patient is safe. The monitor showed an almost unchanged and regular heart rhythm, the oxygen saturation had remained at 100% and Magdi was giving Catherine some extra oxygen, to make sure the level stayed there. There was nothing to worry about, so I said 'Yes' in a reassuringly loud voice, to emphasise the lack of any concern. The second stimulation was at 184mC. The initial muscle twitches were much weaker, with the face muscles even more incapable after their feeble attempts to contract at the first stimulation. But after a few seconds the arms and feet started twitching, first almost imperceptibly, like a nervous shaking, then more clearly, in coordinated twitches that continued for 48 seconds. This was a good seizure and it was backed by a clear pattern of generalised tonic-clonic seizure activity on the EEG, which stopped soon after the muscles stopped twitching.

At the second treatment, three days later, we gave Catherine a higher electric dose, 253mC, as we need to treat patients with doses well above their seizure thresholds. Her further treatments were uneventful: she had good seizures throughout, and didn't need any changes in the electric charge.

After four ECTs, given twice a week over two weeks, Catherine was still depressed but her reasoning had improved to the extent that she was able to think clearly about her illness. At that point she noticed that the treatment was helping her and signed a consent form to continue with ECT.

It was Catherine's seventh session. I arrived at the department early in the morning. My first action, as usual, was to stick my head into the waiting room for a quick feel of what was going on. An unusual sight presented itself: somebody was reading one of the posters on the wall. It was Catherine. Instead of looking aimlessly around, slumped in a chair, as I remembered her on the previous occasions, she was reading the small typeface of an article that we had displayed proudly in the waiting room. I approached her, trying to hide my joy and surprise. The poster was an article on ECT that had been published in a newspaper. It was one of the rare positive accounts of ECT, even though the central photo showed, as usual in an ECT account, Jack Nicholson on the psychiatric ward in the film *One Flew Over the Cuckoo's Nest*. Catherine looked back and smiled at me with a soft and charming smile, that suited her face and seemed to be her natural expression.

'Interesting article, and they mention you.'

I had indeed been interviewed for it - that's why we had displayed the photocopy in such a prominent place! I was even more stunned by this level of attention and interest from a person who had been unable to think clearly a week earlier. She was feeling well now and agreed that ECT had helped her. The memories of her illness were patchy. She was bemused to hear that her speech and her movements had been slow and that she had insisted that she could not get better. The suicide attempt felt strange and inexplicable to her and she showed no interest in discussing it, beyond admitting that she knew the femoral artery would be the biggest one she could get hold of. She tried to describe how she had felt: 'Deep despair, depression, sadness, befuddled.' 'Befuddled' was a new word for a non-native speaker like me – ah, the joys of the English language! She was so impressed by her transformation that she was writing notes about her experiences. I wanted to hear the acknowledgment again. Did she appreciate how much she had changed? Did she really attribute this to the ECT?

'So you are surprised by how well you are responding?'

'I am shocked!'

The smile confirmed the joke.

I explained that we should now space out the treatments, instead of stopping them suddenly, in order to reduce the risk of relapse. She found the idea very sensible. I mused why a patient who had been psychotic until a week ago found this idea sensible, while so many sane people, and even some professionals, didn't. Only 15 years ago the official guidelines suggested that 'treatment should be stopped when a response has been achieved'.

Catherine had four more ECTs. She became so ebullient and full of energy that somebody on the ward worried that she was becoming manic - she was painting her toenails for the first time in many years, for goodness sake! I wasn't so sure there was anything to worry about, although this can indeed be a side effect of ECT. When you come out of Hell, you can be excused for feeling excited about life. Where does happiness end and mania or illness start? At what point does elation spill over into excess? Mood normally goes up and down in response to events, and it must be a great feeling when the joy of being well again kicks in. Was it abnormal that Catherine wanted to get a car or plan a holiday? No, I argued, this was not mania. She had made a complete recovery, and was back to the bright, happy person she had been previous to her depression. But there was no need to continue with ECT and everybody agreed that it should be stopped.

Catherine started taking Lithium and remained well during our one-year follow-up period. She even volunteered to speak publicly about her experiences with

ECT, a brave offer that will be taken up. If every ECT course was so straightforward, and every patient recovered, there would be less controversy over this treatment. And I wouldn't have much to write about.

ANXIETY

I was about to attach my memory stick to the computer in the lecture theatre of the Postgraduate Centre. It was a routine talk to junior doctors, and I was just pausing to think of an introduction, when I was interrupted before I could come up with a single line. Sarah, one of the senior registrars, took me to one side and said, 'We might have a postnatal woman for ECT.' Talk at once forgotten, my attention was now entirely focused on her. Postnatal psychosis! This rare but very distressing and serious condition amounts to a medical emergency – and tends to respond very well to ECT. It affects between one and two women in every thousand and is different from postnatal depression, devastating though that can be. Postnatal depression often involves sadness, tearfulness, and a feeling of not being able to cope, whereas psychosis can include hallucinations, delusions, mania, and severe confusion. It poses a real risk to the wellbeing of mother and baby alike. I have to admit to some selfish professional interest at this point. I had already noted that this topic was missing from my stories, as we hadn't had a postnatal case for years. Perhaps this was going to be the right one. Maria, the deputy ECT consultant, now joined us. She reported that the young woman, Elinor, had given birth a month ago and was feeling highly anxious.

'Is she psychotic?' I asked hopefully, as postnatal psychosis should respond easily to ECT. She wasn't, not a hint of it, just anxious and agitated. I tried another line. 'Is it just anxiety, or is she pacing around, asking for reassurance?'

I was trying to find reassurance myself, rather too hopeful that she had an agitated depression, as pacing and agitation can be part of the acute mental turmoil that comes with psychosis - but no, she was only anxious. 'But she is in hospital, separated from the baby, surely she must be quite desperate?'

I was now getting slightly desperate myself to find a good prognostic feature. It was clear that both Sarah and Maria were not sure if the patient was a good ECT candidate. Elinor had been suffering from anxiety for many years. She had felt more depressed during her pregnancy but had improved quite a lot with Mirtazapine since her admission to hospital. 'Perhaps we should wait until Monday and see if she continues to improve,' Sarah suggested. This sounded like a good plan and I was allowed to start my teaching session, just in time. I didn't see Elinor that day.

The plan was going to fail spectacularly. To be fair, that Friday we were not dealing with a case of post-natal psychosis, perhaps not even post-natal depression. The pregnancy and birth could not quite be ignored, of course, but what we had heard of Elinor's case sounded more like psychological factors: problems with coping and adjustment rather than the storm of hormonal changes after birth that is blamed for the sudden onset of post-natal disorders. Alas, my glib expectations were to receive a reality check.

Monday came and Kara greeted me with a well-rehearsed conspiratorial air, but her smile was strained.

'Um – a bit of news. Elinor, the mother with the new baby - she tried to strangle herself over the weekend.'

Great start to the week. Poor Elinor had used a dressing gown cord and had tried to tie it around her neck. Perhaps the attempt was half-hearted, or maybe she was too frightened to carry it through properly, but this didn't sound like a mere cry for help. After all, she was already receiving help. This act suggested a real desire to kill herself, despite the recent arrival of her baby, which was well planned and anticipated with joy by the whole family. Kara and I went to see her.

Elinor behaved and spoke like a completely normal young person. She was able to reason well, her voice was low, but fluent, and she made appropriate eye contact. But there was no joy in her eyes, which were scrolling around, as if searching for help, and I could sense fear in the background. She looked so helpless and sad, fragile to the point of looking like a child. Everybody was full of empathy, with a desire to help her and to feel her pain with her. I asked Elinor to describe her problems. It was anxiety, she told us. Such strong anxiety that she was afraid of it. She had experienced panic attacks for many years, although up until recently she had been able to cope with them. A few months into the pregnancy, though, she had started fearing them so much that her mind had become consumed with worry that an attack might strike.

I was sceptical because I don't believe in giving ECT for panic attacks or anxiety alone. But there was something more here. Elinor was suicidal. She couldn't feel close to her baby. And there was the urgency of the situation: we couldn't wait a few months for her to try a couple of antidepressants, while she was such a risk to herself, and while she would be missing vital time to bond with her baby. I didn't know for certain whether ECT would help, but I felt that it was her best chance. By now I had started thinking aloud and stating my arguments to her, to her husband and to the rest of the team. The more I mused on the pros and cons of it, the clearer the options became: Elinor should either have ECT now and hopefully get well within three weeks, or she should wait and hope it would pass without any changes to her treatment. We left her to think about it. Later that day Kara contacted me to say that I should come into the unit the next morning if I wanted to supervise Elinor's first ECT.

Elinor scored a massive 40 points on the Hamilton Depression Rating Scale (HAM-D). Kara was pointing to the score, claiming that it confirmed her severe depression. I was still sceptical. Some patients with anxiety can score very high levels on this scale, while the really ill ones might score fewer, especially if they hide symptoms or are mute.

Elinor was lying on the treatment bed, and I remarked that she appeared to be calm.

'No,' whispered Danielle, our nurse. 'She's very frightened, she kept talking about it.' We gave her a low electric charge to start the titration, in line with our protocol for people under 30 years: 46mC. Methohexital[3] was the anaesthetic and Glycopyrrolate was added to prevent bradycardia (overly slow heart rate), which I feared due to Elinor's existing prescription of beta blockers. The seizure was very good, nearly a minute long. There were no complications.

---

[3] Methohexital is the most suitable anaesthetic for ECT, but world-wide production stopped soon after this case, and you will not hear much about it in other chapters.

Some fifteen minutes later, Elinor was waking up and correctly answering some of the questions on orientation. And then she started weeping uncontrollably. 'Why is this happening to me? I always wanted to have a baby!'

Despair and sadness were pouring out of her eyes and infecting people around her with compassion. I don't enjoy other people's suffering, but at this point I felt some relief. These were her true emotions. She was unable to control or conceal them, as she wasn't yet fully awake. She was depressed! At last I felt hopeful for the outcome. Unfortunately, the many years of anxiety disorder amounted to a poor prognostic sign, but even if she only improved to the point of her usual low-level anxiety, Elinor would be able to lead a normal life, like so many people out there. Elinor lay on the bed for another 20 minutes, surrounded by several compassionate young female nurses, who had children of their own, or were looking forward to having them. We had not chosen them on purpose, it just so happened that morning. She was in the right company.

Two days passed and I was thinking hard about how much to increase the electric charge for Elinor's next session. Normally we would double the dose or raise it by 50% if the first seizure was good, and there seemed to be no apparent reason why this shouldn't work for Elinor, too. Surely nothing medically wrong could happen to a young woman who had gone through the much tougher challenge of giving birth. But what if her heart overreacted to the massive cholinergic discharge during the seizure and developed bradycardia or arrhythmia? But if we didn't increase the setting, we might miss a seizure, as the previous one had been weaker. As a matter of fact, I was not thinking entirely rationally. Like everyone else in the team, I too was affected by the overwhelming feeling of compassion and the desire not to harm this fragile young mother. I settled for 69mC, still one of the lowest treatment doses we had ever used for a treatment dose.

My increasingly obsessive ruminations were interrupted when I met Elinor herself again. She was calm and assured me that she was feeling better already. This had started soon after the first session. There was no fear in her eyes and at one point I even noticed some playfulness in her expression as she talked with her mother. This was too good to be true, but I was easily - perhaps too easily - persuaded of her progress. Another very good seizure took all playfulness and focus from her eyes for a good half an hour.

Another three days have now gone by, and I am cycling, exerting more pressure than usual on the pedals, in order to get to the centre early, before they give Elinor her ECT, as I want to see her myself before the treatment. I am half-hopeful that she will be well. The other half of my mind is already worrying about what to do if she has slipped back. Now, ironically, despite my initial relief at her good results, such a quick recovery makes me worry that it's all too good to be true - or maybe it just awakens the dormant pessimist in me. When I arrive, ECT hasn't started; in fact, I have to supervise the junior doctor, so they were going to wait for me anyway. Elinor had scored just three points on the HAM-D (better than me that day! I had been sleeping poorly for a few weeks, enough to give me five points, before even thinking about the questions on anxiety). Her improvement no longer excites remarks in the office, it is now accepted and reported as a matter of fact.

So I get my time with Elinor. The transformation is startling. There is a sparkle in her eyes as she scans her surroundings and wonders how to make a joke of the situation. Her voice is up a few decibels from the whispers of last week and projects confidence. Her husband tells me that she now feels better than she has done for years, and she even told him that she is looking forward to life. They are excited and I am trying to hide my own excitement and to look professional. Not too difficult, as I am thinking ahead and once again weighing the doubts born of my long experience of patients in the ECT field. Already I am mulling over what will happen once Elinor stops ECT in the next couple of weeks. (Should I get another point on my self-HAM-D score for 'Intermittent doubts that things will improve but can be reassured' I wonder?) I suggest that Elinor has only one ECT next week, and perhaps another two spaced out after that, if she remains well. It is clear that she and her husband will be happy to accept whatever I suggest, so I am trying to ensure we get the balance right. Short duration of illness, quick recovery, first severe episode: surely this predicts a very low relapse risk and no need for a long course? Elinor decided to stop ECT the following week, after just four sessions.

Ten days later I was regretting my optimism. Elinor had relapsed. She was not complaining of depression, she was looking lively and smiling, but her anxiety had come back and so had her panic attacks, in turn making her frightened of having even more anxiety and panics. I was reproved for my frivolous speculations regarding my own potential HAM-D score: Elinor's own score was a frightening 36. The anxiety had not diminished when she came back for her sixth session. My own anxiety was mounting to comparable levels. She was not feeling depressed any longer; this was simple anxiety and panic, and anxiety disorder is not meant to respond well to ECT. In fact, it's not meant to be treated with ECT at all. Elinor's anxiety disorder had been present for years, but in the past had not disrupted her life. Now it was making her life unbearable, but further ECT looked pointless. Or did it? Given that we don't quite know how ECT works in any case, how do we know exactly what is happening in the brain and which faculties are being affected by treatment? And was the anxiety worse because her depression was still in the background? Not to mention that everybody is different and that typical reasonings about anxiety and ECT might just not apply in certain cases.

Over the next few sessions, Elinor gradually settled. I didn't. I was worried about the effectiveness of ECT and was unable to suggest a clear plan. Instead of relying only on ECT, I recommended exercise as well, explaining how this would help get rid of the excessive energy that otherwise presents with symptoms such as palpitations, rapid breathing and sweating. In other words, my usual advice for addressing somatic anxiety. Elinor was in agreement when we spoke about this, but never followed up with any action. Perhaps at that stage the prospect of exercise was simply too much for her. Unlike me, though, she was optimistic about the ECT, convinced that it was helping her and willing to continue despite the incomplete effect. She was right. After 11 sessions she was back in remission, and her anxiety had gone away completely. We spaced out the last three sessions, and after the 14th she went back to work part-time. Relief!

We had a couple more meetings over the following few months. Elinor remained well, although understandably worried about relapsing in the future. She was enjoying looking after her baby, and her bonding with her child was unaffected, as far as I could tell. Elinor works as a musician and, always interested in the effects of ECT on musical abilities, I was keen to learn whether it had affected her memory for melodies or her ability and skill in moving her fingers across the keys and strings of her instruments. She was clear that it had not affected her performance.

3

A WICKED MAN

He was a wicked man, he said so himself. I'd seen his stern face through the window of the interview room, focused on a cognitive test he found impossible to complete, despite the gentle prodding of our nurse Danielle. Even at 80, he should have been able to finish the test within two minutes. Yet he was clearly pre-occupied with some other, immense concern. His eyes were remote; when asked a question, he would think for a long minute, then revert to events that had happened long ago in the past. He seemed to be carrying some huge burden of guilt; the hints he let drop showed that he was worried about being dirty. He would ask nurses to sniff him, to check for smells. He feared that they would see how dirty he was if he tried to take off his clothes for a shower.

'I am a wicked man,' he stated. 'I am dirty.' He was a man of God. Being wicked was against his beliefs, perhaps the worst feeling he could experience.

What could an old man have done to be carrying such guilt? Our patient believed he had done something wrong but he couldn't say what it was. I'd first seen him while doing my usual scanning of the rooms when I arrived at work. Through the window of the interview room, on my way to the treatment area, I had noticed the new silhouette. I slowed down. An old man was bent over a piece of A4 paper covered with circles, the Trail Making Test - part of our cognitive testing - done before and after an ECT course. This had to be a new patient, being assessed prior to his first ECT session. The aim of the test is to connect the 24 numbers and letters in the correct order.

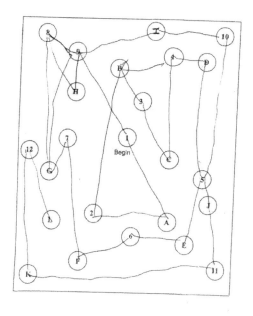

Time taken: 5·13

Trail Making Test, part B, completed by our patient with some mistakes, in just over five minutes.

Danielle was sitting next to the old man, holding a stopwatch. The score for completing the test is the time it takes to connect the circles in the right order. Young people usually complete the task within half a minute, while older folks take longer. But the old man hadn't moved for a few seconds. This caught my attention, so I stopped in front of the window. He was concentrating. He was focused on the paper, but the hand holding the pen wasn't moving.

'No, what goes after H?' Danielle nudged him. She looked at me with despair. She was stuck doing one of those 'slow' cognitive assessments. A few minutes later she came to debrief, exhausted by the patient's slowness and relieved I had seen it for myself. She needed a break, but I was already hopeful. Our new patient was showing psychomotor retardation, one of the best positive predictors for response to ECT. I swapped places with Danielle: there was some time to spare.

Mr W, our new patient, made surprisingly quick eye contact when I came into the room, and almost got up from his chair once I was introduced as the consultant. He was keen to fill me in with details, although he had to weigh every statement before uttering it. His depression had started only a few months ago - another good sign, I thought. He didn't remember ever having been depressed in the past. I jumped ahead, hoping to find some delusions in a person with such severe depression.

'Are you medically well?' I asked. No, he wasn't. Or perhaps there was something wrong: he had difficulty passing water. And his penis wasn't right, he volunteered. I was filling in the story with bits from the hospital entries that somehow had been placed in my hands. Yes, he was worried about passing water - this had been documented already - so much so that he believed he was dirty and smelly.

He had been drinking less water, to prevent him from passing more urine and was down to one glass of water a day. This, he felt, would also be a proper punishment and would help him to die. Just as well he had admitted this because it had sounded the alarm bell for his doctor who had signed an emergency section for ECT treatment and had referred him to us the previous afternoon. This explained why I knew nothing about him when I arrived in the morning. He was not yet dehydrated; his pulse and blood pressure were stable but another few days' delay, and the picture could have been different.

He had been told about ECT and understood what it involved but was not able to make rational decisions. The sectioning under the Mental Health Act was appropriate. He objected to the treatment but had accepted the decision and was complying with instructions. We proceeded with ECT after a short discussion with the anaesthetist about his heart function, which had been an issue during a previous admission to the general hospital. Despite his age, his 32-second seizure was long enough at the first stimulation on our emergency protocol (184mC, bilateral, with Thiopental). And for somebody whose heart performance had been questioned, his vital signs remained unremarkable after the seizure.

'Just a small increase in dose next time, 253mC', I suggested. (The first seizure in older people tends to be better than subsequent ones. He had no complications, so a gentle increase felt reasonable).

As he was prepared for his second ECT session, we tried to explore his feelings of guilt. After some reflexion he murmured something. There was a problem, he admitted, a big problem. His voice was getting so low that it was drowned out by every distant sound in the corridor. We closed the door in order to hear him better. He had expressed anxiety about passing urine, so we asked if his problem concerned this. He repeated more assertively, 'No, it is not the urine.'

We didn't get any further. Mr W was sinking into thought, his face becoming more concerned, in deep deliberation, his eyes staring in front of him, the wrinkles above the nose getting higher and deeper, in the classic Omega (Ω) sign of depression. We continued with the preparations. As the anaesthetic slowly made its way into his blood through the cannula, his voice became louder.

'There is a problem... a problem.' He seemed about to confess something, his face was full of anguish and sorrow. But there was no time, the anaesthetic had reached his brain, his eyes closed and his eyelids did not react to the touch of the anaesthetist. He didn't share his secret. I turned round to the nurse who had accompanied him: 'He feels guilty about something?'

'Yes, he believes he has done something wrong but he hasn't said what.'

The seizure was very poor, with some EEG spikes but no muscular twitches. I had shown weakness and at the last minute had decided not to increase the electric charge from the previous 184mC. I knew this was going to be a mistake, as I had argued for the correct dose so persuasively three days ago, but then preferred to be cautious, worried about his age and his previous history of heart problems. Well, no harm done. He was not in any immediate danger and we would increase the dose next time. Staff had already noticed an improvement in his depression after the first treatment, but it had gone after two days. This was promising - he should pull out of it soon.

At the third session the dose was increased to 253mC. Mr W responded with a 53-second seizure, but the EEG wasn't great, so I planned 299mC for the next session. He still lacked understanding of his illness and seemed immersed in another world, which was not a kind one.

ECT No.5

I had been away for session No.4 and was relieved to see a change. Not just any change, but one that provoked a now familiar excited murmur in the department. 'You should see him! He looks so different today!' Everybody who knew him had to pop into the waiting room to see him. The transformation was one of these miraculous ones that convert people into ECT believers. He was smiling, he greeted people in a polite and gentle manner, and modestly remarked that he was glad he could please us with his appearance. He happily agreed for the two medical students to be present at his treatment. He still didn't know why we thought he was better, or that there had been a problem before. Then, when lying on the treatment bed, he offered his arm to the anaesthetist and even cracked a joke. The whining and crying of the previous days had disappeared. This was great, but we couldn't see any hint that he would consent to ECT, once he regained capacity. And this was imminent. I had left the junior doctor to assess his capacity to give consent for the treatment, without giving her any background, in order to see how a newcomer would judge his condition. If she felt that he had capacity and he then refused treatment, we would have to honour his decision. This would not exactly be the end of the world: he was so much better and not in any danger any longer, as he had resumed regular food and fluid intake. The SHO had no hesitation, however, 'He doesn't have capacity - he cannot weigh the pros and cons of the treatment, and he doesn't recognise that he has any problem.' I was glad to hear this and didn't argue.

ECT No.6

Mr W was still detained on a section, much to my annoyance as I had assumed he would have regained capacity by now. I couldn't dodge responsibility any longer, so I started the capacity assessment myself, joined by the SHO. Our patient was pleasant in his manner and engaged in discussion; he spoke fluently and was able to listen.

'I just can't understand how giving somebody a shock of electricity would make them feel better,' he opened the argument, clearly not showing any enthusiasm for the treatment that had just pulled him out of his misery. He obviously understood the nature of ECT and made his opinion clear.

I was already thinking about what would happen if he stopped his treatment today. He might relapse, then there would be a delay before he was put on a new section. He might not even be ill enough to be sectioned, even though he was still feeling depressed. If he had the treatment today, he would almost certainly continue to improve and realise what ECT had done for him. Did he have capacity to make the decision himself? So far he had passed three of the four criteria for capacity: he understood the information relevant to the decision; he was able to retain it; and he communicated his decision. The only criterion in the capacity assessment that was left to explore was his ability to use and weigh the information available to make a decision.

'Do you remember how unwell you were?' I started probing. 'When I first saw you, you were worried that you smelled.'

'Really?' He looked bemused. He had forgotten his feelings of guilt and was showing no insight. After some thinking he reasoned that he occasionally dribbled urine, so had to wear a pad. He was wearing one now. 'But this is okay, I am not worried about it.' He still couldn't appreciate how unwell he had been. 'People keep telling me how much better I look, but I think I am the same. Perhaps it is the very good diet on the ward that helped.' I couldn't prevent a burst of laughter escaping through my lips, and he joined in with a smile. The food in NHS hospitals is not known for its healing properties.

'Do you still blame yourself for something?' I persisted.

'Let's not dig into things,' he sighed. There was still a problem that he would not divulge, but it was no longer held with such passion and desperation.

We needed a good discussion with the SHO. Mr W was able to reason but was completely unaware of the extent to which ECT had helped him. He was denying the severity of his illness and had forgotten some of his delusions and his refusal to drink for fear of becoming smelly. He still had some feelings of guilt that he wouldn't share. Surprisingly, though, he entertained the possibility that the electric shock could somehow have an effect on his mood: 'I guess it is theoretically possible.' I could see how with a bit more insight he could accept that this treatment was making him better. But making an unwise decision doesn't necessarily mean a lack of capacity. This was tricky: I couldn't be sure what decision he would take if he was well.

According to the law, a patient either has capacity or doesn't. But the way to recovery is gradual, and at certain points, to some extent, capacity can be variable. There is rarely a sudden point when the patient shouts out, 'Oh my God, what happened? I must have been mad, but now I am well!' Mr W had been deluded, slow, and unable to make decisions. Very soon he would be back to his normal self, a clever and highly responsible member of the community. Somewhere between these two extremes his mind had to traverse a grey area of hesitation and uncertainty, and this is where he was now. To make things even more delicate, capacity can fluctuate even during a single day, as can the patient's mood. This is the reason why, in our unit, we have decided to re-test capacity in the morning, just before giving each treatment, even if this has been already done by the patient's teams the previous day.

The real question was what his decision would be when he was well and had full capacity to decide. Had he reached that point? It is our duty to accept such decisions. I could see that some colleagues might feel that he had capacity to decide about ECT, while others would not, so I looked around to assess the mood in the room. Kara and the SHO were clearer in their minds that he lacked capacity, and they probably felt that he was worse than I had judged him to be. I concluded that he still lacked insight into his illness and that this was impairing his capacity to make a rational decision about his need for treatment. We would treat him today, but we would warn his team to have a new discussion tomorrow and hope that he would consent to further treatment if he had capacity. If he didn't consent, we would stop ECT. Most importantly, Mr W was not objecting to having the treatment. If he had done this more forcefully, we would have accepted his refusal. In fact, he looked relieved when I suggested that we start walking towards the treatment room. He himself was in two minds about the need for ECT and looked relieved that someone else had taken charge of the decision that he wasn't able to make. Before lying down on the treatment table, he welcomed the two students who were there to observe his treatment. He made a joke which provoked laughter in the staff closest to him. I couldn't hear it.

ECT No.7

'Ah, here you are,' Kara greeted me when I popped my face through the door of the treatment room, a bit late for the start of the session. 'Can you consent our patient?'

'Ugh, what has happened, has he agreed?'

'Dr Isaacs has taken him off the section.'

Things had proceeded fast and as predicted. On Tuesday after the last treatment, our patient's doctor had replied to us, saying that Mr W still lacked capacity, but that he had had another chat with him the next day, and had accordingly stopped his section. He should have obtained the patient's consent for ECT too, but had probably got distracted. This is why Kara asked me to obtain consent. Luckily, I didn't have to use any persuasion skills. Mr W was different today. He admitted that he had been ill and that it must have been the ECT that had made him well. 'What about the diet?' I teased him, just to be able to enjoy his laughter. He still wondered how it was possible that passing electricity through one's brain could make a person feel better, but it is a strange thing, which most people do not believe anyway. I reminded him that the electricity elicits a seizure. Indeed, I had to give him all the information before he gave consent. He looked slightly unhappy and thoughtful but seemed to accept this further illogical and worrying element of his treatment. We went through the remaining points of the consent, including warnings about confusion, memory, dental damage, and he accepted everything. He only agreed to have three more treatments, though, as he didn't see the point of having more once he was well. I didn't argue, as his history didn't suggest the need for continuing ECT after remission had been reached. My conclusion that he lacked capacity earlier in the week had been correct: he was now in a clearer state of mind and his decision had shifted along with his capacity.

This might have been my last chance to find out what had made him feel so guilty. I started inquiring very gently, suggesting that severely depressed people can feel very badly about themselves and may even imagine they are guilty of something. Had he felt like that a couple of weeks ago? He tried to think but couldn't remember such feelings. I probed more, but he looked puzzled as to why I was suggesting this. He had forgotten his ideas of guilt, just as we forget our dreams, if we don't write them down straight away. Had it been some childish prank that had been magnified to a sin through the lens of his depression? Or perhaps when he felt he was wicked, he was trying to remember the misdemeanour that justified the description, but couldn't find it, as it didn't exist.

'What about your body? Something was not working properly a couple of weeks ago.'

'Well,' he contemplated, 'I can't really run a marathon, but other than that I am all right.' As he started to walk towards the treatment room, he asked me if 'this young lady can attend the treatment', pointing charmingly to a student nurse who had come with him. Surely she could, I myself had been about to ask him for his permission. There were two medical students waiting in the treatment room, and Kara asked him whether they were allowed to stay as well. 'Yes, of course they can,' he said in the same generous tone, then pointed at me and added, 'But I don't want Professor Kirov to be present,' and gave a cue that this was a joke, before lying down on the bed.

Mr W made a complete recovery after this session, scoring just three points on the HAM-D. He had only one more ECT. I didn't recommend continuation treatments, as I had no reason to suspect a high relapse risk. One month later he came for a follow-up and a repeat of cognitive tests. They were all dramatically better. The Trail Making Test time was almost halved and he achieved the best score for his age on the Complex Figure drawing. At the start of the ECT he had been unable to reproduce even a single line of it. A very agile mind had been slowed down by a nasty illness. And yes, he was again a kind and gentle man, as he had been all his life.

I was wrong about one thing, however. I had misjudged the relapse risk, not for the first time. Despite all the good prognostic signs on which I had relied, five months later he relapsed, with no warning. He didn't experience guilt, but otherwise his presentation was a carbon copy of the first one: slow, denying any illness, denying that ECT had worked last time. His bladder was working fine, but this time something was not right with his bowels. His response to ECT was also nearly a carbon copy of the first course: he took six sessions to improve, then he consented to more treatments. After eight sessions he was in remission, and then had four more treatments, reaching a score of just one point on the HAM-D before going back home. I think I know what to suggest if he is hospitalised again.

4

PERSONALITY DISORDER

As young psychiatrists, we used to recognise young women with personality disorder at a glance. Their forearms were covered in cuts of various sizes, their colours indicating how recent they were, often along with holes from cigarette burns. Known in those days as Borderline Personality Disorder,[4] this condition often accompanies a history of sexual or emotional abuse in childhood and is more common in women than in men. Research on people with personality disorders suggests a poorer response to ECT. Indeed, ECT does not change a person's personality and I am quite happy to point this out to my more nervous patients by way of reassurance. However, treatment might backfire with personality disorder - the outcome might not just be lack of success, but downright deterioration. People who do not benefit from ECT, but who experience side effects only, might then perceive ECT as harmful rather than beneficial. This is a realistic premise of which we are fully aware, and we take that into account when deciding whom to accept for treatment. We can do without any more bad publicity for ECT.

So when I was asked to provide a second opinion on Zoe, I was not very optimistic. Zoe had had a difficult life. Her mother had died when she was only four years old,

---

[4] The subtypes of personality disorder have been scrapped in the latest classification systems, with clinicians being asked to assess personality disorder along a spectrum.

and she was then looked after by her stepmother, who had children of her own. Zoe felt that the other children received more attention than she did and that she was unwanted. Later, she would describe this period of her life as one of emotional abuse. It was probably that feeling of being unwanted from as early as she could remember that shaped her adult personality and made her deeply suspicious of relationships. Poor Zoe would go and visit her mother's grave at night, and also developed other, more worrying morbid habits, including self-harm.

Zoe had done well at school initially and had even been happy for a while. She had also managed to stay at college for a year or so but after that could not cope any longer. Her self-harm had started much earlier, when she was 12, and she took her first overdose at the age of 13. Her life at school was marred by drugs, alcohol, and binge eating. And yes, her arms were covered with old scars, some not so old, some reaching her shoulders and encroaching onto her neck, mixed with numerous hallmark pale or pinkish crater-shaped scars, from deep cigarette burns. Over the years the list of self-harm episodes had become longer, and now we were entering the realm of 'near misses': on two occasions Zoe had been found hanging from a ligature. One of these was in hospital, while under 'close observation', which required a nurse to check on her at least every 15 minutes (and to make a record of this). Between two of these visits, Zoe was found hanging from a rope tied round her neck. She had had a narrow escape indeed - she was taken down unconscious and having suffered a cardiac arrest, as can happen after asphyxiation, but was successfully resuscitated. On another occasion she tried to jump in front of the cars on a busy road, and once more from the fourth floor, suffering several fractures. On other occasions, the cuts she inflicted on her arms were so deep that she lost enough blood to go into shock and again only narrowly escaped death.

Zoe was now kept on a Mental Health Act section in a secure ward. Impossible as it may sound, things got even worse about a year after her admission. Zoe would try to stick objects down her throat in order to suffocate herself. Staff had to constantly watch that she didn't get hold of a pencil, a piece of cloth or even a piece of paper. She would scrunch the paper into a ball and try to stick it down her throat, to stop her own breathing. And all the time, this desire to end her life appeared to be genuine; the attempts didn't feel like the 'cries for help' that are sometimes associated with personality disorder. The staff who looked after her didn't think they were cries for help, either. They too believed that she genuinely wanted to kill herself. That was unusual and required my attention. After talking with her, I had the same impression. Zoe just didn't want to live. Apart from her personality disorder, she had severe depression and that paradoxically gave me hope that she might respond well to ECT. Indeed, over the years I have learned that the more severely ill the patient, the more likely they are to respond to ECT, and, frankly, I would rather deal with very severe depression, preferably psychotic, than with a personality disorder. Ironically again, Zoe's prospects would have improved further if she had had some psychotic ideas, but I couldn't establish anything delusional.

A patient with severe depression would normally receive strong antidepressants and probably a referral for ECT. However, Zoe had personality disorder, and this was not just a diagnosis on paper. In addition to her attempts on her own life, there had been several episodes of assault against nurses, fellow patients and even police officers. Not surprisingly, even before ending up in a secure unit, she had spent years in psychiatric hospitals, under 'close' or 'one-to-one' observation. Most recently, she had needed two people to be with her all the time and this had continued for a year and a half. But no one doubted that otherwise she would succeed in taking her life. Zoe had clearly decided to kill herself when she got the chance. Building a therapeutic relationship with her, as with many such people, was difficult, as she was afraid of relationships and highly apprehensive that they would end in disappointment.

Zoe's doctor, however, was fairly certain that she had genuine depression on top of her personality disorder and started talking to her about ECT. This was a brave and unusual step. Throughout all my years in Cardiff, we had not given ECT to a single patient from a secure hospital. After some months, Zoe agreed to have ECT, more than two years after entering the secure hospital. I could easily understand why she had not been asked to have this treatment earlier.

When I first saw Zoe, she established a good rapport, but was shaking continuously from head to toe. Despite the well-grounded doubts as to whether she would benefit from ECT, it didn't take me too long to be convinced that she deserved a chance. Zoe herself clearly had some hope that ECT might help her, and this hinted at something more important: I felt that she genuinely wanted to stop feeling suicidal and to get better. She wasn't pressurised to have ECT, as it was quite clear that she had full capacity to make decisions for herself and although she was sectioned under the Mental Health Act, nobody would force her to have this treatment. In any case, her team's opinions were divided in this respect. It was Zoe who had made the decision to have ECT. I always respect people who do this, perhaps because I don't know how brave I would be to agree to it myself, were I to need it one day.

Zoe's cognitive tests were impressive. She was one of the very few people who managed to copy the so-called 'Complex Figure' from memory without any mistakes. My respect for her increased not least because at my own first attempt to draw that figure, I had not achieved that score. She was a resourceful girl, and I was encouraged to feel that she had the potential to get on with life. I was quick to praise her and noticed that she liked the praise. Don't we all like to be told that we are better at something than most other people?

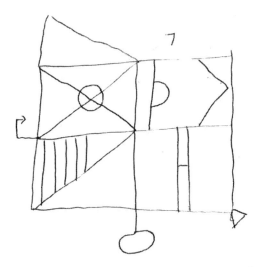

The Complex Figure drawn from memory by Zoe, with no errors.

I didn't, however, tell Zoe what I felt her personal chances for success were: much lower than the figure in our information booklet, which gives the average for our patients. From all I had learned over the years, though, I knew that even people who on paper should not respond, do occasionally get well, proving me wrong time and time again. We would give Zoe 12 sessions and if she did not improve, we would stop. This was only a trial. I rated her chances at 20%-30%. Not bad compared with, say, certain cancer treatments, and the prospect if she was left untreated was just as grim as for someone with a nasty cancer. The difference was that Zoe could theoretically be kept alive for another 50 years in high-secure wards - provided her two guards didn't take their eyes off her.

ECT started and despite the enormous cocktail of sedative drugs Zoe was on, including anticonvulsants, she had good seizures, requiring only rare increases in the electric charge, to keep them over our arbitrary 15-second duration. Her depression rating dropped to 25 after two ECTs, to 22 after four and then to 16 and 12 after the sixth and eight sessions. She had started with 33. This was too good to be true, but it indicated a pattern. I expected a person with a pure personality disorder to fluctuate rather more in her mood: to have high expectations one day and then just to turn back the next day to a dark rejection of everything. Each time she came, I would ask the three members of staff, who accompanied her on the short journey to our hospital, how she was doing (three people now, rather than two, as it was so much easier for Zoe to run away during a car journey, or to jump out of a moving car, as she had done in the past). And each time I heard encouraging news, with signs of improvement and less persistent expression of suicidal ideas. Finally, Zoe came for her 12th ECT. Her depression rating was eight. She had reached remission level. She confirmed that for two weeks she had not had thoughts of killing herself. The fact that she still didn't want to live was a minor matter at this point. Good news continued to arrive. She was allowed a lot more freedom, needed less 'as required' medication, and there had been no attempts at self-harm. She had started to interact with staff and was seen laughing at times. Everybody in her team was now convinced that there had been a genuine improvement, even those who had had strong reservations about ECT at the start.

The depression was defeated, but I didn't want to stop there. We had already analysed our data and found that over half of people who remit after ECT relapse during the following year. And one of the best predictive factors seemed to be the length of the depressive episode. People who had suffered for many years were more likely to relapse. Logical, I always thought, but with the longstanding prejudice against ECT, even in the 21st century, after 80 years of experience, the standard advice to psychiatrists is still to stop treatment when the patient gets well. This is in stark contrast to the advice for antidepressants: continue taking them for at least six months after remission. In our hospital we had introduced a 'continuation ECT' protocol, advising patients not to stop after they get well, but gradually to increase the time between sessions and to stop only if they remained well at three-week intervals. This takes time and patience, especially when the person feels completely well and wonders why on earth they should have more treatments. I wanted to explain the potential benefits to Zoe, as she had already started to miss her appointments and had apparently made up her mind to stop soon.

I decided to make a somewhat dramatic presentation in order to convince her of the value of continuation ECT. I knew that Zoe had a logical mind, and this was going to help her. I needed her to reach the same conclusion on her own, after hearing the facts, in order to collaborate with such a long-term commitment. I gave her the relapse rates in our unit and then drew a parallel with other branches of medicine.

'Does the surgeon remove only a large part of the tumour, or does he make sure that all tumour cells are removed? Do we stop the antibiotics when we feel better, or make sure that all the bacteria are killed?'

Zoe thought about it and said with no hesitation, 'I don't want to feel depressed again, I will do whatever you suggest.'

I shook her hand and smiled. Zoe didn't see that when I left the room, I made a stronger celebratory gesture with a hint of a clenched fist, like a tennis player after a good passing shot. I was really pleased for her!

Elated, I had temporarily forgotten the common wisdom on personality disorder and ECT. I was to have a salutary reminder. Over the next few days, I learned that Zoe had decided not to have more treatment. She found it unpleasant. We had more conversations, helped by the really great team looking after her (by this time everyone had been converted to ECT). Zoe was asking me all the right questions on how long she needed to have ECT, questions to which either I didn't know the answers, or I didn't dare tell her, as it promised to be quite a long period. Above all, I feared that her risk of relapse was very high, and that the continuation was only going to prolong her remission, and that when she stopped ECT, she would still relapse. I hinted to her that she might need to continue for six, or even 12 months. In reality, I could not see how a patient with such a history would change unless she remained well for several years. I had no hope that Zoe would continue ECT for two or three years, even if it was given once a month. Nobody had ever done this after a first course, in my experience. Patients always stop ECT well before this.

In the end, I did in fact tell Zoe and her team that the more realistic scenario was years rather than months, but that it was okay to refuse further treatment now, as she could always come back in the future, and she could be sure that she would respond to it again. The important thing was not to put her off ECT, or to pressurise her, but to empower her and keep her in sole charge of these decisions. She was clearly weighing the pros and cons and I was prepared to wait through months and years of her starting and stopping if need be. In other words, I was in it for the long-term. The great breakthrough had been achieved: she was an ECT responder and this gave us the means to get her well each time. The future was far from clear: there was a long road from a secure unit, with one-to-one observation, to independent living or holding down a job. Neither had been achieved yet. But anything in between, such as not needing someone to be with her every minute of her life, was still going to be a success.

After a four-week gap, Zoe did come for more ECT. She had stayed well but had noticed that her anxiety and suicidal thoughts had increased over the last week. This was more or less what I had expected, I told her. I then started thinking aloud whether her next ECT should be in one week's time, as is the standard continuation protocol, or in two weeks, as she had already had a long gap and had not relapsed. After I had laid these two options on the table, Zoe surprised me again. 'I think it will be safer if I come again in one week, Doctor.' If this was personality disorder, then it was a very unusual kind. Not many people would make this choice in her position.

During the following month Zoe managed to miss another ECT session and became suicidal again. In fact, she nearly managed to kill herself. It was another ingenious suicide attempt, showing again how creative she was. She took the string from her pyjama bottoms and when her nurse wasn't looking (for only two minutes, I was assured), she quickly wrapped it around her neck, twisting it into a knot several times, then pulled strongly at the ends. As the string was twisted a few times, it didn't loosen up when she lost consciousness and released her grip. Clever! And I had thought until then that you can't strangle yourself with your own hands. The nurse spotted her in time, and once again, she survived.

Zoe continued to surprise us, but in a positive way now. She did start coming for ECT regularly, once a week. At times she refused to attend, giving various reasons, but she would be back for the next clinic, so that she never delayed her sessions by more than three or four days. After five more ECTs, her depression ratings dropped below our magic 10-point margin (remission level) and Zoe stated once more that she no longer felt suicidal.

Our continuation treatment protocol suggests extending the interval from one week to two weeks after just two sessions, if the patient is well. But I was still worried about doing this with Zoe. She had already relapsed after fewer than four weeks without ECT, and her depression had lasted for many years. She had 10 sessions at roughly weekly intervals, a record itself for our unit! During these three months she didn't feel suicidal and made no suicide attempts, even minor ones. Her observation level was down to one-to-one, she had escorted walks outside the hospital, and had even been allowed short periods with no observation. And then she asked to stop again.

Zoe joined us for the usual multidisciplinary team meeting and took part in the discussions. She suggested a plan: she would ask for more ECTs if she felt suicidal again. She was also complaining of memory problems, some stretching back a couple of years. One annoying area of memory disturbance was her forgetting the content of her psychotherapy sessions. I felt sympathetic towards her therapist, who was sitting next to her. I wanted to give her all the facts again and make her decide what was best for her. If she stopped and relapsed, we would need to re-start with ECT twice a week, thus potentially causing even more memory problems. Alternatively, we could increase the interval to three weeks, which would help her memory (something we had learned recently). Zoe interrupted my monologue: she agreed with the plan. I thought to myself, 'When was the last time I managed to persuade anybody to change their mind?' And I was not just thinking about psychiatric patients!

Despite all these positive developments, I was still conscious that the prognosis was poor. I couldn't visualise Zoe living independently and holding down a job, although she was fully capable of doing so, as long as she didn't try to hurt herself or anyone else. I felt that I would need a lot of patience and staying power to find out the end of this story.

Three years later

I had put this story aside but can now resume it three years later. Zoe stopped ECT soon after achieving remission. But instead of relapsing, as I had predicted, she remained relatively well - at least, she no longer tried to kill herself. She didn't quite manage to get herself discharged from hospital but had progressed to an open ward. And then, about two and a half years after the last ECT, her suicidal wishes came back. She agreed to have more ECTs. We greeted each other like old friends when she came for her first session. Her mind was still sharp and she was pleasant with staff. The overpowering wish to take her life had returned in full force, however, and she shared it with us during the cognitive testing in her own unique way. The MMSE questionnaire contains one item that tests people's writing but occasionally reveals what is at the top of their agendas: 'Write any complete sentence on the line below, anything that comes to your mind.'

Zoe had written '*This place is a fucking bullshit hellhole. I want to fucking kill myself.*' But she still knew that ECT was helping her and agreed to have it! Hats off to her – for sheer perseverance in a near-impossible situation, Zoe won my admiration every time. This ECT course was again quite successful and her commitment to maintenance sessions extended over another six months.

I might meet Zoe again, or she might continue to improve without ECT, time will tell. But I will stop this story here. Unlike surgery, for example, these stories do not always have a clean ending and are not always resolved. Instead, like everyday life, they tend to go on.

Many of my colleagues will struggle to give ECT to people with personality disorder and in most cases they will be right. However, we may forget that people with personality disorder can become depressed, and in fact most of them will suffer an episode of depression in their lifetime. Depression and other mental health problems respond to ECT. Should we deny such an effective treatment to these people just because they are labelled as having personality disorder? In the case of Zoe, it didn't 'cure' her, but it did give her years of improved functioning. Even if 'only' the depression improved, this still had a significant knock-on effect on other aspects of her behaviour and obviated the need for close observation – in itself a major blessing. I hope she will leave hospital one day and I am not as sure as before that she will kill herself after discharge. I guess we just need to look for the right indications in selecting people for treatment, to keep patients well informed and to give them full autonomy in their decisions.

5

CATATONIA[5]

'New referral today, you need to check it out - she has some 'holes in the brain," Kara greeted me with a wink, including me in the joke as I came through the door of the treatment room. The patient had been referred for ECT by the liaison team from the general hospital, and nobody had asked me for an opinion, so I knew nothing about it. Kara wanted me to look at it, as she had spotted a suspicious MRI report on the system. We don't want to treat somebody with a brain tumour, but what is 'holes in the brain'? I needed to see the scans and dig out more details about the history.

The general hospital computer system stores MRI images, letters, discharge summaries, laboratory tests... There were a lot of these under Laura's entry, and the more I read, the more complicated this story seemed to be as it unfolded.

Laura had first been admitted to hospital about two months previously, with confusion that had lasted for several weeks and that had not abated throughout the admission. She had been given a working diagnosis of hypoactive delirium - in other words, she was confused

---

[5] Catatonia: a syndrome of movement disturbances, such as slowness or stupor, missing or minimal verbal response, grimacing, agitation. It can develop in psychiatric disorders or secondary to general medical conditions. It is treated with benzodiazepines first, but if they don't work, ECT can be successful in over 80% of cases.

and disorientated, perhaps with some psychotic experiences, but didn't have the agitation and over-activity of typical delirium usually associated with severe alcohol abuse ('delirium tremens' or alcohol withdrawal delirium). The diagnosis hypoactive delirium describes the presentation, but conveniently avoids any indications as to a possible underlying cause, which can range from illness or infection to the effects of surgery or medication. Laura had a urinary tract infection, and a pleural effusion was detected on a chest X-ray, (i.e. excess fluid between the lung linings), suggesting an infection in her lungs. Either of these can in fact cause delirium, especially in a frail person. But, despite the strong antibiotics she had been given, Laura wasn't making much progress, so infection appeared a less likely cause.

So far, then, this was looking like a medical illness. The doctors suggested Laura's delirium could be due to possible cognitive decline, that is, dementia. I was sceptical about this diagnosis: the onset of illness was quite sudden, with changes in her behaviour and cognition progressing substantially within a single month. She was also a bit young to develop dementia, although unusual cases do tend to concentrate in hospitals. Laura had had one admission to psychiatric hospital for a nervous breakdown, but that was more than 30 years ago and she had not been treated by psychiatrists since. Recently, she had been talking about feelings of sadness and hopelessness for the future. Reading this account for the second time, I noticed comments that I had overlooked at first, but that were now beginning to fit together: 'Eyes mostly closed … lying still in bed … gripped firmly my hand … speech very quiet … limited answers.' Catatonic elements were offering themselves as a differential diagnosis, but Laura was still holding conversations and was able to move around. So far this was most likely to be purely a severe case of depression. The medical team wanted her transferred to a psychiatric ward.

Then came the brain scans. They showed multiple white matter lesions in the brain. The radiologist wondered if these could be the more usual infarcts from small blood vessel disease, or whether they could indicate multiple sclerosis (MS) or a related demyelinating condition. Another MRI found some similar lesions in the spinal cord as well. Laura had been transferred to a neurological ward and given steroids for suspected MS. But after a few days the neurologists concluded that the changes on the scans were old, left from undiagnosed MS that had flared up many years ago and could not account for the severe mental health presentation and cognitive decline.

One week on and Laura was still in the general hospital. Her condition had been deteriorating; she had stopped eating and was now being fed via a nasogastric tube. She would not open her eyes, even resisting the doctor opening them, and was not responding to questions though apparently able to hear them. ECT was considered, as this now looked more like psychotic depression with catatonia. It was at this point that Kara asked me to check the brain scans. Now, I wondered, was this presentation caused by MS, or some other neurological condition that had been left undiagnosed? Even if it was, ECT could still be indicated if the patient developed catatonia or severe psychotic depression. A third brain scan had been ordered, due to Laura's severe deterioration, but reassuringly, the scan images remained unchanged.

Lorazepam (a benzodiazepine) is the first drug that should be given for catatonia, and with this diagnosis now top of the list, before starting ECT, Laura was given 2mg, followed by another 2mg, intramuscularly. The effect was impressive. She was reported as brighter and she herself described her mind as much clearer and her mood as 'not too bad'. She had started eating again, was able to brush her hair herself and was even smiling. She was happy to see her family. 'I was closing off to the world' sounded like a good description of a catatonic state, where the person feels there is a barrier to movements and speech. ECT was cancelled by a beaming SHO who came to the clinic to share the good news. 'It's the first time I have seen Lorazepam used for catatonia; it's great!'

'Yes, Lorazepam *can* sometimes work for catatonia' was my more sceptical reflection, having treated cases where it hadn't worked.

The euphoria that had spread among the psychiatric liaison team lasted only until that evening. Laura deteriorated again, quickly, her movements slowing down, although she was still talking. Repeated Lorazepam did nothing to stop the decline. A few more days, and she became mute. ECT was planned once more.

One can read such descriptions of medical uncertainties for hours, but you always learn something new when you see the patient. I confess that I had not yet seen her and was getting ready to cycle to the general hospital where Laura was still being looked after, when I received a call from the liaison psychiatrist. It turned out to be almost as informative as seeing the patient. Laura was looking depressed. There wasn't a single neurological sign to suggest acute MS. Her reflexes were normal, the movement of eyes, reaction of pupils, speech (when offered), and muscular strength were all preserved. But she was resisting movements, not answering questions, and refusing food and drink. The picture painted by my colleague was clear and he had no doubt that this was one of these cases that needed urgent ECT. This was catatonia.

'Okay,' I concurred. 'We can treat her tomorrow morning.'

Later that day I wrote down Laura's story up to this point. I added subsequent details week by week, as events unfolded. I didn't know what would happen to this patient, but the build-up intrigued me so much that I wanted to document the details, even if Laura didn't have ECT. I have written a few of the stories this way, happy to take the risk of having to throw them away later, if they proved too devoid of interest. But they never did. Sometimes I had to wait for weeks or months to find out what happened to these patients - occasionally even years - but, to my mind, the interest never flagged, as I tracked the progress of this courageous and varied group. Unlike me, the reader can learn the outcome in just a few minutes, but can still share my uncertainty and sometimes anxiety about the unknown outcome. I quickly appreciated one other advantage of writing 'in real time': I remember more details if I write them down in the evening, just after they happen.

ECT No.1

I was still in two minds about Laura's diagnosis. On the morning of my first encounter with her, however, all doubts disappeared. She was brought into the unit by ambulance, lying on a stretcher. She looked like someone on the point of death: eyes closed, mouth half-open, lying flat on her back, limp and without movement. My first thought was whether the anaesthetist would even agree to anaesthetise her or would instead conclude that she was terminally ill. She certainly gave that impression. But she wasn't about to die, or not yet, at least. Her blood pressure, pulse rate, temperature and oxygen saturation were all appropriate even for a fit young person. Her face was pinkish. She responded to my voice by blinking rapidly and by twitching her lips. I felt that she was trying to answer as I addressed her by name, but she could produce no words. I checked her muscle strength. She was opposing my movements: the more I tried to pull her wrist away from her chest, the more strongly she pulled back, not allowing her hand to move even an inch away. Likewise, when I tested this the opposite way, pushing her wrist towards her body, she was pushing my arm back. The same strong muscular response was present on the left and on the right. Her eyes were shut and when I tried to open them, she resisted. I needed to open them, to examine their movement and reaction to light. These functions were normal. All this was very reassuring: not only was there no obvious loss of muscle tone or any neurological deficit, but the active resistance suggested a name to the presentation (negativism), supporting the diagnosis of catatonia.[6] This clinical picture can be caused by medical or psychiatric causes, but the treatment with ECT was now looking mandatory. By now I didn't have to worry about any possible physical contraindications, a mass in her brain having been excluded after several brain scans.

---

[6] The opposition to instructions or external stimuli is called negativism, another sign of catatonia. You need to have three or more catatonic signs to be given this diagnosis.

Our anaesthetist didn't see much danger in treating Laura either, apart from low potassium that was corrected with a bag of intravenous fluids, and a possible risk of cardiac complications, for which new defibrillator pads were prepared and the defibrillator was tested one more time. We went ahead and delivered the first treatment. Pads were not needed, and a rather poor seizure at 195mC caused hardly any change in pulse rate or blood pressure. This starting dose was according to the emergency protocol, with no titration to establish the seizure threshold, to avoid a wasted session, but even this setting was not strong enough to create a proper therapeutic seizure. The Lorazepam of the previous few days must have increased the seizure threshold. 'Never mind, we will get it right next time,' I muttered to myself. 'She is stable enough and she must respond to ECT.'

ECT No.2

Laura looked unchanged after the weekend. Her face just flickered when she was asked to respond, and once more she resisted any movements. She was still on regular Lorazepam, despite it clearly no longer working. Even worse, it was working against the seizures. I made a note to tell the team to stop this drug, as it was only a nuisance. As it was, we would have to increase the electric charge for the ECT to have any effect. Perhaps a 50% increase was reasonable or even too cautious. To my satisfaction, Laura had a great seizure today, so good that I was surprised and even took a picture of the EEG traces, to have an image to hand of what a good seizure should look like:

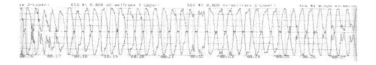

The EEG of a good seizure.

ECT Nos 3, 4 and 5

There was a clear response to the treatment. Laura was reported to be sitting up in bed, talking, and eating toast. After ECT No.3 she started combing her hair herself and was able to smile. After ECT No.4 she was sitting up in bed and talking to staff. Unfortunately, I didn't get to see any of this. Not because I was away, either. Just as her response to Lorazepam had lasted for only 12 hours, so Laura's response to each ECT was also short-lived. After the fourth session she had been talking and sitting up for two days, but on the third day, when she came for treatment, she was again unresponsive. This raised the question of what might happen if we gave her ECT at shorter intervals. Logical enough, but in the UK, ECT is given twice a week only, and an increased frequency is discouraged (although not formally banned), probably due to the same reason for which ECT itself is discouraged – concern about possible cognitive side effects. But in the USA, ECT is given three times a week. If Laura had an ECT a day after the previous session, while still talking, perhaps the next one would bring the further improvement we needed, instead of starting again from level zero. It was all so logical that I was now considering breaking the rules and giving her ECT three times a week.

I decided to probe the views of my colleagues who lead other ECT clinics in the UK. I placed an inquiry with our ECT accreditation service (ECTAS), which distributes such questions by e-mail to all clinics. Very quickly it returned responses of universal support from colleagues for the use of ECT more frequently than twice a week in emergencies. My colleagues know their trade. But I didn't need to make use of this option.

The following Monday Laura had been taken off her section, as she had regained capacity and had provided written consent for ECT. My immediate comment, when she arrived on Tuesday morning, was that the decision had been premature. Laura had stopped talking again and I was just about satisfied that she still had capacity, by leaning over her face and very intently trying to make out the faint words that she was whispering, 'Yes, ECT is helping me... yes I want to continue with it...' Her consultant had heard a much louder voice on the previous day and seen a smiling and chatty lady, I was assured by the nurse who accompanied her.

We could now plan an extra session for that week, on the Friday. But on Thursday evening, I read the following excited note that Kara had posted on our secure communications server, pasted here with no changes: 'She is miraculously cured, chatting away, really lovely lady, spontaneous conversation, interested in what is going on around her, thinks the treatment was great and will recommend it to others. Asked us why she had not been talking, apologising if she had been rude to staff.' This transformation had happened after six sessions. We cancelled the extra treatment planned for Friday.

The following week I finally managed to witness for myself this 'miraculous recovery'. It was exactly that. Laura was not just smiling but was showing such interest in people around her, it was almost as if she was working here! She admitted that she couldn't remember what had happened to her and how she had come to stop talking. The words were quick, articulated at a normal volume and pace, as if she had never gone through her recent dramatic breakdown.

Of course, I wanted to figure out what was the actual medical diagnosis. For example, despite the contradictory evidence, did she in fact have MS? This was still unresolved: the neurological opinion was that she probably had gone through a mild episode in the past, but there was no current flare-up. Despite that view, she was still prescribed steroids for a few weeks, a fact that somewhat further exposed the diagnostic uncertainty. And a few weeks after the ECT course she did have another episode of numbness that raised renewed fears of a stroke. However, a CT scan returned the same uninformative message: 'No change from the previous scans'.

There was one more complication to this medical story. Laura had used a wheelchair for several years, due to poor mobility. Surely because of MS, I assumed. Not really. She told me that it was due to her bad back, which caused her significant pain if she tried to stand up. She had suffered with her back for many years.

The muscular strength in her arms and legs was preserved. Her reflexes were intact, and so were her fine motor skills. 'She should be able to walk, really,' I muttered under my breath. I was annoyed that our ECT hadn't produced an even more miraculous recovery and allowed her to jump up from her wheelchair and walk! I had assumed that her current inability to walk was due to her having been bedridden for so long.

'We will organise some physiotherapy now. I think you can walk.'

But this prospect was not greeted with great excitement, as far as I could make out. Perhaps Laura had already tried and had given up years ago. Maybe she simply couldn't go through the pain and effort again. I changed the subject.

Laura had a total of 10 ECT sessions and was discharged back to her own home. A month later she came for a follow-up and told us that she felt better than she could ever remember feeling. She was still using a wheelchair, but a nurse who visited her at home told me that Laura had opened the front door herself to welcome her in, using a zimmer frame. She was indeed able to get out of the wheelchair, but it was always too much of an effort and probably caused pain. Laura was happy with her life and was doing 'bits and bobs' in the house, the nurse explained. Okay, I conceded, we didn't get her out of the wheelchair, but Laura was happy and certainly not confused any longer: her MMSE score was 29 (out of 30).

Laura remained well during the one year of follow-up. I remained curious as to the cause of her presentation and about a year later visited her at her home to find out more. She opened the door herself, leaning on a frame, as described by the nurse, but moving quite skilfully around the house. She was smiling and assured me that she had not felt depressed since the ECT. She remembered being frightened of everything around her, but the memories of the episode were quite patchy. No surprise there, she had probably not been fully conscious or orientated for some of the time. Although mentally completely well, she was now in physical pain, which stopped her from walking. She sounded quite conversant with the medical terminology: 'This is a neuropathic pain in my legs. It is caused by the MS.' So she did have MS after all, as always suspected. She was having regular neurological appointments and had been told she now had MS that was showing signs of progression, having had a relapsing-remitting form in the past. This explained the numbness in her legs that had occurred a few times in the past but that she had attributed to a prolapsed disc in her back, as well as the numbness in other parts of her body, that had attracted other explanations. The old lesions noticed on her brain scans had indeed been caused by MS, not strokes.

"I know I had catatonia, doctor. I was not talking, not moving. Do you know what caused it?' If she had asked me this question a year ago, I would have been a bit vague. But now everything seemed to fit in.

'Catatonia can develop not only as part of a psychiatric illness. It can also be a consequence of serious medical conditions. You were physically unwell; you were not fully awake. You had two infections: a urinary tract infection and one in the lungs. And perhaps the MS also played a role. These periods of numbness tell us that your MS was active around that time, although mild. I can't see how this could be just a coincidence. Your depression had not got any worse before the episode, so I don't think it can on its own account for what happened.'

Laura was nodding in approval. She knew that she had not been her usual self, and a medical illness made more sense to her in terms of explaining her predicament. Before we said goodbye, she stressed how kind the ECT staff had been to her. I was surely going to pass on this message.

6

PARKINSON'S DISEASE

Elizabeth is one of our regulars, coming to our clinic once every five weeks. As she has trouble walking, she uses a wheelchair. Her hands and fingers flap around when she is not holding them together on her lap. Her face looks a bit stiff and her skin is always pink and warm, due to the constant, involuntary body movements caused by her Parkinson's disease. But she always smiles warmly and tells us that she is doing all right and enjoying life. Eight years ago, nearly everybody had given up on her treatment and she was nearly discharged to a nursing home with a diagnosis of dementia. However, her psychiatrist had other ideas.

Parkinson's disease is about dopamine, a neurotransmitter in the brain involved in the fine regulation of movements. It also controls our drives, our reward-motivated behaviour, and our addictions, increasing sensations of pleasure. If the neurons stop secreting enough dopamine - around 80% less than normal - the person's movements become stiff, they start shaking and walking with small steps, their faces may become mask-like, and they may even freeze, suddenly unable to move or even speak for a while. The disease can be treated with drugs containing dopamine, but occasionally these drugs can cause hallucinations and psychosis. In fact, people who suffer from schizophrenia are treated with drugs that block dopamine receptors, called antipsychotics, which can actually lead to symptoms of Parkinsonism, although modern antipsychotics cause considerably fewer of these side effects.

As you can see, we are already setting the scene for a problem here. A person with Parkinson's disease who develops psychosis will be given antipsychotic drugs, which will exacerbate their motor symptoms. Thus the two drugs work against each other, and we are pushing the same system from two opposing sides.

Somehow ECT fits very well into this scenario. During seizures there is a sharp release of dopamine in the brain - so much so, that the dopamine release can be used as a test to check whether a person has had a real epileptic seizure. So not only is ECT very effective in the treatment of depression and psychosis in Parkinson's disease, but it can even help the motor symptoms. Granted, ECT might not lead to the production of more dopamine or the synthesis of more neurons that make dopamine, so it shouldn't really make a change to the motor symptoms of the disease, but this effect has been noticed in many reports. These theoretical considerations and many observations of real patients have resulted in ECT being promoted as a valid treatment of depression and psychosis in Parkinson's disease. But as usual, things do not follow the script. Elizabeth was a patient who almost missed out on this treatment.

Her first symptoms started just before the age of 60, when she was bothered by a tremor in one hand. It was starting to become embarrassing, although not yet affecting her functioning. A brain scan was normal, but the neurologist diagnosed Parkinson's disease, and over the next few years she gradually progressed from beta blockers to drugs that stimulate the dopamine receptors

(Ropinirole) and eventually to dopamine itself: the drug Madopar delivers levodopa to the brain where it is changed to dopamine. Eight years later her movements were still excellent, 'No falls, cognition intact, symptoms well controlled' read a hospital appointment letter. In fact, she was fully independent and even continued going to dancing classes! The need for Madopar was, however, increasing.

At this point Elizabeth became psychotic. It happened suddenly. She believed that she was a wicked person who had betrayed her friends, that her flat was bugged and that the television was transmitting programmes about her. She was depressed, unable to concentrate, she wished she were dead, and had no energy. She was admitted to hospital, tearful, paranoid of people around her, wringing her hands, that were at the same time jerking uncontrollably with shakes. Her delusions were expanding: she now felt that she was emitting a nasty odour. Her Mini Mental State Examination (MMSE) score had dropped down to 23 out of 30 (22 is an accepted cut-off for dementia). Her psychiatrist correctly suspected that excessive dopamine from her current drugs was responsible for the psychosis (more dopamine > more psychosis), so Madopar was stopped. She improved and was discharged home, only to be readmitted two months later in an even worse condition. This time she believed that her food was contaminated and she was refusing to eat. She complained that her belongings were missing and even that her legs were missing. Visual hallucinations of people walking around ignited further worries among her doctors about incipient dementia. Indeed, dementia occurs at an increased rate among Parkinson's patients, with the typical type recognised as Lewy body dementia, presenting with visual hallucinations in 80% of cases. Lewy bodies are abnormal protein deposits in the brain, named after Friedrich Lewy who first described them in 1912, although the disease was not recognised until many years later. This diagnosis was not firm, as her CT scan returned a fairly intact image of her brain, but as it is not possible to get a brain biopsy, nobody could be certain.

Elizabeth was treated with antipsychotics this time, despite the risk of inhibiting her movements further. A few 'atypical' antipsychotics were tried first, as they have a lower risk of worsening the symptoms of Parkinson's disease, and very soon she was tried on the best choice for this condition: Clozapine. Not only is Clozapine the most effective antipsychotic, but it is also the least likely to cause Parkinsonism. But it didn't work. Not only did it not work, but Elizabeth continued to deteriorate. Her MMSE dropped to 15, suggesting severe dementia. Her behaviour was becoming increasingly odd too: she was shouting, stripping, and walking backwards or on tiptoe. She kept repeating the same words. And then she stopped moving, started freezing on the spot, and at times she was incontinent. In fact, she stopped communicating completely. Placement in a nursing home with a diagnosis of untreatable dementia was looking very likely. Her consultant psychiatrist didn't give up, however. He wanted to try ECT and asked me to support his view with a second opinion.

It was at this point that I first saw Elizabeth, entering this story a number of years before writing it. Elizabeth clearly had Parkinson's. Her muscles were stiff, if we exclude the severe tremor of her fingers and some lip movements. Her face was immobile, like a mask. She could not communicate with me but instead kept repeating the same phrase over and over again. Initially I couldn't understand what she was saying, but after a few repeats figured it out: 'I can't do anything.' I was struck. She realised that she was locked in by her illness, unable to move or talk. She was describing her condition correctly, and I had to assume that she was also aware of everything that was going on around her. This was not just the immobility of Parkinson's disease: she was also catatonic.

We had a bit of a dilemma. Elizabeth seemed to be developing Lewy body dementia and there was nothing anyone could do about that. She was psychotic, but if we increased her antipsychotics or stopped the dopamine, she would become more immobile. If we did the opposite, she could become more psychotic. Dopamine had already been stopped by this point, resulting in her frozen presentation. We were caught between the devil and the deep blue sea: a frozen state, with Elizabeth aware but unable to communicate or move, or psychosis, with all its tormenting illusions. When I presented her case at our weekly academic meeting, there was one sole view among my colleagues: her best chance of survival was ECT. Even if Elizabeth was developing dementia, ECT could still provide her with a better quality of life, eliminating the psychosis and allowing her to have the dopamine that would unlock her movements. The literature was also clear: ECT is effective in treating depression in Parkinson's disease and even improves the motor symptoms. Dementia is not a contraindication.

By the time we started treatment, contact with Elizabeth was impossible, so she was treated on a section of the Mental Health Act. The treatments were uneventful and after five ECTs she was able to talk and feed herself.

However, she still appeared demented: she was unable to complete the MMSE and displayed inappropriate behaviour with angry outbursts on the ward, that were quite out of character, I was assured. After 10 ECTs we had another discussion with her psychiatrist and the neurologist and agreed that it was safe to restart a low dose Madopar.

After 12 sessions it was time for the miracle! This was eight years before I sat down to write this story, so for this account I have to rely on what I wrote down in her notes at the time: 'Dramatic improvement, MMSE=27. Consenting to ECT, agreed to continue ECT twice a week until full improvement has been reached. Diagnosis of dementia seems unlikely.' Elizabeth was now smiling and talking in a kind, soothing voice. She had never been demented, only slowed down by her illness. The persistence of her psychiatrist had paid off and literally saved her. Her shaking was much reduced, but she still couldn't walk unaided, due to her Parkinson's disease. With her psychosis no longer standing in the way, the neurologist was able to increase her Madopar to proper treatment doses. I did my bit by stubbornly keeping her ECT at a frequency of twice a week.

On the morning of her 19th ECT we witnessed her somewhat triumphant entry into the treatment room. She was almost upright, still holding onto a frame but walking on her own, unsupported by anybody. She was smiling, looked at each one of us and greeted us in a soft but clear voice. Her depression score that morning was just three points: she was in remission. Later that week she was discharged to her home, with the occupational therapist confirming that she could look after herself. ECT was stopped after a total of 22 sessions.

Of course, the story didn't finish there. Three years later Elizabeth relapsed with very similar symptoms of psychotic depression, telling us that her legs were broken and that she was killing 'everybody in the world'. Six ECTs in quick succession were enough to bring her back into remission. It was not that difficult to persuade her that she needed maintenance ECT in the future, and we settled for giving it every four weeks after a gradual increase in the interval between sessions that did not precipitate any relapse. She stuck to this regime and now, as I am writing her story another four years later, she is still free from depression, coming to our unit every five weeks, and with no doubts in her mind that this treatment is keeping her well. Unfortunately her shaking is becoming more pronounced with advancing age and is at times so severe that it warms up her whole body. Her walking is also deteriorating, and she needs help - but she still manages most activities at home independently, and her carers only visit her during the day. She is able to enjoy little things, like television and outings in town. And what about her dementia? Well, her MMSE eight years after the presumed onset of dementia was still 28. Just like mine. Yes, I got two items wrong last time I tested myself. I was always bad at naming nearby streets, but why did I get the date wrong?

7

NOT RESPONDING TO ANYTHING

'Dear Colleague,

I would value your opinion on this patient of mine who is suffering with treatment-resistant depression and has not responded to anything…'

I get these letters all the time. Here in Cardiff, we provide an academic second opinion service, and I deal with the referrals about depression. These come from colleagues who have tried hard to treat people in a variety of ways - different medications, cognitive behaviour therapy (CBT), admission to hospital, stopping all medications, etc. My heart sinks when I see these letters, as most options are usually exhausted. Only rarely is there a glaring omission in the treatment list or some relevant medical condition that has been overlooked. Overall, when my colleagues have already prescribed eight or nine drugs, I know that my 'clever' suggestion for drug number 10 is also likely to fail.

I carried on reading the letter. There was a strong family history of depression. The lady herself, Margaret, had been a cheerful and confident person all her life, had brought up her children and had later enjoyed the company of her grandchildren. She had first become depressed around the age of 50, had been given an antidepressant and had improved straight away. She had stayed well for another 10 years without a hint of a problem and had been cheerful and liked by everybody. Then came a diagnosis of breast cancer, which was treated successfully. Margaret was told that she was cured. That should have been the end of the problem, but the stress appeared to have lodged inside her mind and remained stuck there. Two months later her depression came back. She was given the same antidepressant as during her first episode but this time didn't get better.

The reading became more and more gloomy. 'We have tried her on the following medications: Quetiapine, Mirtazapine, Olanzapine, Duloxetine, Lithium, Pregabalin, Sertraline, Paroxetine, Trifluoperazine. She had combinations of Mirtazapine + Lithium + Venlafaxine and Olanzapine + Duloxetine + Mirtazapine. She is now on Lithium + Quetiapine + Mirtazapine + Venlafaxine.'

This list was longer than usual and hinted at desperation. My options for advice were shrinking. My best hope was to spot the glaring omission. I scanned down the letter to see if she had been given ECT. If she hadn't, then I could recommend something. Bad news: 'Last year she received a course of ECT but did not respond.'

I interviewed Margaret and her husband. She established good eye contact and even managed to produce a few smiles but was clearly depressed. She looked rather restless, fidgeting and wringing her hands. She described her feelings as terrible mental torture - she kept worrying about everything and was not interested in anything. She felt like a different person. Life was not worth living for her, in fact, she would rather be dead, but was not planning to do anything because of her children. I asked them about the ECT course: did it really not work at all? Her husband made a clear statement, 'Yes, doctor, I couldn't see any difference whatsoever.' This was only a slightly worse account than that written by her doctor in the letter, which suggested some mild but unclear improvement.

I looked back over the medications and tried to see what she had been taking during the ECT course. It seemed possible that it had coincided with the time she had been on Pregabalin, a drug used to combat anxiety but an antiepileptic in origin, which would have mitigated against good seizures under ECT treatment, potentially cancelling it out. Did she have good seizures? I knew I was clutching at straws, but there wasn't much else to clutch at.

I suggested that her psychiatrist try her on a tricyclic antidepressant. Tricyclics are the oldest antidepressants, the name coming from their chemical formulas that contain three rings of atoms. They remain the most effective antidepressants but have worse side effects than the newer ones. Margaret also needed a course of cognitive behavioural therapy (she had declined a previous offer) and Modafinil, an activating medication used to treat excessive sleepiness. I also stated that my colleagues should organise a brain scan: what if secondaries from the old cancer had spread to the brain? And of course, they should review the ECT course, seizure quality and duration, and perhaps persuade her to have another one... (I suggested a few ways to improve seizure quality). I sent off the letter and heard nothing back.

I forgot about Margaret. Four years later, I received a letter asking me to provide another opinion on her condition. She had remained virtually unchanged. Her HAM-D was 22 (practically the same as the 24 points from four years earlier). She had tried three more medications, although my advice on tricyclics and Modafinil had not been followed. 'Drugs have done nothing,' stated her husband, and I couldn't add anything to his conclusion.

On this occasion I received a detailed breakdown of her ECT course. Nearly all seizures had been just nine seconds or even shorter. It was not just the effect of the Pregabalin; the problem was probably made worse by the Propofol used as the anaesthetic. The electric charge was high enough, with doses of up to 750mC being used at the end, towards the upper end of the machine range.

There was only one realistic chance for her - to respond to better seizures. This could only happen if we stopped all drugs that might interfere with the seizure quality. First, I had to persuade Margaret that she could benefit from another course of ECT. I also explained that she had to stop her Diazepam and Lamotrigine (another anticonvulsant used also as a mood stabiliser) and to stay off these drugs for two months. I was taking no chances of giving her another series of marginal seizures. It was easier than I expected, as Margaret and her family had no other suggestions or hopes left. I also promised that we could arrange her treatments at our unit, so I could supervise them myself and make sure the seizures were good.

Just over two months later, Margaret presented herself for ECT. She had hardly managed to survive without Diazepam, with the anxiety increasing after she reduced the dose. Her first stimulation was at 184mC with Thiopental, on the higher end for a titration session, as I expected a high threshold. The seizure was very poor, but it gave us a clear threshold. The electric dose was doubled for the second ECT, but annoyingly and surprisingly, the seizure lasted only 11 seconds visible and 16 seconds on the EEG. I want to see at least 15 seconds of visible seizures before labelling them as 'good'. The third was just nine seconds, despite the dose now reaching 426mC. I could see where this was going - we were following the pattern of her previous course. I didn't experiment with Thiopental any longer and at the fourth ECT she was given Etomidate, while keeping the electric charge the same. Changing the anaesthetic to Etomidate is not popular in the UK, but in our department it nearly always solves the problems of poor seizures, bringing the seizure threshold down by about half and invariably prolonging seizure length. However, the seizures improved only marginally, lasting for just over 15 seconds. The stronger ones provoked some extra heartbeats, but these didn't cause any real concern, and they became more isolated with time.

A more persistent problem was slowly building up and would gradually take priority: Margaret's memory was deteriorating. The complaints she listed got worse and worse. She had already experienced problems before the start of ECT, and her MMSE was fluctuating between 22-25 points. Her husband told us that the memory gaps were becoming a family joke, though he wasn't sure how funny they really were. And then I was treated to a rare example of retrograde amnesia, dispelling any doubts that this was real: Margaret appeared to have forgotten completely that she had had breast cancer, that same cancer which had triggered the avalanche of her depression some seven years previously. She would not even believe it had happened, until her husband pointed to the scar beneath her breast. But even more convincingly, she had remembered another operation many years earlier, that had also left her with an operative scar of a similar size. The retrograde amnesia had spread back over at least seven years!

But for now, all such problems seemed insignificant to Margaret. She was improving and after 14 sessions was scoring close to remission, although not quite reaching it, as she was still having problems with anxiety and sleep. Her husband was delighted. Margaret was sharp, witty and cheerful, even laughing at her own memory gaps. She was chatting to everybody, following people with interest, her eyes sparkling with life. I even wondered if she could be getting slightly hypomanic, only to be reassured by her husband that this was her true self.

This was a success. We had lifted the depression in a person who had been ill for seven years, who had moreover tried over a dozen drugs and had had an unsuccessful previous course of ECT. So our ECT protocols were good and yes, this was yet more proof, if it were needed, that seizure quality does matter. Maybe I was a bit too chuffed at it all! But, really, deep down I knew all too well that the hard work had only just started. These treatment-resistant patients are the ones most likely to relapse and I had no idea of Margaret's long-term prognosis. We quickly moved to weekly sessions in order to reduce her memory problems. Then after a total of 18 ECTs, we tried to go to two-week intervals.

This is where everything started going downhill. Margaret's mood was already dipping three days after an ECT, and the two-week intervals proved too optimistic. We went back to weekly ones, but the momentum had been lost. Margaret was now clearly suffering from poor memory. This had been laughed away by her when she was well but was magnified when her mind was overcome by the pessimism of depression. Now it became too much of a problem. Her memory loss was real and the gaps were spanning years back. We tried to minimise the problems by switching to right unilateral ECT (with the two electrodes placed on one side of the head, over the right, non-dominant hemisphere), as this method has been shown to cause less confusion and fewer memory problems. She had six of these at weekly intervals and after a short improvement, relapsed again. I was not surprised: she had not responded to poor bilateral seizures in the past, and unilateral ECT is slightly less effective than the bilateral type, where the electrodes are placed on both sides of the head. We had to switch back to bilateral and after just two sessions she was well again, scoring one single point on the HAM-D.

Deep vein thrombosis necessitated another break in the course. Thrombi from the legs can be dislodged by the muscular contractions during the seizure, and while there are ways of preventing this, we were advised to wait. It took six weeks for her depression to come back, and another six before we could treat her again. After three weeks of ECT, given at a rate of two sessions per week, her smile returned. Eventually we moved to weekly sessions again. But this time Margaret wouldn't reach the single-digit scores on the depression scale that signify a remission. Gradually, she was losing faith in the treatment. Memory problems were dominating our conversations. After just three sessions spaced at weekly intervals, she refused to continue. I found it difficult to insist: by then she had had a total of 48 sessions over a period of nearly one year.

Margaret remained depressed over the following year, although not as severely as when she had first come to see me. It was painful to know that although ECT had brought her back to her usual cheerful self, we were unable to keep her well. I am not sure what we could have done better. With a more intensive course she might have stayed reasonably well but this would probably have been at the expense of worse memory problems. When Margaret was very well, she was willing to ignore these, but once anxiety and doubts returned, her memory became more important. If ECT was spaced out to every three weeks, we might have solved the problem, but her depression didn't allow it. A fine balance that we were unable to strike.

Epilogue

Two years after I wrote this story, I did another follow-up on Margaret. I didn't expect to see much good news in the hospital computer records, so I was surprised and pleased to read an entry stating that she had been feeling very well, smiling and enjoying life. Her doctor seemed equally surprised and had asked to what she attributed her improvement. 'Perhaps it is the Chlorpromazine' she had suggested. I browsed back through the entries on the screen, going a few months back. Indeed, this drug had been started while she was still depressed, to reduce her severe anxiety. She found it helpful and the dose had been increased. She had then improved and was now very well.

Good old Chlorpromazine! Almost unused now by older psychiatrists, almost never encountered by the younger ones, this was the first antipsychotic, discovered by coincidence in Paris in 1952, by Pierre Deniker and Jean Delay. Its potential use in psychiatry was first recognised by a surgeon, Henri Laborit, who was looking for a way to reduce surgical shock in his patients. He tried various antihistamines, among them a new substance, Chlorpromazine which, he noted, caused indifference in patients facing surgery. Chlorpromazine's clinical use was further investigated by Delay and Deniker, who reported, 'The results were stunning. Patients who had stood in one spot without moving for weeks, patients who had to be restrained because of violent behaviour, could now make contact with others and be left without supervision'. These patients were suffering from schizophrenia, not depression, but an effective antipsychotic had been found and the trend was set.

Over the years, Chlorpromazine has been replaced by new antipsychotics, but with the exception of Clozapine, they are not more effective than the original, scoring better only on side effects. A sobering thought: three drugs discovered in the 1950s – Chlorpromazine, Lithium and Imipramine (a tricyclic antidepressant) - are still on my list of recommendations today, when I review patients who have not responded to anything. ECT was introduced even earlier, in 1938. Did it have a role in Margaret's eventual recovery? I can't quite exclude it.

8

TO HELL AND BACK

As the years pass, new referrals to the clinic are often likely to be people whom I already know, having treated them in the past. The name of our latest referral, Rashid X, was familiar. Although he had been admitted to hospital, this was almost like a self-referral: he himself wanted to have ECT. He didn't like the side-effects of his medications and wanted to decrease them. For some reason he had retained better memories of his ECT course. He came for initial assessment and we at once recognised each other and recalled the success of his previous treatment. He had stayed well for several years but recently had noticed the signs of illness again. These weren't difficult to recognise: his speech was hesitant, he was ruminating about his health, and crying at times.

My memories of his previous course were patchy. I checked my notes and was disappointed with myself. They didn't contain enough detail for me to reconstruct his story in full, despite him presenting with 'severe psychomotor retardation' during that first episode. Kara also reminded me that he had been very slow, but also that he had been an 'extremely nice chap, who did so well with ECT'. She clearly remembered more, having seen him many more times, and I sensed that his story would have been a good one to include. Pity I didn't write a better account at the time.

Trying to salvage something, I resorted to going through the electronic hospital records. This is a chore I hate and try to avoid whenever possible. I just spend too much time navigating the computer screen, and most pathways end in something irrelevant. Everybody who makes contact with a patient in the hospital leaves an entry: nurses, dietitians, occupational therapists, doctors. The more unwell you are, the more people interact with you. Rashid had at least four entries for each day and I had to negotiate my way through them one by one, trying to find the relevant statements and observations. As I was doing this, though, it became clear that these entries themselves were shaping into a story and I didn't need to do much more than just pick out the right moments and phrases and let them build up the story. It gave a different angle of observation - the views from the psychiatric ward, instead of my own perspective from the ECT unit. I could have summarised it, but felt that I should leave it to you, the reader, to follow the unfolding of events and the gradual worsening of symptoms, and to feel Rashid's story taking shape from these rather stark entries. I have refrained from making too many comments and only corrected some typos.

26.10 Admission avoidance assessment.[7] Actively suicidal, GP referral.

Middle-aged male. Born in XX. University degree in the UK. Self-reported issues with OCD since around 1980, when he was placed in a hospital for treatment due to a mental health breakdown.[8] Issues with OCD re-emerged 20 years later. Returning to XX to live with family until two months ago when he returned to the UK. Symptoms started a month ago.

---

[7] The community psychiatric team is trying to avoid admission to hospital.

[8] The later notes indicate that he had ECT during that admission, but this was not known to the team.

Since being back in the UK these symptoms of OCD and anxiety have exacerbated and he describes racing thoughts. Describes poor sleep due to these thoughts. Finds that when carrying out rituals at home he becomes overwhelmed with these thoughts, which increases his levels of anxiety. Objective evidence of low mood and anxiety throughout assessment. Hard to ascertain what is happening currently with Rashid. No historical documentation available, presented alone, no family or friends here, unknown to GP.

27.10 Hard to gain a reliable history. Quite distracted with poor focus and concentration with evidence of mild thought block. Managed to inform us that he has been hospitalised in XX for a 'breakdown' that was similar to how he is feeling now - at this point he was medicated with an antidepressant, Sertraline? Visibly anxious with poor concentration, easily distractible. Tearful and distressed throughout. Says he is very afraid. This seems to be generalised - afraid of everyone, had to leave city centre yesterday due to overwhelming feelings of fear. Expressed being worried about a couple of clinicians he encountered in the Day Centre - afraid they were going to harm him. Seemed essentially acute anxiety-related and not psychotic.

27.10 Expressing he cannot cope. Asking to be hospitalised as he is constantly very fearful and cannot take it anymore. Told us repeatedly throughout the assessment that if he was to go home he would wander the streets as he couldn't bear to sit at home acutely afraid - informed us he was having strong thoughts of taking an overdose.

27.10 Conducted emergency review with Dr. J. Attempted to persuade Rashid his anxiety would reduce if he took some Diazepam and Olanzapine and offered urgent review in outpatients with Dr. J tomorrow. Rashid unable to tolerate this, very distressed and tearful, fixated on his 'fear', referring to taking an overdose, asking for hospital admission.

27.10 Referred to CRHTT,[9] they will see him later. Possibly could have been managed with CMHT[10] with a decent support

---

[9] Crisis Resolution and Home Treatment Team

network such as close friends or family to stay with him, manage medication etc. However, very isolated and struggling to rationalise everything due to acute distress.

27.10 Says he may take an overdose due to fear and needing to be looked after. Admitted to Crisis House.

29.10 Staff reported that he'd not slept at all last night and appeared extremely anxious. Wringing his hands, variable eye contact. Long pauses between questions and answers - seemed to find it difficult to concentrate.

30.10 He told me he couldn't stay in his bedroom as he would contaminate everything he touched in there and wanted to stay in the lounge for the rest of the night.

30.10 Rashid stated that he is constantly fearful; afraid of leaving his room and going outside; this is due to him believing everything is 'dirty' and 'contaminated'. Rashid is also afraid of making his own food and drinks due to this belief, resulting in him not maintaining a good food and fluid intake.

1.11 Diet is poor due to OCD thoughts of being unclean therefore struggled to prepare food and drinks for himself. Rashid explained that when in his flat, and he thinks of dirt, his OCD symptoms and thoughts become so overwhelming he 'freezes' and can't concentrate on what he needs to do. This then triggers him to panic.

2.11 Very slow gait, long time to respond, sitting in chair, squeezing hands/fingers, making fists, minimal eye contact, took time but some rapport built and engaged.

Speech: very, very quiet, softly spoken.

Mood: 'scared, anxious' objectively dysthymic and anxious.

Thoughts: some thought block - takes a while to answer any questions. Has too many thoughts going through his head, cannot make any decisions because of the thoughts - it takes him a long time to do anything because his thoughts are going around in circles, back and forth. Feels paranoid and suspicious of others on the ward, does

---

[10] Community Mental Health Team

not feel like anyone is out to harm him. Feels he is 'going to have a mental breakdown', 'scared to go into my room', 'going from bad to worse'. Unable to say whether he has any suicidal thoughts.

Psychotic experiences: denied any hallucinations.

Insight: has some insight.

Found the ward environment very frightening and that he felt the staff tried to push him to do things that he wasn't ready to do: get out of bed, go for breakfast, and he found it a bit intimidating. He said that he had not been eating and drinking much.

3.11 Rashid was sat up on his bed with the lights off. He was dressed casually in clean clothes although his hair was dishevelled. He was sat with his cheek resting on his right hand, staring at the floor. He did not respond to any of my questions and remained in this pose throughout the review. Neither did he respond to touch.

4.11 Rashid told me that there is no point in living and he should be dead. He was not suggesting killing himself but more wishing he was not alive. He told me that he wished that the floor would swallow him up. He was trying to talk and tell me about his problems but I was unable to understand him due to him crying. Doctor spent 90 min with him. He has no confidence and noticed OCD symptoms from childhood. He explained that when he touches things (i.e. coins) he would feel that his hands are dirty, then when he touches other things, they would become contaminated by the germs.

6.11 Continues to isolate himself in his room, observed to be either sitting on the edge of his bed or standing by the door. Movement continues to be laboured and slow.

7.11 Isolating himself, slow. Stated has trouble swallowing things, however appears to swallow fine when eating. Later came to medication room asking for a clean cup, saying that all the cups are dirty, he also requested water that was not contaminated.

13.11 Every movement and action extremely slow. Incontinent of urine.

14.11 Rashid was slow walking/moving throughout the activity, conversation was made difficult by Rashid mumbling and talking quietly.

14.11 At Rashid's home he struggled with the most basic of tasks i.e. opening the door, climbing the stairs, entering the property he nearly fell over the doorstep. Inside his flat he remained very anxious, not settling the whole time we were there. On the journey back Rashid was upset at returning to hospital and cried, stating, 'I just want to sit at home in peace'.

14.11 Appears to need prompting ++ to eat small amounts of a meal.

14.11 I questioned him about his request for ECT yesterday, he voiced that he has no hope, he will get better and doesn't see 'a way out'. But wants to go home. Diazepam calms him down for a few hours. [Each entry over the last few days states that his movements were extremely slow, so I will spare the repetition.]

16.11 Rashid would often point at his throat and state he is having trouble breathing.

18.11 Discussed ECT. Moving around in a wheelchair but walking at other times.

19.11 Rashid stated that he has so many thoughts and things rushing through his mind. I attempted to explore this further, however Rashid stated, 'I cannot explain'. He stated he is so weak, he cannot even open the doors. Understands what ECT is and he stated he has had it before. I asked Rashid when this was and he replied, 'When I was very young'. I tried to speak with Rashid further regarding this and what his thoughts were in relation to this treatment. He stated he is struggling to feel things, that he doesn't know when he is hungry or thirsty or when he needs to go to the toilet. He stated he is in pain because his body feels so weak and can barely walk from his bedroom to the lounge.

24.11 I got an ECT information booklet to go through with Rashid. On approach Rashid stated 'I know what it is'. Consented.

24.11 Rashid didn't accept any food or fluids this evening. I encouraged Rashid to write his feelings down on paper. Rashid wrote **'I feel like I'm in hell'** *and 'It's too late'. Requested ECT. Assisted to go to bed, as his movements are too slow.*

26.11 Unsteady on his feet, swollen ankles. 'There is nothing left inside me, no feeling'. Talked about feeling that his brain is not working, he cannot move himself out of bed without help, observed to be very delayed in his responses.

29.11 Rashid continues to portray psychomotor retardation/almost catatonic - observed to be sat in same position for prolonged periods.

30.11 Seen in ECT clinic: Rashid explained that he is unable to do anything as he has no strength. He described his legs as weights and said they were weighing him down. Rashid reported that he needed nursing staff to help with daily things such as washing and dressing, and nursing staff also reported that he only eats and drinks if they bring it to him. There was obvious retardation during the assessment but Rashid did know why he was at the clinic and what ECT was. Rashid reported that he did not believe that things would improve. He stated that he had feelings of guilt but would not elaborate on these. Rashid reported suicidal feelings, but no energy to do anything.

[HAM-D on the day was scored at 33 points, but several items could not be scored, due to poor communication, so the real score was presumed to be higher].

2.12 [After first ECT]. A bit brighter for a few hours, then back to baseline. He doesn't find any improvement.

4.12 Spending some time in the communal areas. Getting into bed with no assistance.

5.12 [After second ECT]. A little brighter on the ward. 57kg (3 kg loss since admission.) Doesn't feel different.

My notes show that HAM-D after the second ECT was 44, higher than at the start, as he answered all the questions that could not be scored before the first session.

6.12 More responsive, eating and drinking. Approached staff later in the morning stating he was feeling lost and did not know what to do with himself on the ward.

8.12 [After third ECT]. *He stated that life is terrible, and he feels everyone is able to get on with their lives while he is stuck and unable to live. He said he does not see the point in anything.*

9.12 Definite improvement noted, Rashid is more reactive and able to articulate his words.

10.12 Appeared a little brighter.

13.12 [After four ECTs, approached a nurse and asked to talk about financial matters. The nurse wrote]: *His speech was coherent, tone and volume normal. He was able to maintain good eye contact throughout our conversation. Stated that today he is feeling in a positive mood.*

14.12 Complains that his legs are not as fast as usual. Adequate diet taken and mobilising independently.

16.12 [The day of the fifth ECT. There are very few entries by staff in his notes, as if he is not causing any problems. My notes show that his HAM-D is 17].

16.12 Rashid spent a settled day on the ward. Bright in mood, good diet intake, spent majority of time in the communal area, interacting well with peers and staff.

19.12 [ECT No.6 given in the morning]. *Despite the great improvement he is not sure that ECT has helped him. Asked me if his recovery was due to the ECT, I explained it is probably a factor, along with his medication. Told me: thinks he looks better because he trimmed his beard. Discussed long-term plan and I have a feeling he will refuse c-ECT (continuation ECT) but is accepting the idea of having further sessions if he gets unwell again.*

23.12 Feels bored on the ward.

24.12 Much brighter in mood and displaying good humour.

26.12 Explained that he now only feels he needs it once per week. Recalling struggling to walk, and he was having trouble speaking.

29.12 Rashid played chess and appeared pleasant throughout the two games. Bright in mood and jovial.

30.12 [ECT No.7 given this morning, HAM-D is 11]. *Dietician: His weight has increased by 5 kg over 4 weeks, currently he is within a healthy BMI at 62kg (BMI 21.5). He no longer requires a food record chart as he is eating well on the ward.*

[Entry after entry now contains the expression 'good humour' in it.]

5.1 Wants to go home and have ECT as outpatient.

9.1 Discharged.

I am picking up the story from here. On 12th January Rashid had his ECT No.8, as an outpatient. His HAM-D was just five points, well inside the remission level of 10 points for this scale. Two weeks later he had a meeting with his consultant, and it was agreed to stop ECT. His weight was 67kg, a gain of 10kg in two months after starting ECT.

One month later he came to the ECT unit for follow-up and repeat of cognitive tests. The tests were extremely good, and he remained in remission. He had bought a laptop and was spending a lot of time on the internet. He was fully independent. He had started a course that he hoped would help him give private lessons when he went back to XX. A few months later, he finished the course and passed the exams. I will now add the entry from a follow-up with his consultant, another few months later. The entry would feel standard and almost boring, if one didn't know the condition of this gentleman six months earlier:

26.6 Rashid presented as a smartly dressed and well kempt man. He made good eye contact and it was easy to achieve a rapport with him. There were no psychomotor abnormalities. He was polite, pleasant and co-operative throughout. His speech was fluent and spontaneous, slightly increased in amount, normal in rate, rhythm, volume and tone. His affect was euthymic and appropriately reactive. No psychotic symptoms. He has good insight into his illness.

Rashid remained well and after another year was discharged from the psychiatric service.

A few years passed and I met Rashid again, as stated at the start of this story, when he was referred for another course of ECT. The deterioration had been picked up at a much earlier stage of his illness, before any severe signs could develop. He had no psychomotor retardation, speech was spontaneous, although he was struggling to articulate exactly what he meant. Medication was tried for only two months, but the antipsychotic Olanzapine was too sedative for him. It made him groggy in the morning, and he found this intolerable, as things were hard anyway. The memories of his previous experience with ECT were still fresh, and they were also fresh in the minds of those who looked after him. He had made it clear that he needed to get better quickly, and he and his doctor had concluded that there was no need to experiment with other treatments before using ECT.

ECT was started one week after referral, and five weeks after his deterioration was first spotted. Two and a half weeks later, after five sessions, his HAM-D had dropped from 31 to five points, remission level.

He was clearly somebody who appreciated the effect of ECT, and I started talking with him about the poor public perception of this treatment. He offered to help and was happy to talk, not just to other patients who were contemplating the treatment, but also to journalists. By some coincidence, the need to respond to a journalist arose only a couple of months later, when I was approached by the media, something that does happen from time to time. This made Rashid the first of our patients to speak to the press.

9

ACADEMICS

'Do you intend to generate genetically modified fish?' The question is staring at me from the computer screen. In my other life at Cardiff university, I do research in genetics. But I don't work with fish. Or with birds, or with any other animals. This morning I am pushing myself to fill in some of the hundreds of such entries and questions on the website of a grant-giving organisation. I am writing a grant, aiming to analyse certain genetic findings - in humans. The question on genetically modified fish is real. It has to be answered by everybody applying for a grant, even by those who do not do genetics. Aargh, I am struggling. Thankfully, at this point the phone rings and saves the day. I click the 'save and continue later' tab on the screen and pick up the receiver. It is from the ECT department, about a very depressed colleague of mine. I immediately feel more alert.[11]

I like treating academics. I see bits of myself in them, my worries, my obsessions. We have treated several of them. I don't know whether depression is more common among academics, or whether there are simply disproportionate numbers of them in a university town. I

---

[11] I can disclose that the grant I was applying for was rejected. I know this for sure despite the passage of time because I haven't had any grant funded for a few years. If this book gets published, my chances might drop further. And I will have an interesting annual performance review meeting with my boss.

address them as 'my colleague' or 'my friend' and assume they will take my joking on board. Academics provoke questions in me, sometimes uncomfortably close to home. Would I resemble them, if I were to fall prey to a nasty form of depression, or to madness? I am fascinated by their anxieties, even by their delusions, as they tend to involve the insecure life at universities and to hint at things that worry many of my colleagues - for example, losing their job, or missing the chance of getting a better one, where their full brilliance would have shone forth. There is always a better place, where they would have so many more opportunities to succeed. But I shouldn't talk about my own anxieties…

I was looking forward to this consultation with feelings of self-importance and vanity mixed with a healthy dose of self-doubt. I was going to see a senior lecturer. Somebody had advised him to have ECT and had suggested that he should discuss this with a colleague. Selfishly perhaps, I was rather hoping that he might be severely ill, as in this way he would have a better chance of improving with ECT. I was preparing myself for a detailed scientific account of the pros and cons of treatment, remission rates with exact percentage points, statistics with odds ratios, discussions of the theories on mode of action and, surely, minute details about the effect on memory. I could cope with all these but was less sure what to say about the possible effect of ECT on his academic performance: would he remember the contents of his lectures?

Nothing like this happened during the consultation. My academic friend was not asking questions about ECT. Instead he was narrating his story. He had stopped work about two months ago. His main complaint was that he was feeling 'overwhelming regret' for having taken up his current job instead of going to another university. But this decision was not a recent one - it had happened nearly two decades earlier. He was now worried that he would lose his current job, and that his wife would leave him. Or even worse, that he would remain trapped in this job, that he hated so much and that this would go on for another 30 years with 'no way out.' As his age by no means suggested a clear prospect of working for so many more years, this worry did seem a bit unreasonable to me, although I felt unable to call it a psychotic idea. But it was the first hint that his thinking wasn't entirely rational, and that his depression might turn out to be at the severe end of the spectrum. This evidence was gradually piling up. He wasn't eating or drinking, he had lost over a stone in weight in just two months. His sleep was poor, although his estimate of just one hour per night was probably also unrealistic. His speech showed some mild slowing, and he clearly displayed obsessional thinking, reverting several times to his 'wrong decision' to turn down the offer from that other, higher ranked university, although he had made this point quite a few times already. Was this a colleague who was ruminating rationally about his career, as perhaps we all tend to, and what more he could have achieved in life, if only...? Or was he developing severe depression, which was clouding his judgement and should respond to ECT?

He had thought in some detail about killing himself. He had put a belt around his neck, to see what it felt like, but found it too painful, and so had been weighing up other options. He even researched it on the internet, as he didn't want to be unsuccessful and leave himself disabled after a failed attempt. I hadn't thought about this before, but perhaps we should take academics even more seriously when they talk about suicide; after all, they are resourceful people and want to succeed in life (or, in this case, death).

Past history can resolve many diagnostic problems, so I switched the interview to my colleague's psychiatric history. He had been depressed many years ago for nearly one year, and had responded well to Dothiepin, an old tricyclic antidepressant that has many side effects, but is probably more effective than some of the newer drugs. This was at the time he refused a PhD offer from the other university and came to Cardiff instead. He stopped Dothiepin after a few months and remained well for several years. Then another depressive episode developed, that sounded very similar to the current one, where he was tormented by doubt about the choice he had made on his academic path. In fact, it sounded like an identical picture to the one now in front of me.

But did he really have good reason to doubt his choice? The other university was a bit higher in rankings, yes, and there might be various reasons for living in another town. But after all, he was a senior lecturer in his current job, a long-term appointment with a clear path to progression, hardly a bad outcome. And our university is not doing too badly in the rankings, either. Perhaps on each occasion the depression had come first and magnified an old and insignificant event into a major disaster? I questioned him about how he had felt between the episodes. Had he always regretted his choice? It sounded as if, on the contrary, he had been doing quite well and had no problems with his mood or negative feelings about his job. It seemed inappropriate to get an independent opinion from anybody in his department, and impossible anyway, without infringing on his confidentiality, so I decided to continue trying to figure things out myself. During his second episode, he had been depressed for six months and again had responded to Dothiepin. Now he had developed a third depressive episode and again was fretting about a decision taken two decades ago, which seemed quite irrelevant to me.

Could he be on the verge of psychotic thinking? If so, I would expect him to respond to ECT. But talking to him, I saw a completely rational person, reasoning clearly, responding coherently, looking like... well, just like any other academic discussing a problem with a colleague. If he is genuinely unhappy in his job and has made a truly wrong decision, then ECT has no place, I mused. Or does it? We now had two ruminating academics talking to each other. He had downloaded the Hamilton Depression Rating Scale from the internet and self-scored himself at 48 points, but this was clearly an over-estimate. Perhaps the true score was only half that - still a moderate level of depression, just about enough to allow ECT, on the grounds of treatment-resistant depression.

Academic quibbling apart, I felt that the suicide risk was real, another reason to give serious thought to ECT. But surely, he should try Dothiepin again first, given that he had recovered after taking it on two previous occasions? Nowadays however, my colleagues are more likely to avoid the old drugs, as they are dangerous in overdose and cause more side effects. He was on a triple combination of Sertraline, Mirtazapine and Quetiapine - not ideal, but not a bad choice either.

At this point I managed to gear the conversation towards ECT for the first time. We discussed the possible side effects. He explained that in his teaching he had to rely more on logical reasoning and ideas, rather than on memorised facts, so any memory gaps might not be important. I had no worries about ECT causing problems with logic. And he should be fine in terms of examining students and marking their work. I explained that for a person with his type of depression, we achieve about 50% remission rates. Mistake. He interpreted this as a 50% chance of not improving, as a pessimist would regard a glass as half-empty, rather than half-full. He looked disappointed.

Later I realised that I had actually been wrong in my estimate, in any case. When I went back to the computer to double-check the success rates achieved in our own clinic, I noted that non-psychotic patients still had an impressive 57% remission rate (provided they completed 12 sessions). The psychotic ones remitted in 58% of cases. Some patients took longer to reach remission. If we included those who needed up to 24 sessions, 67% of the non-psychotic patients and 72% of the psychotic ones reached remission. Should I contact my colleague with these updated numbers? Should I quote 58% or 67%? And why do I still believe that psychotic depression responds so much better, despite looking at my own results, which showed little difference between this and non-psychotic depression? Doubtless these 'non-psychotic' patients were also severely depressed; we don't really give ECT to people who do not suffer with severe illness. The real question should be whether he was severely depressed. I was ruminating again…

A couple of weeks later, I learned that my colleague had decided against ECT. My turn to be disappointed now. Deep inside I wanted him to have it, not only because I felt there was a risk of suicide, but, apart from this very real concern, I was also genuinely interested to discover whether his type of depression would lift with ECT. I was also curious to hear how a highly functioning academic might describe the experience of ECT and how he would judge his memory and functioning afterwards. But of course I didn't want my curiosity to interfere with his decision and wasn't going to encourage him in any way merely out of academic interest! My role was to give him the exact facts, so he could make up his mind. But perhaps his depression prevented him from making the correct decision? What if he was becoming psychotic? What about the suicide risk? Perhaps I should be more assertive. Now that he had decided against ECT, I sat down to read through his notes again. The more I thought about it, the more worried I became, as his suicidal thoughts seemed to have been picked up on more than one occasion. If I had told him that his chance of getting well was 67%, would this have changed his mind? I don't want to sound too upbeat with patients, though, as there is another story behind these numbers: one year after an ECT course, over half of those who get well relapse back into depression. So the overall outcome after a year would be below 40%, unless they have additional sessions. Should we state these numbers at the outset, or discuss the problem only after patients get well?

The next day I got so worried about my colleague's suicide potential, that I alerted his treatment team. Whether because of this, or because he was deteriorating anyway, he came back to the department a week later, to talk about ECT again. I met him in the morning for a chat, hoping to provide more information, but ended up trying to consent him. He looked different. He was holding his head in his hands and rubbing his face, so that it looked red and sore. He was constantly pulling his hair, and rocking on his seat so that his head almost touched his knees, his eyes scanning the room in desperation. He kept repeating his line about the wrong path taken all these years ago; indeed, he could not talk about anything else. It now looked as though he was not just suffering from agitated depression, but on the verge of becoming psychotic, developing ideas of guilt that seemed highly inappropriate.

I stated that I had to revise all my predictions and that he needed ECT straight away and that I was as certain as possible that he would recover. Each time I thought that I had convinced him, he would revert into ruminations: 'Even if I get well, the terrible mistake I made will come back to me and will bring me down again'. I could see some logic there. It is hard to argue with people who have obsessions, or with people who have entrenched negative thinking. But when such people earn their living by exploring the pros and cons of scientific evidence, arguing their point by making complex logical arguments, and usually believing, correctly, that they know things better than the rest of the audience, this raises the concept of ruminations to a different level. My colleague was proving impossible to persuade about the need for ECT, so I gave up after an hour, asking him to come back the following day, or perhaps the following week, as I was not sure I had the resources for another exhausting talk the next day.

But at least in my mind there was no doubt left: he was now a good candidate for ECT and could even end up having it on a section if he continued to deteriorate.

We met a week later. I asked our nurse Lorraine to repeat the statement with which she greeted me in the morning: 'He is actually worse than last week'. I asked her to confirm the identity of the patient. Surely this was not him. How could he be worse? He had been so agitated, a picture of misery. Lorraine has worked in our unit much longer than I have, in fact she is retired and comes to do extra sessions for us. She is always right in her judgements about patients. The nurses had been so worried that morning that they had called the duty doctor to assess our patient's suicide risk before I arrived. It sounded as if everybody had been through enough discussions with him, and they were all looking a bit drained emotionally, so I ended up doing the talking. He still didn't want ECT, 'because it will not change my horrible situation'. (Yes, the same idée fixe.) I didn't rate my chances of persuading a senior academic to change his mind; I have tried in the past. But somehow, at the end of our chat, he did exactly that and agreed to have it! Perhaps it was my clear approach about the benefits, expressed in more reassuring numbers ('I now rate your chances at 90%; my goal is to get you back to work'), perhaps my question about what was there to lose if he did try ECT, compared to the chance of getting better without having it, which he conveniently rated as zero - probably not far off the truth. At any rate, something about the numbers and the logic of the arguments persuaded his scientifically trained mind. The ruminations about his past 'mistake' were still filling any pause in the conversation, but he signed the consent form and had his first session later that morning.

I was slightly worried whether my 90% remission mark and the prediction for a return to work was too optimistic, or whether he might suffer some terrible complication that I hadn't discussed during the consent process (such as the very small risk of death, for example). But this was swept away by the sense of success and by the uneventful ECT session. Now we had to wait for improvement. 'Four weeks on average to recovery', I had told him, emphasising the 'on average', that implies a distribution of cases on either side of that number. I wasn't prepared to offer a prediction on the time to recovery, I still had enough realism left to avoid doing this.

I had told him during the consent process that he would be confused for 20-25 minutes (*on average*) after the seizure, and it would then take an hour or so before he would be allowed home. So after 25 minutes I checked up on him in the recovery room. I had been a bit too optimistic. He hadn't yet woken up properly and was still completely disorientated. His eyes were looking around in perplexity and with lack of understanding. His scientific mind had been switched off by the electric current and the seizure, and he was lost as a result. I felt rather sad for him. If I was an opponent of ECT, I would no doubt have stated, 'Look what you have done to this bright mind!' It felt unfair that he had been reduced to such a helpless state, unable to make any sense of his surroundings, or to recall where he was and why he was there. I allowed myself this brief sentimental diversion; perhaps it was a sign of respect. Then I switched back to reality and wondered if this confusion was going to wipe out the constant rumination about his 'error' that was tormenting him. Or maybe that would fade away later, after his mood started lifting. I would have to wait.

Three days later I was surprised to see so much improvement in such a short space of time. He was not rocking or pulling his hair. The redness on his face, caused by the anxiety and hand-rubbing, had also gone. But my compliments on his improvement were rejected: no, he felt just as horrible and hopeless, he assured me. Such a terrible person he was, to make that awful mistake, with such disastrous consequences... Should I now be calling this a delusion of guilt? And it didn't stop there. He told me that his throat wasn't right - he had been trying to clear it and had damaged it somehow in the process. So now he had lost the ability to swallow spontaneously and had to do this consciously. I was wondering what medical advice to offer, perhaps more fluids? It sounded so natural and believable coming from him, that the truth reached me only when I told Kara and Sam, who were waiting for me in the treatment room. Their minds were clearer: he was developing a hypochondriac delusion. Just like those patients who thought they couldn't breathe spontaneously, he couldn't swallow spontaneously. I felt relieved that he had consented to have ECT. I couldn't imagine how we would treat him against his consent even if he was clearly psychotic.

We were now treating a psychotic depression, and this made his prognosis better. In a quirky way, this was good for him. But in another way it was not so good for my story line of an academic who was obsessing about moot points, as some academics do, bringing his ruminations to the level of a mental illness.

When he arrived for the third ECT, he looked worse: he was rocking and pulling his hair again. A red eye glanced at me through a gap between the fingers that were covering and rubbing his face. He told me that he had damaged his throat for life, and that the damage was beginning to spread down into his internal organs; there was no hope. He couldn't accept any reassurance that this was just a sore throat and would get better. All optimism had now left him, and again he looked terrified, obsessed and overwhelmed by this new problem. The hypochondriacal delusion was all too obvious now. So he should respond to ECT. As his seizure last time was not perfect, and the EEG waves had waxed and waned a few times, I increased the electric charge to 253mC and he had a perfect seizure of 27 seconds visible and 54 seconds EEG trace, with a clear endpoint and post-ictal suppression (an almost flat line that follows the waves of the seizure). Some 30 minutes later he was awake and chatting, although he got the year wrong - and didn't know that he had just had ECT.

On the morning of the fourth ECT the throat problem had disappeared. He stated this as a matter of fact, somehow ignoring his conviction of a few days ago that he had incurable throat damage, which was going to spread and eventually kill him. And despite this massive problem having vanished, he still insisted that he was no better. The mistake he had made 20 years ago was still colossal and irretrievable.

By the fifth ECT, he had improved further. The redness on his face had completely gone. He was sitting calmly and engaging in rational conversation. His HAM-D score had fallen to 18, down from the 38 recorded on the day of his first session. 'Yes, people have commented that I look better, but this is just because I've had my hair cut.'

'Sure, you are now unable to pull your hair,' I was tempted to joke, but refrained - he wasn't ready for it.

I was away during the next four sessions but received encouraging information. After six sessions, his HAM-D dropped down to eight points, and the following week to six. This meant he had reached a sustained remission and I was looking forward to talking with him at the end of my summer holiday, which now seemed too long.

The meeting took place after the ninth session. He smiled when he saw me enter the waiting room, jumped up, and came to talk with me in a side office. His handshake was firm, the mark of a confident person. He felt well and admitted that the ECT had helped him. And what about the horrible error from the past? 'Ah, that doesn't matter really, it's not important.'

'So life is okay now, despite this?'

'Yes, the job is fine, life is going well!'

He was in remission. This had indeed been depression all along, not a rational appraisal of his academic life. We talked about him going back to work and I expressed my interest in how he would manage with his teaching activities, if there were to be any memory problems. He was now so confident that he easily dismissed the problem: 'My lectures are more like discussions, I don't rely too much on facts. I use some prompt words and guide the discussions according to them.' Yes, he had forgotten a password or two. I shook my head in understanding and grinned, thinking of the several notebooks where I had written my passwords, having long since given up any hope of remembering them. I still asked him to rehearse his first talk on his own beforehand, to check how he was performing. We agreed that he should start the next teaching semester on a half-time basis. The new academic year was starting in just four weeks but we both felt that he could do it.

Of course, I had no idea if he was going to relapse, and I shared this uncertainty with him. He had had a short duration of illness, had suffered only two previous episodes many years ago and had functioned excellently between them. This suggested a good prognosis and no need for continuation ECT. But you never know with depression. It tends to get worse with advancing age, and he could be less lucky this time. We chatted about this and I noted that we were sharing the same thoughts and concerns. We agreed equably to start spacing out his sessions and to observe how he progressed but not to stop yet. It can be nice treating colleagues, despite the common preconceptions.

After the 12th session it was time to repeat his cognitive testing. I did expect good results but he really had to do extremely well to allay my worries about a possible drop in performance (I still worry about this, despite my own research). So when Sam phoned me and said, 'Your colleague came for his cognitive tests... Oh my God!' - I was anxiously waiting for the tone she would pitch for her next phrase. Sam enjoys creating suspense. 'He was amazing!' Phew, thank goodness. Indeed, he had scored better on all the tests, compared to his pre-ECT testing. He achieved the top possible scores on several tests and most impressively, finished the Trail Making Test part B in 22 seconds. I had seen students complete it this quickly, but this test shows an unkind correlation with advancing age, becoming worse all the time, so for somebody in his 50s this was easily the best one we had seen and annoyingly, better than my score! And I have to share what he wrote for the Mini Mental State Examination test. One of the items on this test asks people to write down one complete sentence, any sentence that comes to their mind. The most common phrases people come up with are the standard, 'The cat sat on the mat', followed by something like, 'Today the weather is nice'. Our patient wrote: 'Jung approaches objectively a realm intermediate between religion and psychology'. I had to read it twice, to make sure that I had no clue what it meant. Two days later he gave a talk at a conference; it went very well, he assured me. If there is cognitive impairment after ECT, it spares some people.

My colleague's continuation treatment lasted longer than we had anticipated, finishing after a total of 24 ECTs, spread over more than six months. We couldn't stop earlier because on two occasions his mood threatened to drop. He had been working since the autumn and went full-time during the spring semester, while still coming for treatment every three to four weeks. ECT didn't affect his performance and nobody was aware of the treatment he was receiving. He was also reviewing papers for journals. I trust he is not that nasty Reviewer #2, who rejected an excellent paper on genetics that I submitted that spring, despite the lack of funding!

10

EMERGENCY

It was Thursday evening. I had arrived home and was checking my e-mails. There was a cryptic message from Kara: 'Dr Jones will come at 9:30am tomorrow, so you can go and see that emergency patient on the ward'. It was the first time I'd heard there was an emergency on a 'ward' in our hospital that involved a 'patient'. I knew nothing and had to read between the lines. We can't share patient information on e-mails between the hospital and university, so Kara is hardly allowed to say anything if she writes to my university e-mail. I can't access my hospital e-mail from home, so had to resign myself to leaving the mystery until the next day. I'm sure our university e-mails are secure, as our IT geeks are pretty good. But I complete an information security course every year, so I know the rules.

I arrived at the unit at 8:30am. One patient received treatment soon after, but there was nothing complicated, so I was able to fill in the missing parts of the history of our new 'emergency patient' by reading the hospital notes on the computer system. Ana was from one of the Middle Eastern countries that has been ravaged by conflict in recent years. She couldn't speak much English. She came to our hospital just the previous week, transferred from another hospital in Wales. She had been found sitting on a bench next to the bus station in a nearby town, looking around aimlessly. She was sitting there rather too long, so the police were alerted. They tried to help her, but she was unable to give them much information and was admitted to the local psychiatric hospital. Eventually the hospital found out her correct address (in Cardiff) and after a few more days managed to transfer her to us. The story was not summarised in a single entry and I had to piece it together from the various entries. There was a suggestion that she might have been trafficked from her country, but no details and no relatives to contact.

This was beginning to shape up as a case of an unfortunate asylum seeker whose mental state had crumbled after some horrific experiences. I resolved to keep all options open. Somewhat hidden between the lines were entries stating that she was not eating and drinking much on the ward. This was surely the reason for the urgency.

Dr Jones arrived at 9:30am sharp. He filled in more of Ana's history but my prevailing sense was still that we didn't know much. An interpreter had arrived, but we were warned that the girl hadn't said much to her either. Dr Jones explained that the patient had been mute but had started to communicate a little after she had received 5mg Haloperidol. She had also eaten a slice of toast and had drunk something after the medication. This sounded quite positive, perhaps we should put her on antipsychotics without delay? 'Yes,' we agreed. Then we briefly considered one potential danger. This looked like a first episode of psychotic illness: the patient was mute, the history was poor. What if she had a brain tumour or some other nasty brain disorder? No, this had already been sorted out: the previous day she had had a brain scan, which was normal. I opened up the images on the computer and looked at them myself, to be absolutely sure, as we had recently seen a patient with a brain tumour. 'Her prolactin[12] is 3,000,' noted Kara, looking at a

---

[12] A hormone produced by the pituitary gland that promotes lactation. This level is several times above the norm.

second computer screen. Another short discussion followed, but in the absence of a pituitary tumour on the scan that could produce excessive prolactin, or breastfeeding, there wasn't much else either to worry us or to provide an explanation. The most likely reason for an increased prolactin level on psychiatric wards is the intake of antipsychotics. Could it be the Haloperidol? She had had several doses of it before the blood test and possibly had received more in the first hospital. I wished they had sent us all the notes…

'So I can't see a real urgency, Dr Jones,' I concluded at around 10 am. 'It looks like she could still respond to medication, as she only started it a few days ago. We can observe her, and there is no reason to rush with ECT.'

Deep inside I had a nagging instinct that I was avoiding responsibility and not doing what was best for her. If this was psychotic depression, then surely ECT would provide the fastest treatment. Medication was likely to help but would take longer, so she would only suffer for a longer time. I am always lecturing about the likely benefits of using ECT first in such cases, and here I was, leaning towards a longer wait, perhaps fearing I might be reprimanded for not exhausting other options first, or because I was not 100 per cent sure that we had enough information, and had not excluded some organic cause that might put her life in danger during an epileptic seizure. Natural caution, but was I right?

I couldn't gather any more background information, so it was time to see the patient. We walked down the corridor to the ward and were shown into the interview room. Ana wasn't there yet; she was still in bed, we were told. I followed the two nurses who went to fetch her, so that I could observe her walking and communicating as she got up from her bed. And this is where my plan started changing. Ana was not talking; she was staring at people, but with a face that showed no emotion and without uttering a sound. But more importantly, her movements were slow. Her gaze shifted slowly from person to person, she hesitated before walking and once she was in motion, it took over a minute to reach the interview room, a distance of no more than 20 metres. Ana was in her early 20s. A slim and obviously fit lady, she should have been hopping around. I knew that I had little excuse left for delaying ECT, as psychomotor retardation and stupor or catatonia are probably the best predictors for response.

We sat down with the interpreter, who was trying her luck at eliciting some answers.

'I know her from a couple of years ago. I translated for her when she had her asylum application assessed,' she explained. 'She was so different then. She was a bubbly lady, full of life.' This clearly weakened my theory that stress, abuse and psychological damage in her country of origin were all responsible for Ana's mental state, as she had indeed been through this but had remained 'bubbly' for some time after leaving. The idea of a sudden and nasty mental illness was now emerging. Stress was probably still the trigger. One of the nurses looking after her told us that a few days ago, Ana had mentioned hearing voices, adding even more credence to the picture of psychotic depression, if more evidence were needed.

With my mind almost made up in favour of ECT, I got up and walked towards the girl, to check her pulse. This was just instinctive, a routine check I always perform, being a bit obsessed with heart rates, as there was no reason to suspect anything in this fit young girl. It was then that the case became an emergency.

The pulse rate was 120, about twice what I expected. Was she frightened? Possibly, although her face didn't show any emotion. She certainly had not exerted herself too much during her slow, awkward walk, and she had been sitting in the chair, absolutely still since then, in a state of near stupor. The tachycardia was not caused by thyroid overactivity - there were no other signs of this, and a thyroid function test had returned normal results. What was going on? Blood pressure was 140/100, high for such a young and slim woman. It could also be due to anxiety. 'Let's check the pressure with a manual cuff, perhaps the monitor is wrong.' '140/100,' confirmed the nurse after a minute. The idea that Ana could be dehydrated was beginning to cross my mind. As the notes had stated, she had not been eating and drinking much. 'Let's check the blood pressure after she stands up, to see if she has postural hypotension, in which case it would drop.' The blood pressure remained the same, but my fingers struggled to keep pace with her pulse rate, which went up to around 130. If Ana was dehydrated, why was she not feeling faint or collapsing on the floor? She kept absolutely upright and steady, showing no distress, paleness, sweating, or anything else to indicate discomfort. Her lips were not cracked and the skin on her arms was tight, no indication of dehydration, but she was too young really to show such signs, so this didn't help much.

'Can I see the fluid chart?' I requested. She had been put on a fluid chart due to her poor fluid intake. With the help of the nurse I figured out that the previous day, the 22nd, she had drunk one bottle of nutrient drink with a lot of prompting - 200ml, confirmed the nurse.

'Anything else?'

'No, she refused.'

'What about on the 21st?'

'Looks like she refused everything.'

Indeed, next to each drink offered during the day, the chart stated '*refused*'. The same information was recorded for the 20th. No chart was filled in for the 19th. I was staring in disbelief. For the last 72 hours this woman had taken no more than 300ml of fluids. But as she looked physically fit and was not complaining, nobody had raised the alarm. Well, I am unfair, they did: the patient was referred for emergency ECT because she was not eating and drinking well, but the extent of the problem had not been fully appreciated. She was still strong, standing up, not fainting, and keeping her blood pressure high. But this was because she was young and fit, so she was able to compensate for the lack of water in her body with a high pulse rate and high blood pressure. But for how long could this go on?

'Let's give her ECT now.'

I had changed my mind. We all nodded in agreement. Dr Jones had been correct all along in asking for emergency ECT. If she had been left over the weekend with no fluids, at some point her heart could have tired and slowed down, and her blood vessels would finally have run out of sufficient fluid to keep enough oxygen reaching her brain, and she would have fainted. If this had happened during the night, she could potentially have died, if nobody had noticed her. She was not going to express any discomfort; she wouldn't complain or alert anybody; she clearly felt no thirst. Perhaps I was going over the top: anorexic girls survive for years on a few sips of fluid per day. I don't really know what could have happened, but I did know that there was a real danger to her life.

I was so impatient to see the outcome that I wrote down my impressions after each ECT:

ECT No.1

Most clinics have an emergency ECT protocol. The idea is that when it is vital to achieve a quick improvement, then considerations about confusion and memory problems become secondary, as one should treat the patient straight away, with a proper therapeutic dose, avoiding the delay of titration with increasing doses. I was certain that Ana would have a seizure on 46mC, our usual starting dose for titration of young people, therefore 80mC would have been twice seizure threshold, surely a good treatment dose. I stepped this up to 103mC, to account for the few Diazepam tablets she had received and the urgency of the situation, while resisting the temptation to give her an even higher dose, worrying that her cardiovascular system had been put under strain by dehydration and that she might react with a drop in blood pressure after the seizure. One litre of saline solution was dripping quickly into her vein while she was waiting for the treatment. Her pulse rate dropped to 90 with this single measure.

The seizure was good, although the EEG traces could have been better for such a young person. The EEG activity didn't stop after the muscular twitches fizzled out at the 23-second mark. Low-level seizure activity continued and at three minutes we gave her 5mg of Diazepam to terminate it. It did the job, and everything was uneventful after that. I wasn't worried about the prolonged seizure: young people do have longer seizures and the first one is sometimes the longest. I was going to increase the electric charge the next time and expected, somewhat counter-intuitively, that this would produce better organised seizure activity, with a clear endpoint, followed by a flat line, indicating the post-ictal suppression.

I was more interested to see if this single seizure was going to produce any 'miraculous' changes in her behaviour. This didn't happen. Ana remained mute over the weekend. Perhaps there was some small change: she started eating and drinking more. Dr Jones ensured stricter monitoring and encouragement of fluid intake, by putting her on one-to-one observation, i.e. a nurse stayed next to her all the time, to supervise and record her fluid intake. Whether this did the trick, or whether it was the

ECT, I don't know, but she had taken about 800ml of fluids each day over the weekend.

ECT No.2

On the Monday morning I was pleased to see Ana's weight increased by 2 kg (all fluid, no doubt) and her pulse rate at a normal 70 beats per minute. The chart of her pulse rate was even more impressive. Over the weekend it had gone down each time it was measured, three times on each day, and had reached 67 on Sunday evening. Blood pressure had also reached a healthy 117/77. Dehydration had indeed clearly been the cause of the previously high pulse rate.

Was that a smile? It looked like a smile but a stiff one, and nobody knew what she was smiling at. She had been doing this since Saturday. Perhaps it was an attempt to show us that she was better, whilst still struggling with her inability to show emotions. Or maybe she was smiling at something not evident to us. Staff suspected she was listening to voices. Incongruous smiling or a response to voices, this was yet unclear.

For the second ECT, I increased the electric charge by about 30% to 138mC. This produced the desired improvement in EEG quality, with a clear endpoint at 47 seconds. We were back in business.

ECT No.3

Ana keeps throwing problems at us: this morning before the ECT she vomited, causing more discussions about a possible organic disorder (another personal look at the brain scan images to reassure myself). And then she has another prolonged seizure, that has to be stopped with Diazepam after two minutes. But there are more signs of improvement: she is now eating and drinking well and has exchanged a few words with staff, in English. She maintains eye contact with me, with a somewhat inquisitive look, but still offers no speech.

ECT No.4

It is unusual to find something to write about for each treatment, but Ana is keeping me busy. Today I increase the electric charge again, to 195mC, hoping that this will result in better organized seizure activity. This happens indeed and there is clear endpoint at the 54th second. I indicate my delight with a hint of a clenched fist and the SHO smiles appreciatively. For about 30 seconds the ECG shows the unmistakable pattern of bigeminy: an irregular heart rhythm whereby one normal beat, initiated in the sinus node of the heart atrium, is followed after a shorter interval by a beat which originates in the ventricles of the heart. This is followed by another pair of sinus and ventricular beats, in a striking continuity. The pattern disappears just as suddenly as it starts. Blood pressure and oxygen levels stay normal, the ECG pattern remains regular. We are used to bigeminies after seizures and have stopped worrying about them. Young and fit people seem as likely to develop them as the old and frail. Strong seizures are more likely to induce this type of arrhythmia and I prefer to regard this only as another sign that this was a pretty strong seizure. 'She should pick up now,' I hazard. I wait for her to wake up completely and attempt another assessment before she leaves the unit, while the interpreter is still here. Ana is making more slight progress. She is trying to answer my questions, slowly, hesitantly, although in such a low voice that only the interpreter is able to pick up the words. I learn that over the weekend she asked to have her make-up done. She couldn't remember where she was or how she came here. Walking is still slow, but the pulse rate is now 63.

ECT No.5

I was not surprised to see Ana smiling and answering the nurse's questions almost fluently when I arrived in the morning for her next session. She was giving us some details about herself. The slowness in her speech and movements was more apparent now that she was actually speaking and moving. This time, though, her smile looked natural, coming from both eyes and lips. She was so well that the SHO needed some time to decide whether she had capacity to consent. Ana told him that ECT was helping her and agreed to have more, but I was skeptical that she understood what was wrong with her and what ECT was. No complications this time during the ECT, no extra beats on the ECG. A few more sessions like this and she should be back to her usual self, surely. And perhaps we would know whether she had become ill in reaction to some horrible experience. We had treated other asylum seekers previously. One turned out to have developed schizophrenia, and although he had experienced horrific things back in his country, the stories of persecution by the same group of people after coming to the UK were the fruit of his morbid imagination. We knew that for sure, as he could hear them talking to him while we were in the same room. Another one, from a North African country, did very well, somehow managing to forget the horrors he had been through.

ECT No.6

Walking into the clinic in the morning, I caught Ana's eye through the window of an office, being assessed by a nurse. I was glad to have made it to the clinic before her session started, so that I could see how she was doing. 'Good morning doctor, how are you?' That was Ana speaking, smiling at me. Yes, in English. I shook her hand and tried for a longer conversation. This was still difficult, and even the interpreter couldn't understand some of her statements, occasionally concluding, 'That didn't make sense.' But Ana told me about her parents who still lived in their country. She couldn't figure out what had caused her illness and when her depression had started. Her slow improvement was continuing, however, and her ECT session was uneventful. We still didn't know whether she had gone through some traumatic abuse, but I wondered whether there might be a less violent explanation, one more rooted in psychosis.

ECT No.7

Our interpreter couldn't make it this morning. A replacement offered to travel from London and charge us for eight hours of work. I declined. In fact, I welcomed the opportunity to gather some information without interference and to see how much Ana could converse in English when there was no help at hand. Ana greeted us with a smile and hugged the nurse like an old friend. 'She has been a bit inappropriate on the ward, disregarding boundaries with staff,' confirmed the staff nurse after the interview. Clearly this friendliness was seen as unusual. We sat down for an interview. Ana's English was poor for a young person who had lived in this country for several years. She was raising her eyebrows after every long word and struggled with every answer. But there was no depression, and she was feeling really well. Was she still ill? I wondered whether her English would improve further after more ECTs. Or maybe this was the level she was going to reach, as her illness was interfering with her cognitive performance. (Staff were now sure that she was listening to voices, making schizophrenia the most likely diagnosis.) I broached the question of her past history. Why had she come to England?

'Life is not good back home. My uncle was killed. I want to find a better job.' That made sense.

'So how did you travel, by plane?'

'No, in a lorry, with other people.' Whoops, I had gone too far. Her case was still being investigated by the police, and I understood that it was not really for me to get involved. Ana was an illegal immigrant and was probably lucky to have survived the journey. My job was to concentrate on getting her free of mental illness and she was making one huge step forward with each ECT. She had one more of these today.

ECT No.8

This morning Ana appeared more guarded; she kept staring at me and the others, and her movements were a bit slower. She smiled spontaneously, but the smile was not a natural one, her mouth was slightly twisted to one side and she had no words to accompany the smile. She told us that she did hear voices – two voices, a man and a woman - but they just called her name. She still didn't know why she was here and what treatment she was receiving. She didn't ask anything, and it was a struggle to get anything beyond 'Yes' or 'No' from her. The interpreter confirmed that she was not back to her usual self. I asked Ana whether she watched television, and she replied that she watched the news, adding that she had watched the recent story about a model abducted in Italy to be sold as a sex slave.

I then spoke further with the interpreter about Ana's history. It transpired that Ana had been living in Cardiff after arriving from the Middle East. The Home Office had refused to grant her leave to stay in the UK. She had experienced conflict and had lost relatives, but her parents were well and still living there, apparently reasonably safe now. Clearly a hard life, and one that would unsettle most people, but she had been coping despite all these problems, doing a voluntary job, attending English classes and remaining lively, as remembered by the interpreter the last time she had seen her a couple of years ago. From a psychiatric point of view, it was clear that her current communication problems could not be explained by poor English, and the conversation confirmed that Ana was not back to her usual self.

ECT No.9

Ana was still slow and not saying anything spontaneously. I tried to figure out whether she really heard voices. She said 'yes', but it then turned out that she was referring to my voice! I tried posing the question in different ways, but her answers remained conflicting. I was struggling to work out whether this was all due to poor understanding. The interpreter also remarked again that she couldn't understand what Ana meant at times. Was this thought disorder, a symptom of schizophrenia? But this didn't change the need for ECT, as an acute psychosis will also respond to this treatment. I asked Ana to step on the scales. She had put on 5 kg in four weeks.

ECT No.11

The interpreter told me that she had not noticed any confused speech today and had had a normal conversation with Ana. She had seen her talking on the phone with her parents and the conversation had been fluent. However, I still found Ana's smile unnatural and she was still unaware of what she was doing in the hospital.

I was away for the next two weeks, as it was August, holiday time. Ana had finished the course of 12 ECTs and no more treatments were given. Dr Jones wanted to see how she got on without ECT. The reports I was getting indicated a lack of further improvement. When I came back, I went to the ward and tried to assess one more time whether she was psychotic. Ana was smiling but remained passive. Was she frightened of anything? Yes, her asylum application. Was she hearing voices? Yes, mine. Not much of a psychosis there. Her face remained immobile, her smile somewhat twisted. But could it be that the lack of spontaneity and her blank face were due to her medication? She was on an old-fashioned antipsychotic, Haloperidol, she had Parkinsonian gait, her arms were kept flexed almost at right angles in the elbows. I took her hand and moved her wrist up and down. There was stiffness and it was yielding to the gentle pressure in a stepwise fashion: this was cog-wheel rigidity, a sign of excessive blockade of dopamine receptors in the brain by old-fashioned antipsychotics. This is similar to the problems experienced by people with Parkinson's disease, when they start losing the neurons that make dopamine in the brain. It can also cause a lack of facial expression and can reduce the person's drives. I wanted to stop the Haloperidol and see how Ana was and how her movements appeared when free of the side effects. I looked at the medication chart and noticed with approval that Dr Jones had already started the switch to a more modern drug.

Overall, Ana's illness was proving difficult to treat. Only a week later, (two weeks after the 12th ECT session), she stopped eating and drinking again, and her speech and movements slowed down. After a brief discussion, the decision seemed easy: she was relapsing, so we restarted ECT. Just after the first treatment, she spoke more, asked when she could go home, and her English appeared better. The next day I noticed good spontaneous speech, smiling and she even initiated a 'Give me five' slap with her hand with me, to celebrate her good mood. Food and fluid intake were also back to normal. Perhaps monitoring the level of her English was as good a way of measuring her condition as any complicated psychiatric rating scale - or even better. If somebody has psychomotor retardation and their thinking is slowed down, perhaps a newly acquired language does suffer disproportionately, as one has to make an effort to find the right words.

So perhaps she wasn't fully cured yet? Should we give her an even higher electric charge this time? Her EEG traces were nearly, but not quite perfect. She was young, she should have a perfect EEG pattern, so perhaps her seizure threshold had increased further, and she was not receiving the optimal ECT? This case had drifted away from being a medical emergency, but Ana still continued throwing questions at us. If she didn't recover, she might spend the rest of her life in chronic psychosis. Now was the time to prevent her from becoming chronically ill. This was an emergency of a different type, just as important as saving her life had been two months earlier.

Over the next few weeks Ana had ECT twice a week. Her condition was changing very slowly, but for the better. She was phoning her parents regularly, and was eating and drinking well. But something still wasn't right. There was still little spontaneity, apart from her asking to be discharged. The light in her eyes had gone out, she was not smiling as genuinely as before, and would not say anything unless she was asked a question. When asked to subtract seven from 100, her answer was 10, and that was after some prompting. Was the ECT making her confused? But she was relapsing without it and getting even worse, so I couldn't resolve even this question.

Time passed. I had nearly given up on Ana, fearing that it was too late and that she did indeed now have chronic psychosis. I was just about holding onto some hope of her further improvement. We continued with ECT, more out of desperation than anything else. Ana and her doctor seemed more positive about it, though, so in the absence of any objections or side effects, it was only natural to persist a bit longer. It was just as well we did. After a total of 20 ECTs there was clear improvement at last. Ana's face looked natural, she was smiling and talking quite well in English. She had regained her capacity to make decisions about her treatment and given consent for more ECTs.

Ana had a total of 30 ECTs. She achieved stable remission at around ECT No.22 and continued to improve after that. We spaced out her treatments, firstly to one per week, after that, every two weeks, and then every three weeks. The last ECT was given after a break of one month. A total of six months had elapsed since she started. Each time Ana came for treatment, she looked better. She started a voluntary job and resumed English classes. She was smiling and full of life and exuberance, as the interpreter had remembered her. Her English turned out to be quite decent, as I had suspected.

Ana remained well. She did not have schizophrenia - or perhaps had a mild form and recovered from it completely. I have little doubt that she became ill due to stress, and now that she was receiving so much support, her prospects looked brighter. Her application was still not approved by the time I lost contact with her. I don't know what one has to go through to deserve asylum.

11

MAINTENANCE TREATMENT

It was just another day at the clinic, with only three patients going through their routine treatments. Nothing to report; I just had to check for any new e-mails before leaving. A piece of paper with something scribbled on it was placed in front of me. It was a short message, asking me to ring a doctor. Her telephone number was there and the name of a patient. I knew the name - everybody who worked in our department knew it as well. I had expected something like this. Florence was an old friend, but without ECT she simply didn't stay well. We all knew that she had started to deteriorate after stopping her maintenance ECT nearly four months earlier. For her this was a long period without ECT, the longest she had had. The fact that she had stayed well for as long as three months was most unusual for her. I rang the doctor straight away to sort out the problem. To my surprise, the person at the other end of the line didn't sound familiar with the story.

'I've got this patient called Florence X who is very unwell. She is eating very little and will only take sips of water. I understand she has been under your care?'

'Don't you know her?' I asked, puzzled that a psychiatrist in our hospital should never have come across her case. My slightly condescending tone was unjust. After a few more exchanges, I realised that I was talking to a medical registrar. 'Right, so she is on a medical ward,' I concluded, rather embarrassed, having realised my mistake. 'Yes, we know her very well. She needs ECT. She will get well very quickly. I will sort it out, we will get the psychiatric team to take over and we will treat her very soon.'

I was not being over-confident. I knew for certain that Florence would get well. I knew this because I had observed it so many times. She had deteriorated countless times in the past after missing sessions and had improved each time after just a few ECTs. But on this occasion, I hadn't grasped the seriousness of the situation. As usual, it was the end of the week, and it was another few days before Florence came to us for treatment. Or rather, was wheeled in on an intensive care bed. She looked like a person about to give up the ghost. Her body was immobile. Her eyes flickered open only briefly, full of anguish. Her mouth stayed open, her lips were very cracked and her cheeks sunken in. She was nearly 80 and reminded me of certain patients I had seen a couple of decades previously as a junior doctor, when called out to see old and terminally ill patients by their nurses, who suspected that the end was near and felt that the duty doctor should familiarise themselves with the situation and agree with the 'Do not resuscitate' decision. Some of these visits were followed by the writing of the death certificate the next day.

I had never seen Florence in such a poor state. In fact, the last time I had seen her, four months earlier, she had been cheerful, with a spring in her step, going out in town, enjoying life. She had even looked young for her age. In fact, this had been the problem: she was so well, that she couldn't imagine how she could ever get ill again and hence had decided to stop treatment. Mistake. I knew however that she would indeed get well again after two or three sessions. I had seen this transformation many times before, when she had stopped ECT over the years. But this time she had left it far too long, refusing to come for maintenance sessions. And now such was her state, that I started seriously doubting whether she would survive this time. She was older, weaker, and her body might not pull through, unless her depression lifted soon, which would allow her to start eating and drinking again, and getting out of bed.

I had met Florence for the first time at the very beginning of my work at the ECT clinic. She was to become our longest-serving ECT patient. Our first encounter took place in an old psychiatric hospital, one of those Victorian red brick buildings, surrounded by vast and beautiful gardens, that were built all over the country during the 19th and early 20th centuries to improve the care of psychiatric patients. Florence was lying in bed, looking frightened and responding to very few of my questions. Her eyes were shut, her face frowning, as if she couldn't bear to see the frightening world around her. She believed that she was guilty of having done something wrong, something she didn't want to share with me. And although she realised that she was depressed, she felt that she would never get better again. Her team almost shared this view. After all, they had tried many drugs, including lithium, antipsychotics, combinations of two antidepressants, and other cocktails of medications. ECT had also failed: the notes stated that she had had it about a year earlier and had got better with right unilateral treatment, but that the effect was short-lived: this too was rated as failure. She had been an inpatient now for eight months, she was eating less, her feelings of guilt had become more serious as time progressed, and recently she had stopped getting out of bed.

I had been asked to provide a second opinion on her treatment in my capacity as lead of the local clinic for treatment-resistant depression, rather than because of my specialist knowledge in ECT, which was still quite limited at that stage. When even ECT has not worked, I am usually left with very few options. But had it really not worked? Some 20 years earlier Florence had had a first course, which had in fact been successful. Ten years later she had had a second course, again successful. And her last course seemed also to have worked temporarily, but she had relapsed back into depression almost immediately. The advice I offered was to try ECT again. It seems trivial to me now and sometimes I feel a bit of a fraud for being paid a consultant's salary for providing some obvious advice regarding ECT. But at the time it was not that obvious, at least to a novice like me. Everybody knew that many patients who had responded to antidepressants or to antipsychotics in the past, stopped responding to them when they tried them after a relapse some years later. Was ECT different, does it lose its effect? I didn't know, the books I had read didn't make it clear, and the available guidelines of that time advised against prolonged use of ECT.

My notes from that time read, 'A great and sudden improvement on depression scores after the sixth ECT, with remission achieved after the ninth ECT'. The word 'sudden' indicates some degree of surprise on my part, but also reflects the rather miraculous change from deep depression to a state of well-being that can only be observed after ECT. This sudden change is sometimes seen after a single session, leaving even an ECT critic with an open mouth and changed beliefs.

Florence had 12 sessions during that course and three weeks later had already relapsed. This time we gave her ECT without another long wait, resuming it just two weeks after the depression returned. It took only five sessions for her to get well again, and another three weeks for her to relapse once she had stopped. Three months later, she had another course, when she recovered after eight sessions. Common sense started to prevail in me, in Florence, and in everybody involved, so the next time we didn't stop ECT, but suggested that she had continuation ECT (progressively increasing the time between sessions), hoping to prevent relapse. Things did not go smoothly, though. Florence kept relapsing too quickly, even when having regular sessions just two weeks apart. At times she stopped because she didn't want it, or because she felt well and thought she didn't need it. And each time she relapsed, she started looking around with fear, pacing up and down and always thinking that this time she would not get well again. And each time I shared a little bit of that fear, not knowing if ECT would stop working. But, conversely, each time Florence restarted ECT, it worked again, and if anything, it worked faster. With time we learned that we didn't need to treat her twice a week when she relapsed, as she would get well even after a single session, as long as she had not left it for too long.

We were now into what should be called maintenance ECT, i.e. uninterrupted ECT given to maintain remission in the longer term. I was reading case reports that came my way about it, and while they were all reassuring, there were still not many such reports. The patients described in these papers were having ECT at intervals ranging from one to six weeks, and some had accumulated hundreds of sessions. Florence was clearly one of the most treatment-resistant cases, and while she was an astoundingly good ECT responder, her relapses were also astoundingly quick. She would not stay well for more than a week without treatment. Whenever we tried to space out her treatments to two weeks, she would relapse within a couple of months. Finally, we gave up and settled for weekly sessions. This pattern continued for about five years.

Eventually we began to wonder how long this intensive treatment could continue. Florence was only in her early 60s. Her veins were hard to find and sometimes she needed multiple attempts at finding a venous access. The seizure quality and duration deteriorated with time, the electric charge had gone up to 611mC (by comparison, in America the ECT machines can only deliver up to 550mC, due to local regulations). And she complained of memory problems that seemed to be getting progressively worse. Surely, we risked harming her brain with each session, and surely, we couldn't go on for ever? Each session was a struggle – it was a relief that we had given her another week of good quality life, but with this came the underlying thought that there weren't that many weeks of good quality life left.

After about four years, however, still nothing untoward had happened. On the contrary. Florence continued to get well with ECT after each break from the treatment. On most occasions she greeted me with a smile and not only remembered everybody perfectly, but also accurately recalled the various discussions we had had, news items, family stories, and so on.

We had already introduced a long battery of cognitive tests for our patients, as part of a trial. We were repeating

Florence's cognitive tests on a yearly basis and I was worried to see that her performance on several tests was worsening. After this initial scare, I realised that the performance also depended on the length of time since her previous ECT, so perhaps the initial deterioration we had noticed was due to acute effects, and my pessimism was hopefully misplaced. Indeed, her test results plateaued and when at last we managed to test her on a day when she was not depressed and had not had ECT for two weeks (it took a long time to catch her on such a day), I realised that she performed just as well as she had done at the start. So after about four years of more or less weekly sessions, we all learned something very reassuring, which was going to influence our practice in the future: repeated ECTs did not cause cumulative cognitive problems, and therefore patients could have ECT over a long period of time, perhaps even for life, without the risk to brain function that we had been fearing. The frequency of treatments appeared to affect the cognitive performance more than the total number of ECTs over a lifetime. The literature claimed similar conclusions - but it is different when you observe it yourself. Yearly cognitive tests are now a requirement for long-term maintenance patients.

Whether psychology was also playing a part or not I don't know, but once we all accepted that Florence could have ECT for the rest of her life, everything seemed easier. The anaesthetists started to find her veins more easily, or perhaps found a couple of tiny but reliable veins, their locations recorded and shared. The seizure quality stopped deteriorating. The cognitive tests stabilised, despite her being older at each subsequent test. And Florence started accepting that she would get better again when her depression returned after the usual break or attempt to increase the time between sessions. And then we noticed that even the pattern of her illness was becoming milder. After about five years she managed to stay well with ECT every two weeks. After eight years, this could be increased to every three weeks.

Florence's life was transformed. She was able to go on foreign holidays, her activities increased, her memory improved - or at least, she stopped complaining about it. Her last MMSE score was 28 out of 30 (her best score since I had met her) and some of her other cognitive tests were also the best she had achieved during the years we had been treating and testing her. She had not been an inpatient since I had first met her in that old psychiatric hospital, and her attendance at the day centre had gradually been reduced.

So it was with some dismay that I now looked down at Florence on the stretcher, after all our shared history. Here we were today, more than 15 years after I had first met her, after about 400 ECTs, and she looked like she had at our first meeting, but much more physically frail, as if at the end of her journey. There was a short discussion about consent forms. I asked Florence whether she wanted to have ECT. I was concerned about what to do if she refused it. Sure, we would put her on a section and treat her, but would we manage to complete the paperwork that morning? Another 24-hour delay felt too risky. I wasn't about to delay a life-saving treatment whatever happened, I explained to the two medical students attending. All of us were leaning over her, trying to catch her whispers and understand her wishes. It was a clear 'Yes', no matter how faint. I produced the consent form and asked her if she could sign it. A faint whisper came through the cracked lips, which was beyond my abilities to grasp.

'She said that she can't,' explained Sam, whose hearing is better than mine. Florence was too weak to hold a pen but was consenting to the treatment. Well, a signature is not legally required for consent, although it is the best practice, and there is a provision for people who are unable to write down a signature but consent verbally: a witness can document that fact on the consent form. With a few witnesses present, this was not a problem.

There was a more pragmatic problem, however: Florence's veins, always difficult even for the most skilful anaesthetist, had shrunk even further due to dehydration. Attempts to find a vein were failing one after the other; even the jugular vein wouldn't yield blood. We could give her Sevoflurane, an inhalatory anaesthetic, through a mask, but we knew that this would reduce the quality of seizures. We had observed with other patients that Sevoflurane approximately doubles the seizure threshold compared to her usual anaesthetic, Etomidate (thus accordingly reducing the likelihood of a seizure). Her last session had been given at 922mC, close to the ceiling of the machine, so there was not much room for any increase. We might not even elicit a seizure. And as we needed to give her a muscle relaxant intravenously, we needed a vein for this.

What about treating her without a muscle relaxant? I started pondering the risks. After all, the whole point of relaxation is to reduce any muscular pain and prevent injuries during the seizure. Florence was so weak, she was not going to injure herself. But if something went wrong, I could be asked in court why we gave ECT without a muscle relaxant, even if that was irrelevant. While I was obsessing about these heretical options, Sam recalled from her time in general surgery that Sevoflurane relaxes the veins, so we could administer it easily and painlessly through the mask, and then perhaps find a vein for the muscle relaxant when Florence was asleep. I grasped at this idea. There was, indeed, nothing else I could think of.

The plan then improved even further. We could wake Florence after the needle was in, to allow some time for the anticonvulsant effect of Sevoflurane to evaporate, so that she had a better chance of a seizure and successful treatment. I didn't know whether this would work, or how long we needed to wait. Our anaesthetist insisted that Sevoflurane wears off quickly, but I wasn't sure if the same applied to the anticonvulsant effect. But this was the best option, so we proceeded. When Florence was asleep, the anaesthetist tried the jugular vein again. Finally, blood coloured the plastic tube. One of the nurses from the general hospital left the room, crying (she was too distressed at the procedure to stay). The rest of the team was feeling more positive. With the venflon finally in place, we allowed Florence to wake up for a couple of minutes, then proceeded with Etomidate and Suxamethonium to induce the usual anaesthetic effect, increasing the electric charge to 1001mC, for good measure. There was a seizure, only eight seconds of observable muscular twitches, but with decent complexes on the EEG that continued for 23 seconds. This was a success. The effect of the inhalable Sevoflurane had almost gone, we had learned something, and we were hoping that Florence would have her usual miraculous response.

At the next session, Florence was tearful, holding her head in her hands. She looked miserable, but this was an expression of emotions and a clear sign of improvement. Indeed, she had walked into the treatment room on her own – a far cry from the forlorn figure on the stretcher I had seen a few days earlier. The vein was easier to find - or the anaesthetist was having a lucky day. Once Florence was well again, we would continue ECT every three weeks and would greet each other like old friends for many more years to come... But I will wrap up this story here.

12

SHE IS QUITE POORLY

Medics have their own code for describing patients who are very ill. Instead of saying, 'This patient is critically ill,' or, 'He is about to die,' a junior doctor might ask a colleague for advice with an understatement: 'Can you have a look at this patient; he is a bit unwell.' If a nurse doubts whether a patient will make it to the morning, a phrase that could be related to the duty doctor might sound something like, 'She is quite poorly.' This avoids panic, especially among relatives who inadvertently intercept the communication.

So when our lead nurse Kara sent me a series of messages on my phone, I knew that we had a patient in a critical condition. 'Just had a phone call from liaison. They want you to look at a person in the general hospital. … I said you were not in the country … Person quite poorly.' Kara could not give me more details on the phone, as it would have meant leaking confidential information. I had to read between the lines. 'Quite poorly' sounded like a quote from a nurse on the general ward. It might mean the highest level of urgency. The 'quite poorly person' was most likely on the point of death.

I typed back a message: 'I will take a plane now, will see patient tomorrow morning.' I was appreciating the irony of the situation. I was actually sitting on a plane just about to leave for London. I had not yet set my phone to flight mode and had just been making a last check, when

Kara's messages had started popping up. Quite a coincidence, and I couldn't wait to get back to work to help deal with it all. At least I knew my timing was impeccable.

More messages arrived before the captain had a chance to lift us off into the air. 'Secure portal is down. You will not be able to see the referral letter until tomorrow.' This was annoying. In order to protect patients' confidentiality, we share medical details via hospital e-mails or a secure server. Kara is not allowed to send such information to my university e-mail, so I was not going to see the details that evening.

I had to wait until I arrived at work the next morning before I could read the letter. The patient was a middle-aged lady with a previous psychiatric history that had switched a few times between depression and bipolar and schizoaffective disorders (a combination of symptoms of schizophrenia and mood disorder, hinting at the overlap between our diagnostic entities). Sarah had been admitted to a psychiatric hospital in the past but for many years had been doing well in the community. Two months earlier she had been admitted again, having become suicidal. She had been expressing paranoid ideas about relatives and members of staff. She couldn't look after herself and was neglectful of her personal care. She was reported as hearing voices and feeling very depressed but still eating and drinking well. About a month ago she had had a fall, after which it was noticed that she had slurred speech and weakness in her left arm.

This suggested a stroke, so Sarah was referred to a neurologist. But then things became less clear. The neurologists didn't find any evidence of a stroke. A CT scan of the head, and just in case a clearer picture might help, an MRI scan, did not visualise a stroke, or a brain mass, or any other brain pathology, that could explain her presentation. A lumbar puncture excluded encephalitis. Various blood tests were done, first for common conditions, and then moving into increasingly more obscure ones, but all kept coming back as normal. Meanwhile the patient was deteriorating. She stopped talking. Then she became unable to eat or drink, so a nasogastric tube was inserted. A series of X-rays narrated a story of poor tolerance of the tube, which was eventually removed. A small pleural effusion (excess fluid around the lungs) was deemed irrelevant because her oxygen levels, pulse rate, temperature and blood pressure had remained stable throughout her hospital stay.

After all conceivable causes were excluded, somebody raised the question, 'Could this be functional?' (codeword for a psychiatric illness). The liaison psychiatry team was called in. Sarah was able to communicate with them only by nodding her head. Some posturing and slow movements were recorded. The head of liaison psychiatry raised the possibility of catatonia. The patient was put on her previous psychotropic medication: a combination of an antidepressant and antipsychotic that had kept her well in the past. However, a medical cause still remained high on the list of possibilities.

The medication seemed to be working. Over the next few days Sarah started talking again, showed good eye contact, and denied unusual thoughts or voices. But still she could not get out of bed. The improvement lasted only a few days. She reduced her food intake, and communication with her was lost once more. The liaison psychiatrist now considered whether she might respond to ECT. This is when I saw the urgent request to give a second opinion. Ten minutes after I had received the message, my plane took off from the runway on its way to the UK.

Nothing from the notes prepared me for what I was about to observe at the patient's bedside. The closest picture was painted by the nurse who had seen the patient last: 'She is quite poorly.' So she was. She reminded me immediately of those terminally ill patients that I saw years ago as a junior doctor, who all too soon required death certificates.

Sarah was lying motionless on her back. Her mouth was open and her chin was loose and drooping down. She did not respond to my greeting. She looked indeed as if she were dying. But she wasn't. At a gentle squeezing of her shoulder and louder inquiries from me, her eyes opened and moved quickly in my direction, too quickly for somebody who is only half alive. They continued to follow me and to react to my questions. Sarah was trying to communicate. She was moaning in response to questions, as if telling me how deeply she was in trouble and how unable she was to explain it. She tried to squeeze my fingers when I asked her to do it. It was almost imperceptible, but the movement was there, and it was the same on both sides. Her tendon reflexes were intact and the pupils reacted well to light. That was all I could find from the neurological examination, but it reinforced the neurologists' opinion that her condition was not caused by a stroke.

Was this catatonia? I didn't see much movement of her limbs to help me identify more signs supporting the diagnosis, but the junior doctor who had looked after Sarah for a few weeks, confirmed that before she became immobile, all her movements had been extremely slow.

She demonstrated this by giving me a display of a slow-motion film. 'Everything is slow, it is not unilateral weakness,[13] just every movement is very slow,' she assured me. There was some rigidity when I tried flexing Sarah's wrists and elbows. In fact they yielded in rhythmic, slight jerks, as if she was resisting or as if I were trying to turn a rather stiff cogwheel - the so-called cogwheel rigidity associated with Parkinson's disease. This could be a feature of catatonia, or the result of antipsychotic medication that can cause Parkinsonian side effects. And then her skin looked greasy, the 'oily' face of catatonia described in the old textbooks.

If this was catatonia, she would respond to ECT. But what if it was a medical illness? What if she had some terminal illness and died on the table in the ECT suite, as a result of the additional stress of the electric shock? I was reminded of an episode when I was a medical student. My father, then head of psychiatry in my hometown of Sofia, trying to interest me in his trade, called me to his department to see a patient who was causing diagnostic problems among his colleagues. He was lying motionless on a bed with his limbs stretched out in a somewhat uncomfortable position. We were shown red marks on the side of his body: he had burned his skin lying next to a radiator a few days earlier, being unable to move away, or failing to react to the pain. 'How many times are we going to lose a human life because we delayed ECT?' My father addressed his colleagues who had assembled in an office to debate the case, some still desperately trying to find a

---

[13] Muscle weakness on one side of the body, commonly associated with stroke that has caused damage to only one side of the brain (the opposite side).

medical disorder that could explain the presentation. I remembered his confidence and the image of the man lying motionless on the bed, not uttering a word. I hadn't understood at the time what was going on, what was meant by the word 'catatonia' and why this strange treatment, ECT, should help an apparently dying man.

The next day I was talking about these very points, this time with the anaesthetist in the ECT suite. 'If this is catatonia, we are likely to save her with ECT,' I observed. 'If we don't, what are her prospects? She is refusing to eat or drink; she is kept alive with intravenous drips; she is likely to develop pneumonia or other complications as she is bedridden. She will probably die quite soon, and as it is, she already looks half-dead.' The anaesthetist didn't need much persuasion: 'If you think this is a psychiatric disorder, let us treat her. Her vital signs are stable; oxygen, pulse, blood pressure are all fine; she will not die on the table.' A certain degree of risk was involved, but also it was clear that this was Sarah's best chance of survival.

We used the emergency protocol of 195mC bilateral ECT (not waiting to establish a seizure threshold, as time was of the essence). The seizure was long enough (21 seconds), but the quality of the EEG traces was not very good. With hindsight, she could have had an even higher dose. The trouble was that Christmas was approaching. Christmas Day and Boxing Day had conspired to fall on two of the normal ECT days, so the next session was going to take place a whole week later.

'Keep her alive until after Christmas and we will get her well,' I advised the nurse who accompanied her from the general ward and who was herself wondering what to make of the strange treatment she had witnessed for the first time.

Christmas passed and I was back in the unit, looking forward to another meeting with our patient. We were told that she had done quite well. She was talking more freely, had started to eat and drink a bit, and appeared orientated. This was after just one session, so she must be a good responder. This was the good news. The bad news was that she had diarrhoea and this prevented her being transported to us, the usual procedure to prevent the spread of infection in the hospital.

Two weeks had passed after the first ECT. It was Friday and we were finally set to give her the second treatment. But Sarah wasn't in the unit. We received a message from the general ward that she couldn't come, as she was not well. More understatement. 'Not well,' as I found out later, did indeed mean something very serious. Bedridden people, especially in hospital, can develop infections. The diarrhoea and poor food intake had exhausted the body's defences, and Sarah had developed a chest infection. It was so severe that on Friday they had called the resuscitation team, as they thought she was going to die. She was indeed not very well.

The anaesthetist's view was that with a severe chest infection, she might not survive the treatment. It is his decision to judge who is safe to be anaesthetised and the risk was real. It was now up to intravenous antibiotics to save her life, not ECT. We had to wait for the infection to clear.

Sarah survived her infections and came back about three weeks after her first ECT. After the third ECT she started answering questions, but with just single words, giving mostly wrong answers. It was hard to understand or even hear her. After five ECTs she was much improved, able to speak and to answer questions about her depression. She had started to eat and drink. After eight ECTs I was told that she had been sitting in bed on the ward and watching people around her. This was all very good, but each time she came to treatment, I found her in the same state, lying in bed and not making any attempt to lift her hands or her head, staring at the ceiling, her mouth half-open. Each ECT was keeping her better for only two days.

While I was starting to wonder whether we should give her ECT three times a week, events overtook us again. Sarah developed another infection, this time from the central line inserted into the vein on her neck. ECT was stopped. Her mental state slipped back. She was kept in a separate room, as she had started screaming and upsetting the other patients on the ward (still a general medical ward). A nurse told me that she couldn't understand where Sarah found the energy to scream non-stop for 24 hours a day. Three weeks later, when we were trying to organise more ECT sessions, she was again 'too poorly'. This time she had suspected peritonitis (infection of the lining of the abdomen), but this was not confirmed by the X-ray. Her electrolytes were unstable, with her potassium levels going down. It sounded as if her whole body was going downhill, too. Being bedridden doesn't help your prospects.

One morning, exactly a month after the last ECT, an ambulance brought her back to our unit. I knew she had arrived when I saw that one of the beds was cordoned off with curtains. I entered the enclosed area, curious to see how she was. I didn't know that I was in for a surprise. Sarah wasn't looking at the ceiling; instead, she looked at me and said, 'Hello, doctor.' Her voice was very low, so perhaps I didn't hear correctly? A louder chatter was coming from the other side of the curtains, where two or three nurses had gathered around the bed of another patient.

'Do you remember me?' I insisted on clarifying.

'Yes, I do.'

'Do you know why you are here?'

'To have ECT.'

I was still unsure about the degree of her orientation, so proceeded to the next level.

'Do you know where you are? What is the name of this place?'

Now for somebody who is bedridden, who doesn't talk, who is brought in an ambulance, unable to see where she is travelling, I expected an answer such as, 'In the hospital,' or, if she was really that good, to give me the name of our hospital, as the one she came from was in another part of town, some half-hour drive away. She mumbled something, which I couldn't understand, but that didn't sound right. I looked at the nurse, hoping that he had caught the words better. 'Hafan-y-Coed,' he related to me. I was wondering what he was talking about now, and then it clicked: Hafan-y-Coed was the not-so-easy name of our unit! I had been unprepared for this precision.

Sarah had really improved, and I felt that she now had capacity to consent. Until now, due to her inability to show understanding of the treatment and even inability to say anything, she had been treated under the Mental Capacity Act. If she had capacity to consent and she refused, she couldn't be given ECT. I took a capacity assessment form and a consent form and started going through the criteria. I first asked if she wanted to have ECT. She said, 'Yes.' That was a good start. I then asked what ECT means. She proceeded in her low and slow voice. I couldn't hear her well, the nurses beyond the curtain were still talking about something. I hate telling people to keep their voices down, so I popped my head out between the curtains and made faces, indicating how sorry I was to interrupt them but that the patient was so weak, I couldn't hear her. Silence followed and I could now discern the answers of our patient:

'Electroconvulsive something... electric shock.'

'When did you have the last one?'

'Several weeks ago.'

'Why are we giving you ECT?'

'To make me feel better.'

'Is it helping you?'

'Yes, definitely.'

I was more and more astonished by her clear answers and wanted to probe deeper. Was she really feeling better? She was still bedbound and looking poorly, did she have the understanding to appreciate that she had been very unwell, that she had stopped moving, talking and eating?

'So you are saying that ECT has helped you. Can you tell me in what way it has helped you?'

Very slowly and very quietly, these words made their way between her dry lips:

'I...can...talk...now.'

This poor patient, who had long-term mental health problems, who had almost died twice, had realised that she hadn't been able to talk and that her abilities were coming back, due to the ECT. Perhaps this was why she had been screaming earlier, unable to verbalise her distress. I felt a certain wetness in my own eyes and my voice went a bit shaky. A few weeks later she gave me an even better description. She had felt as if she was being crushed by rubble - that was why she was screaming all the time. A good account of what catatonia might feel like: an inability to move or talk.

A couple of minutes later Sarah was signing her name on the consent form. The pen was going up and down very slowly over the paper, drawing one letter at a time, but the letters were being formed correctly and resulted in her name. I was humbled. I had underestimated her ability to have insight. She had raised the bar of my expectations. I now thought that we should aim to get her back to supportive accommodation, walking, dressing and washing herself, and enjoying the little things in life. Very wishful thinking, surely, but my emotions were running high. The seizure that day was very good, as I expected it to be, after one month without Diazepam. Just as well I had reduced the electric charge by about 20%.

Another three ECTs later, a total of 18 sessions so far. I had not seen Sarah for a week. She came again by ambulance, on a stretcher. Her face was beaming with smiles and she burst into speech. Her eyes were not merely focused on me but were assisted by a pair of glasses that seemed to have been useless until now. The conversation was so fluent and reasonable, and her emotions were so well preserved, I began to doubt the severity of her previous psychiatric illnesses. But why was she still in bed? I asked her to pull my hand towards her with her right hand. She was applying reasonable force. 'Not strong enough!' we both joked. Her left hand produced similar pressure. She wouldn't be able to do a pull-up with this strength, but she should be able to do most things that are needed to function at home. Now for her legs, which had been nearly motionless only a week earlier. She managed to lift her leg a couple of centimetres off the mattress. Then she managed to lift her knee, flexing the leg nearly to a right angle. Physiotherapy staff had been to see her daily and had managed to get her to sit in a chair. She had taken a couple of steps with support but told me that she was too weak to stand up. But the goal of making her walk again seemed that little bit more realistic.

Sarah continued with weekly ECTs for another two months, before being discharged to a rehabilitation unit. Another two months later she came for a follow-up. She was smiling and had no complaints. She felt happy and was clearly enjoying life. The ECT had stopped her voices, that had kept telling her to kill herself. Physiotherapists had been visiting her regularly and, just as I thought, were confident of being able to fully mobilise her. She was managing her first steps, after months of being locked in by catatonia, still leaning on a frame but moving around unaided. I could count Sarah as one of our miracle outcomes.

13

A PROMISE

I'll never forget my first meeting with Christine. She was an in-patient referred for ECT, so I was asked to see her. I duly went to the ward and the staff kindly found a room for us where we could sit down. But I was the only one who managed to take a seat. Christine was totally unable to settle - she was running around the room like a frightened animal caught in a trap. The room was quite small, and this probably exacerbated the effect this had on me. Not only could Christine not sit down, she could not stand still either and exhibited a kind of perpetuum mobile, pacing around the limited space throughout our entire meeting. At the same time, she talked in a loud voice, likewise without stopping. Strange to say, she was not psychotic and was fully aware of what was happening. She knew this behaviour was inappropriate but was unable to stop. She had enough awareness to ask me why she was like this, and whether I could help her. She was also able to tell me her story, while circling around the armchair I was seated in. The chair was positioned almost in the middle of the room and I was sitting there in a semi-reclined position, pretending to look like the calmest man in town, in the hope that this behaviour would be infectious and slow her down a bit. In vain. At the moment, there was no reaching Christine. But while her mind was overactive, her mood was depressed: she was displaying the features of agitated depression.

In fact, she was in a 'mixed state' as described by Emil Kraepelin in the 19th century, with her mood one of depression, but her thinking and movements like those of a manic person. Sometimes known as mixed depression, agitated depression includes symptoms such as acute restlessness, racing thoughts, and occasionally, irritability and angry outbursts. Christine had had several episodes of depression in her life, starting many years ago, and each lasting for about one year. But she had never been like this. Her condition had deteriorated and about four months ago, her team had felt that she needed to come to hospital. Despite this, her condition had continued to worsen, although she also had periods when she was calm. Each time she needed to discuss anything or make a decision, her agitation would come back and the shouting and pacing increased. Meeting a doctor to discuss ECT was clearly anxiety-provoking.

I looked through Christine's notes, to assemble the history of her treatments. Agitated depression should be treated with both antidepressants and antipsychotics. Antidepressants on their own can be stimulating, as they are meant to lift mood and boost interest in activities. But in some cases, their activating effect can lead to hyperarousal, exacerbating agitation and restlessness, and so should be combined with antipsychotics that will slow down motor and psychic activation. Christine had been on one such drug (Risperidone), but her doctors suspected that it was causing akathisia. This is a condition we don't see that often these days, as it is largely a side effect of the old antipsychotics. Patients can't sit still, feel restless, keep tapping their feet, and have to stand up and walk around to reduce the tension; it is also described as 'restless legs'.

How do you distinguish this side effect from the depressive agitation that Christine had? This can be difficult. In practice, it is not unusual to increase the doses of these older antipsychotics in akathisic patients with the good intention of reducing their symptoms, which in turn further increases their agitation. To avoid this potential problem, Christine's Risperidone had been stopped. Her agitation had increased: this hadn't been akathisia.

Christine was a picture of misery, and I had no doubt that she needed ECT. But what were her chances of success, I wondered? Even in depressive stupor, the illness that best responds to ECT, we do not reach a 100% success rate. Christine's symptoms varied quite significantly from this and also fluctuated from day to day. What success rate could I reasonably promise her? Anxiety on its own does not respond very well to ECT, and there can be a fine line between anxiety and agitated depression. I would have to persuade Christine to have ECT. I started talking about the treatment and her prospects of responding to it. To my surprise, she listened to every word I was saying and asked all the right questions. Although her body wouldn't stop moving, her mind was clear, she was fully orientated and maintained insight into her condition. She had always been a determined and ambitious lady, and her speech reflected this.

Christine had almost made up her mind to have ECT. But she had one more question, and she asked it in her loud, desperate manner.

'Doctor, will ECT make me better? Promise me it will make me better!' She repeated this a few times, still walking quickly around me. I don't normally make promises. I try to give patients my best guess as to how likely they are to respond. Our ECT information booklet of the time stated that at least 50% of patients recover with ECT.[14] Not entirely reassuring in terms of giving me the confidence to promise Christine a complete recovery. Knowing as I do that some conditions respond much better to ECT, I am more optimistic with such patients and able to state that I am 'almost sure' they will get better, although I can never give them a guarantee. In the tension of this narrow room, bemused and slightly giddied by Christine constantly circling around me, and disconcerted by her wide-open, frightened eyes, I gave a different answer, which was honest, but probably way too optimistic. I said, 'You have a 95% chance of recovery with ECT.'

She stopped circling for a second. 'Ninety-five percent? You promise?'

'Yes, I promise.'

This was a gamble – and I wouldn't be able to look her in the eye if she didn't then respond to treatment, despite the high likelihood of success. Already I was regretting my rash promise...

The next day I learned that Christine had agreed to have our full battery of cognitive tests. I could not imagine how she could sit still in order to connect the 24 numbers and letters of the Trail Making Test or to copy from memory the Complex Figure. But she managed! She had to get up and walk around between each test, but she found the will to concentrate and finish them; in fact she achieved very high scores. So Christine was able to think clearly and make decisions. She believed in ECT. This was

---

[14] We have since improved this to 58%, and for those who continued up to 24 ECTs, the remission rates reached 69%.

probably not caused by the calmness and composure that I was trying to convey, nor by any eloquence on my part, as I don't really shine in that area either. It might have been due to my confidence in portraying ECT as the treatment with the best success rate - or the unfounded promise I had given her! There was one other possible reason that I didn't know about yet: Christine's mother had been treated with ECT many years earlier and had responded well. Had I been preaching to the converted? Years later, I would question whether the high rate of positive family history that I noticed among our ECT patients was due to a bias. Could it be that depressed patients with a relative who has responded to ECT in the past, tend to be more willing to have it themselves, while patients who don't know of such a person, are more likely to refuse it?

There was nothing to report for ECT No.1. Christine had a seizure at the first stimulation of 80mC. ECT No.2 was given at 161mC, double the threshold dose, as our protocol prescribed. At ECT No.3 she had a short episode of arrhythmia in the form of bigeminy, lasting 15 seconds. This was too short to make anybody nervous.

On the morning before ECT No.4 her depression rating scale had dropped to 24, from a starting point of 46. This was nearly 50% improvement, but Christine was still agitated, still pacing up and down. Her thoughts were still racing, and her speech was fast, again resembling that of a manic person. When she saw me, she said in a loud voice.

'You said I had a 95% chance of getting well, didn't you?'

I nodded my head in agreement, slightly annoyed that this memory of all others was intact.

'Yes, a 95% chance.' Did she realise that this wasn't the same as getting 95% better, I wondered? Either she would get well, or ECT would fail; this is what normally happens. So if I was correct about the 95% chance - and it was a big 'if' - then out of 20 women in her condition, 19 would get well and one would stay agitated. And, of course, that one could be her. Her chances were not 95% anyway. That morning I promised myself never to make such promises again!

Each time Christine came for her treatment, she would remind me of the 95% chance, and each time I kept my fingers crossed behind my back...

It's day 12, after four ECTs, and I am recording in the notes, 'Possibly first signs of improvement'. And already we need to enter into another pact. Christine tells me that she wants to go to a concert, to see her son performing. She still can't sit still in a chair and the concert is in London, so somehow she needs to get there first. She wonders if I think she will be able to do this and how? By train? At least she can stand up and walk around there if need be. The concert is next week, and she will only have one more ECT before that. I don't give the 95% guarantee this time. All the same, I note that I am thinking that this is not impossible, given Christine's determination and will. The two nurses in the room exchange looks of disbelief: they think I am crazy. I am wondering if we are going to see a miracle. Maybe we need one!

Day 20, after six ECTs, Christine arrives for her treatment and tells me that she went to the concert. In fact, she did travel on her own, by train, and managed to sit still in her seat in the concert hall. She no longer looks apprehensive. She narrates the story fluently and is very pleasant and much softer in her demeanour. No anguish, no restlessness, no pacing around - a completely different person. Some symptoms are still present, so I can't rate her as remitted, but I slightly clench my fist and give her a smile. I got that one right, my promise worked! She's going to recover completely.

It took another week before Christine's score dropped below 10, the remission range. In fact, the score was down to three after ECT No.8. Looks like I would have got the timing right too, if I had been pressed to guess, as the average time to remission in our unit is after eight ECTs.

Over the next two months Christine had four continuation ECTs and then stopped treatment, somewhat to my surprise, as I did advise her to have two more. I was worried that she would relapse and arranged several follow-up meetings. Initially she complained of memory problems: she had forgotten the names of some friends, how to put credit on her mobile phone, some words, the names of some places, and the circumstances of Princess Diana's death. This sounded worrying, as this is one of those events that everyone remembers. She had also forgotten the content of her recent master's dissertation. But overall, she was functioning very well and had started learning a new skill: playing the guitar. We repeated her cognitive tests which remained unchanged, with a nearly perfect Complex Figure, as at the start. I told her that her brain was functioning well and that she should be able to memorise new material again.

Christine remained well and went back to her teaching job. Over the years, she had a few more episodes of depression and anxiety but managed to recover each time and never slipped into the terrible agitation that I had witnessed. Was this the effect of ECT or the long-term effect of Lithium, which we prescribed for her after the ECT course - another strange and archaic treatment that still works well and has been shown to reduce the relapse rates after ECT? But that's another story...

14

AUTISM

I am hesitating whether to include this story, in case some readers assume that I am suggesting ECT as a 'cure' for autism. I have to state from the start that I am not going to do that by any means, but you have to read the whole story.

Many people connect the term autism with children. There are rare examples of such children exhibiting severe self-mutilating or aggressive behaviour, sometimes described as catatonic features. ECT has been used in such conditions and can be helpful. This is best narrated in a book by the mother of such a child, Amy Lutz, *Each day I like it better*. Lutz describes how her son's aggression drastically improved and he maintained the improvement while receiving 136 ECTs over a period of three years. I can easily think of another situation where ECT can help a person with autism: if they develop a psychotic depression. The story I have to tell is not that straightforward and will not answer many questions, perhaps none at all. But it happened and I wrote it down, so here it is.

Cheryl was referred to me for a second opinion. She had asked to have ECT herself, seeing it as a hope that she could change. She insisted on having it, in fact, and had written a long letter to her doctor requesting a referral. She thought that ECT might 'cure' her autism by re-wiring her brain! I don't think it can cure autism, but this idea is close to my understanding of what ECT does to people's brains. Indeed, there is evidence that ECT reduces excessive functional connectivity between neuronal networks in the frontal parts of the brain, which might underpin the ruminations and increased vigilance commonly found in severe depression. And the creation of new synapses has also been observed. It sounded as if Cheryl had researched the literature in as much depth as I had. I was looking forward to meeting her and hearing her story. Cheryl was not a child; in fact, she was in her 30s. She had not even been diagnosed with autism as a child, as one might expect. This had been done only a few years ago by a doctor in a general hospital, where she was admitted after an overdose. That doctor had not been a psychiatrist. A shame, as he would make a good colleague: I agreed with the diagnosis. Cheryl had also agreed: the diagnosis helped her understand and make sense of her experiences.

Cheryl told me about her problems. She had never had friends, had never understood emotions, and had been unable to show emotions or even to feel emotions for others. At school she had persistently run away, had tantrums, and would sometimes curl up on the chair or walk out of the classroom. She was unable to listen to the instructions given by her teachers. But she managed some good GCSEs, and her cognitive abilities were never in question; indeed, she had a good university degree. And more recently she had got married. Asperger's would have been the more accurate diagnosis for somebody who was functioning so well, but we tend not to use this term now, as all forms of autism were recently combined under the umbrella term 'autism spectrum disorder' (ASD), and we would probably rate her as 'high functioning' instead.

During the consultation, she demonstrated a quick and logical mind. We had a very detailed conversation about ECT and the wiring of the brain. She clearly had done a lot of work on the internet and had developed her own theory as to how ECT could help with autism. Up to that point, I must admit that I couldn't see why she would want it or for what reason she would need it.

Cheryl painted more problems that had interfered with her all her life. She felt that she suffered with 'sensory overload': images, videos and memories going through her mind, that she was unable to push away. Her brain would feel increasingly overloaded, to the point that she had to scream with frustration and anxiety. 'My mind is absolutely racing, I can't focus.' For several years, she had continuously felt that life was not worth living and had already taken more than 20 overdoses. She had injured herself by cutting her arms with a bread knife, carving words on her skin, and on one occasion, trying to hang herself by tying her pyjamas to the banisters and using them as a ligature. Banging her head on the wall or with various objects to reduce her agitation, was another dysfunctional element in her behaviour. She had seen psychiatrists for many years and had tried the usual list of drugs for depression or anxiety: Prozac, Sertraline, Quetiapine, Risperidone, Diazepam, Lamotrigine, and others that she could not remember.

Clearly her mood was prone to depression, I reflected, before more problems presented themselves during the second 30 minutes of our consultation. Up until that point, she had looked completely well, laughing appropriately and taking jokes well. Her speech was fast and clear, and she responded quickly to my questions. I had just started asking questions about depression from the Hamilton Depression Rating Scale and trying to gather more details about her autistic symptoms. At this point she shut up abruptly, looking grim. Evidently she was annoyed about something. This changed into open hostility; she accused me of not believing she had autism and of not wanting to give her ECT.

'That's it, I'm leaving!' she said, turning to her husband and getting up from her chair. She had misinterpreted my intention: by that time I had seen enough symptoms to believe the diagnosis of autism wholeheartedly, while her obvious symptoms of depression and agitation had led me to judge that she could benefit from ECT. I felt annoyed with her reaction and explained this, perhaps rather sharply, 'I am on your side, I am here to help you and you are shouting at me!' She did stay but her eyes were directed at the floor until the end of the meeting, and there were no more smiles.

Realising that I had effectively told her that she could have ECT, I spent the rest of the time warning her about the memory side effects and the rather limited chances of it helping her - although I didn't want to leave her with no hope at all. But she had made up her mind before she came. She had tried many treatments, and nothing had helped her, and she believed that ECT was now her only chance. I reasoned with myself that the chance was indeed small, but you never know - I have seen so many people get better, when I didn't expect an improvement, that I have given up predicting outcomes. And I admit, I was curious. When I presented her case to my colleagues at our academic meeting, some of them were against ECT, thinking that this was a case of personality disorder, which would not benefit from the treatment. I wasn't going to change my decision and they accepted it.

Cheryl herself felt that some of her behaviour had been challenging for her medical team. She described how she worked with health professionals up to a certain point but then reached 'a big barrier or a block' that prevented her from progressing further and really changing. She would revert to self-harm behaviours such as cutting and head-banging, possibly motivated by a desire to gain admission to hospital. She worried a great deal about wasting professionals' time and would apologise for - in her words – 'creating drama' or being 'childish and immature'. She spoke of her frustration in having a brain that was 'broken,' and felt she was more tormented than many people with autism. Cheryl wanted a treatment that gave her real hope of changing and was able to identify with ECT by comparing it to a more effective version of banging her head against the wall to manage her distress. I spoke with Cheryl's consultant, and we agreed that she could have a trial of ECT, especially as she had such high hopes for it. When people believe in a treatment, it becomes more effective.

Cheryl was impatient to start and came for her first session a couple of weeks later. A few minutes after the uneventful first treatment, I heard screams from the recovery room. Cheryl was sitting on the bed and shouting, looking emotional and distressed. Two of our nurses were standing one step away from the bed, keeping quiet, trying not to excite her further, and looking at me for suggestions. This was not delirium; she was sufficiently orientated and knew what had happened, although she must have been still partially confused so soon after the seizure. The shouting stopped after 20 minutes and then she calmed down and became nice and pleasant. Before she left, she told me that she had been semi-conscious while shouting, which made sense, although she clearly had memories of the event. Over the next couple of months this happened another three or four times and the recovery nurses got used to it. But we were about to have more problems.

At the fourth session, there was another episode of shouting, but this time in the treatment room, before the ECT. It was in response to the needle going into her vein. The screaming was so sudden and loud, it startled everybody. It was quickly followed by Cheryl shouting accusations at the nurses and the anaesthetist. We proceeded with the treatment without further discussion and after that I gathered more information. I had not been aware of it, but Cheryl had negotiated a set of rules with the nurses around her preparations for ECT. Prior to treatment, a few sets of electrodes need to be stuck to various parts of the body, the temples need to be scraped with alcohol swabs to remove any grease that might interfere with the electric current, a needle has to be inserted into a vein and secured with plasters and so on. Normally, these tasks are performed by several people, each one focusing on the individual job. But autistic people can become overwhelmed if things around them seem chaotic. So Cheryl had insisted that only one procedure be done at any one time, and only one person could touch her at a time. She had also requested that the lights be dimmed, due to her autism-related sensitivity to bright light. This had all been agreed, except the dimming of the lights, but the instructions were piling up too quickly for her. Somebody didn't follow the rules and was attaching an ECG electrode while the anaesthetist was trying to find a vein. The lack of order had been overwhelming, and she had started shouting out of frustration.

The next time she came, I felt that I had to confront her about her behaviour. I tried to put it gently but clearly: her sudden, loud screaming had scared the staff, and could she please make an effort and not shout like that again? I had misread the situation. Cheryl was incensed and took her anger out on me, stating that because of her autism she could not control her emotions and that everything had to be done in the right order. She was unable to control herself again, stormed out of the room and wanted to leave the unit. The nurse at the door looked at me to see if she should open the electric lock, and I nodded without hesitation. It was Cheryl's decision and there was no way I was going to use any strong persuasion to make her have ECT. Later we told her that she was not banned from treatment, and she could come again if she wished.

It was more than a week later that I saw Cheryl again, first thing in the morning, sitting in the waiting room. She smiled and we waved at each other. I walked past without trying to engage in a conversation, in order to avoid further confrontation and later gathered the information I needed from her mother. Cheryl had told her that she felt better after the ECTs. She had not harmed herself since starting the treatment, seemed more motivated and clearer in her thoughts, was socialising with friends, and was sleeping better. This was what I wanted to hear, so we continued - only to face another problem the following week.

Cheryl was increasingly complaining of severe pain from the needle, and the following week this escalated again, with her shouting and running out of the treatment room. I was surprised the nurses were still tolerating me when I declared that she could come again and that we would find a solution. I was beginning to worry that I was accommodating Cheryl's behaviour at their expense. By that time, she had started telling everybody what to do in the treatment room, as if she were in charge. She had refused to be assessed with the HAM-D, as she didn't think it was appropriate for her. However, there was indeed a solution for the pain from the needle. It was suggested by the anaesthetist at the next session. The needle could be inserted in the vein after Cheryl was put to sleep with an inhalatory anaesthetic, Sevoflurane. That way she would breathe the anaesthetic through a mask, rather than via injection. The needle is still required for the muscle relaxant but would be inserted when Cheryl was asleep. Neat. There are many reasons why we don't do this more regularly, though: it is more complicated; requires the room to be ventilated; there is an extra anaesthetic risk; and Sevoflurane suppresses the seizures. But, like the nurses, the anaesthetists also tend to tolerate me, and sometimes go out of their way to satisfy my requests.

Cheryl fell asleep without shouting but didn't have any seizure activity under the electric charge that had worked so well hitherto, and eventually we ended up giving her twice the amount of electricity in order to elicit seizures of the same quality. It took two sessions to work out the correct electric charge, so on two days she received possibly sub-therapeutic seizures. But we had finally found a very effective method to anaesthetise her, with her distress minimised and the risk of her shouting fully cut out once the anaesthetic mask was placed over her face.

Everything was sorted out, but there was another slight problem - it wasn't clear whether Cheryl was really benefiting. I had developed my own criteria by which to judge her improvement in the absence of rating scales: I wanted to see her stop getting into arguments when contradicted, become more tolerant of others, stop self-harming and, ultimately, go back to work. A reduction in depression was a bonus, but this was to be expected from ECT anyway, so it had no relevance to the effect of ECT on other aspects of her autism. Cheryl did manage to go back to work, but conversely, I didn't feel she was ready to tolerate a confrontation with me, so I didn't attempt one. Cheryl did have five sessions with good seizures on Sevoflurane. There were gaps, sometimes a week, then they increased to a month. After that Cheryl stopped coming and phoned to explain that ECT was not helping her.

This was clearly a failure, and I was left with many unanswered questions. Cheryl had 16 sessions overall, and they made very little change to her condition. But was ECT unsuccessful because her 16 sessions stretched over four months, and a couple of them did not result in good seizures? Was that a valid ECT course? Would her explosive behaviour settle a bit, and would her self-harming disappear? Would she feel better about herself and tolerate others if she had a better course? Now that I am writing this, I am annoyed with myself that I didn't manage to build a more trusting relationship; that I didn't appreciate more quickly her need for order and minimal interference during the treatments; that I didn't find the solution with Sevoflurane earlier in the course. Would a less disrupted course have produced a miracle? This is probably wishful thinking and any positive effect would have likely disappeared without continuation ECT. Perhaps my colleagues were right to be against ECT in this case and I am only looking for excuses.

15

MUSICIANS

Vladimir Horowitz, recognised by many as the greatest pianist of his day, had two courses of ECT in the 1960s and 1970s respectively. It would appear that ECT didn't affect the fine skills required to transform the intricate combinations of notes printed on sheets of paper into perfect synchronized twitches of the muscles of his fingers, to produce a musical experience unrivalled by any other fellow human. In 1982, Horowitz was prescribed antidepressants but found that they severely impaired his ability to play music, to the extent that his 1983 performances were marred by memory lapses and some loss of physical control. A few years later, in 1986, having come off these drugs, he was a sensation at his Moscow recital, when he returned for the first time to his country of birth. I have to repeat this message, in case it has gone unnoticed: sometimes antidepressants may have worse side effects than ECT.

I thought of all this when I came to assess Mary, a professional musician. At first, her appointment didn't seem urgent. In order to see a specialist in the UK, waiting lists are the norm, and it is not unusual to have to wait at least six months. I don't have a waiting list for patients referred for a second opinion for ECT. This is not because I am very efficient or hard-working. It is due to a more mundane reason: not many people get referred for ECT. It has become a rather rare procedure in the UK with only about 2,000 people treated each year. So I can always make room for an extra appointment slot, should I get more customers. The only time a patient might have to wait is when I am on holiday, which my colleagues sometimes imply happens too frequently.

Therefore when Mary's referral letter arrived, I asked my secretary to book an appointment in about two weeks' time. Job done. Ten minutes later an e-mail popped up on my computer screen. On ringing the hospital, my secretary had been told that the patient was too unwell to travel to see me - could I possibly go there myself? This didn't sound right. The referral letter described a patient who had made a great recovery with ECT and had started going out on walks. The main question that I was asked to help with was how long maintenance ECT could continue, clearly a matter that can wait for quiet consideration. Something had clearly gone very wrong since the referral letter had been sent, just two weeks earlier. The case had suddenly become more urgent. I started to worry about Mary. All the gains from ECT could be lost if she started to relapse and didn't receive more frequent continuation sessions. It was 3:15 pm. I scanned the rest of my e-mails and then looked at my diary. Nothing was happening really: the world was getting by without any need for my input. It was too early for the rush-hour traffic and my car was in the car park next to my office. I could find no excuses - a drive to her hospital was the right thing to do and I left straight away.

Somewhat to my surprise, Mary didn't look that poorly. She was sitting in a chair, greeted me politely, and evidently appreciated a chance to discuss ECT. She said that it had not helped her. I knew she was wrong. The referral letter had painted a dramatic picture of her condition prior to ECT that was clearly different from the kind-looking lady sitting calmly before me. She had been throwing herself on the floor, where she would lie mute, eyes closed, claiming that she could not see, walk or talk. She believed that she had no bones. All this had disappeared, or had almost gone after a few ECTs. The lady in front of me had somewhat more understandable complaints: she felt that her body was not functioning correctly, that something was wrong with her arms and legs, but couldn't quite specify what this was. I wondered how much better she must have been only a few weeks ago, at the end of the acute course of 12 ECTs, if her present condition was described as a deterioration.

Slowly and with some difficulty I pieced her history together. Mary had first had a breakdown in her late 20s when she was admitted to a psychiatric hospital, diagnosed with manic depression. She had been finding the life of a professional musician stressful. It was not the concerts that bothered her, or the associated late nights - she enjoyed those - but teaching schoolchildren, which she found too repetitive. Her sleep began to deteriorate, and then she didn't sleep for a whole week. One night, having stayed awake again, she began moving around the house, feeling excited. She then went out into the street, ringing on people's doors to share her excitement. She kept hearing music in her ears, repeated over and over again. She was manic.

'Musical hallucinations!' I interjected with excitement. 'Like Schumann.' It was the first time I had shared this knowledge with a patient, although I use Schumann's story in my lectures to students on the topic of manic depression. At last a patient with the same predicament! Schumann, whose hallucinations started suddenly at the age of 44, also experienced manic episodes, hearing music more glorious than any heard on earth. Legend has it that he said he was taking dictation from Franz Schubert's ghost. Sadly however as his illness progressed, he increasingly lacked the organisational ability to put it down on paper.

Her eyes lit up, too. 'Yes, and Tchaikovsky. We are both nutters.' This was beautiful and I admitted that I hadn't studied the Russian composer's mental illness, although I should have.

For a long time, Mary's problems were solved by regular medication. The most successful was an old-fashioned antipsychotic in depot (slow release) injection form, which kept her well for more than two decades. Medication did not kill the music. She was able to continue earning a living by it, playing in various orchestras around the country and abroad, with very occasional relapses that did not disrupt her functioning. Unfortunately, her anti-psychotic eventually exerted a toll on her dopamine-producing neurons, or perhaps she also had a predisposition to the illness: she developed Parkinson's disease. The depot had to be stopped and she started taking anti-Parkinsonian medications. Other antipsychotics exacerbated her condition, so they were also stopped.

Mary stayed well for a couple of years, even without her injection, but adverse life events eventually pushed her into the current episode. Her doctors tried other antipsychotics, but these seemed to make 'no change to her presentation whatsoever', as I read in the referral letter with increasing disbelief. Things had been going downhill for the past two years. Mary had moved abroad. Initially she was placed in a nursing home, but when it became clear that she was not getting any better, she returned to her native Wales and was admitted to the hospital where I met her. The overall picture was one of suffering. Lying on the floor, she would complain that she was paralysed, had cancer, had lost her voice, that she couldn't walk and somehow her legs and arms were twisted backwards and the clothes were getting in the way, preventing her from moving. It is possible that the stiffness caused by the Parkinson's disease might have shaped these bizarre experiences in the mind of a severely depressed person. These episodes would alternate with days when she was settled. Perhaps worst of all, her musical instruments had been abandoned. The illness had truly changed her life. Clozapine was then tried. Of all the antipsychotics, this is the one with the least adverse effect on the dopamine receptors. But other side effects prevented reasonable dose increases and after another four months, her team concluded that Clozapine did not improve her condition (the word 'whatsoever' was used again).

Mary finally agreed to have ECT. Her response to the treatment was dramatic: she started going out of the hospital, shopping, and even playing musical instruments for the first time in years.

Now, though, with the course finished, her doctors were worried that she was slipping back, and I could appreciate the source of the anxiety. I wrote an encouraging response to the referring doctor who had enquired about maintenance ECT. They were giving her the right treatments (ECT + Clozapine), she was a good responder and her relapse was not unusual and could be contained easily. I finished by saying, 'It might be best to resume twice-weekly ECT in order to get her back to the best possible level of functioning, and then very gradually extend the intervals, trying to figure out the longest interval that will still keep her well.' I did envisage a long-term need for ECT but in the circumstances wanted to make sure that first she stayed well over the next year.

It is nine months since my first encounter with Mary, and I am in the car on my way to see her again. Her new consultant trained in Cardiff and witnessed extended ECT courses in my clinic. She had heeded my advice for a long continuation treatment, so Mary was still having ECT once every three weeks while living at home, and only coming to the hospital on the days of her treatments. After one year as an inpatient, she was approaching one year of being well. I was looking forward to talking with her and her doctor. Mary stated that she had not felt depressed even once since the treatment started. She showed me her hands and stretched out her fingers. There was a slight shaking that I hadn't noticed until that moment. This was her Parkinson's disease, controlled with dopamine in the form of Madopar, but this medication was not making her psychotic any longer. Her only complaint was of memory problems but she didn't appear to be too worried; in fact, she was willing to continue with the treatment, if I advised her to do so.

'Am I going to have ECT for years now?' she asked us. I didn't think this was necessary. She had been well for a long time and had had Lithium added to her other drugs recently. She had a good prognosis. I wanted to tread delicately in view of her history, and not mess things up with my visit, but I felt that it was time to stop, and we agreed to tail off with a final two or three sessions at monthly intervals.

This agreed, I switched the conversation to music. She hadn't had access to a musical instrument yet but was planning to buy a second-hand piano and a violin. And she was planning to start playing in a chamber orchestra.

Were there too many musicians among my patients, I mused? Probably a coincidence, as music is popular around here. This is Wales, the land of music, of course. There is a whole literature on creativity and mental illness and on artists who have been ill, especially with manic depression. Musical hallucinations form a fascinating subset of this. Uncommon it might be, but well-documented. Beethoven had musical hallucinations after he became deaf. Chopin also had hallucinations, though these were of 'terrors and ghosts' that once forced him to flee from a performance and are thought to be related to temporal lobe epilepsy. The tune for the Beatles song 'Yesterday' is said to have come to Paul McCartney in a dream and for a time he was convinced it had been written by someone else. A rich field of exploration. It was time to get back and to make a note for another follow-up in the future. I still hadn't seen her play the piano.

16

RED ALERT

The very first patient ever to receive ECT was suffering from schizophrenia. This happened in Rome, in 1938. Ugo Cerletti and Lucio Bini anticipated that electrically induced seizures might be therapeutic in schizophrenia, following recent success with drug-induced seizures. They gave the first ECT to a confused patient who had paranoid schizophrenia. After 11 sessions he achieved remission and was discharged from the hospital. Within two years, ECT was used all over the world. The reason for its rapid spread was that it was so effective. Very soon it became clear that the best effect was on depression, but it was the effect on schizophrenia that had made it so popular initially.

During the following decades, ECT was marred by bad publicity and was occasionally misused, so that the trend was totally reversed. Now we tend to use it only rarely in schizophrenia, and opinions on its use are divided. The National Institute for Health and Care Excellence (NICE) guidelines discourage it: 'The current state of the evidence does not allow the general use of ECT in the management of schizophrenia to be recommended'. The Royal College of Psychiatrists takes a slightly more positive stance on the evidence: 'ECT may be an effective and safe augmentation strategy in Treatment Resistant Schizophrenia'. And if the patient has catatonia, it may even be considered as a first line treatment.

The controversy is not without good reason, though, as improvements in schizophrenia are much more modest than in depression. To make matters worse, patients with schizophrenia may have poor insight and refuse to have ECT, while psychiatrists might be worried about being accused of misusing this treatment. The result of all this is that only about 1% of those receiving ECT in the UK have a diagnosis of schizophrenia. We only treat the worst cases: those who have not responded even to Clozapine, (an antipsychotic used when conventional medications haven't worked); those who are extremely agitated; those who stop eating or drinking; and those who have become too violent in response to their delusions and hallucinations.

We had a new protocol on the use of ECT in schizophrenia and, if ever anyone needed a new protocol, it was Nigel. After being forced to stop his medication due to a serious side effect, he had relapsed and was so challenging to manage that the team had to be on the alert with regard to their own safety while around him. Severely psychotic, aggressive, and tormented by the voices he could hear, Nigel was not even allowed a chair in his bedroom in case he used it as a weapon.

Nigel arrived at a good time - just when our new protocol was rolled out. I had been keen to involve more people, as evidence for ECT's effectiveness in schizophrenia was mounting, with some clear indications on when it should be used. These patients didn't fully recover in the published trials - in fact 30%-40% improvement in symptoms is deemed a meaningful effect in the treatment of schizophrenia - but, this can indeed be the difference between staying in hospital or living in the community; between being tormented by hallucinations, or getting on with life, despite still hearing voices.

Our protocol had been circulated to our colleagues five months previously, and we still hadn't had a single referral. This is why I felt some excitement when an e-mail popped up on the computer, asking me for an opinion on a patient with schizophrenia who had relapsed and was now on close observation due to aggression and disinhibition. He fitted our criteria for treatment and I hurried to see him on the ward the next morning.

The emerging story was of someone who had responded well to Clozapine but who had had to stop this medication. Clozapine is a neuroleptic in its own class, superior to everything else and the only medication licensed for schizophrenia that has not responded to other antipsychotics. Clozapine has several side effects, but one which can be particularly dangerous is a lowering of the number of white blood cells, which are used by the body to fight infections. Very rarely, in about one in 100 patients, white blood cells called neutrophils can fall so low, that a condition called agranulocytosis develops, which can render the patient unable to fight trivial infections and is potentially fatal. This is why the white blood cell count must be monitored frequently in patients taking this drug, a process which has vastly improved the safety of Clozapine.

Nigel had committed acts of aggression many years before and had been sectioned in hospital under the Mental Health Act. Contrary to the widespread preconception among the public, aggression is rare among such patients, and is usually in response to paranoid delusions or voices. After the sectioning, Nigel had taken

Clozapine for over 10 years, which had enabled him to live independently in the community for most of that time. He hadn't exactly been in remission: he didn't have a job, and he constantly heard voices, although they didn't disturb him and he didn't obey their instructions. Somewhat out of the blue, over a period of a month, Nigel's white blood cell count started going down, crossing the level of 1.5×10^9 neutrophil cells per litre of blood. This level triggers a 'red alert' warning issued by the testing laboratory: Clozapine should be stopped, and the patient should be monitored for infections. He was transferred to a medical ward as a precaution, and the blood count tests were repeated every day. His temperature, blood pressure and pulse rate were also measured daily. It looked as if the staff had tried hard to maintain the Clozapine, but when the neutrophil level reached 0.7×10^9 per litre, the drug was stopped. The blood count dropped further to 0.6×10^9 two days later, but after that recovered gradually, reaching a very healthy 3.0×10^9 two months later. Nigel did not contract any infections, but this was the end of the good news.

It is very difficult to re-start Clozapine in somebody who has received a 'red alert' - the risk of agranulocytosis is too high. Our patient was put on a different antipsychotic, but his mental state gradually deteriorated. His voices became louder and occupied him all the time. He was paranoid about the police and about random people, fearing that they wanted to kill him. At the same time, he became disinhibited and started lashing out at people. He was admitted to hospital. His medications were changed, then increased, then others were added. But things were getting worse all the time. By the time I paid my visit, Nigel had been upgraded to two-to-one observation: two nurses were standing in front of his single bedroom at all times to monitor him and keep the situation safe.

I entered his room, followed by our nurse Sam, who came with me from the ECT unit, and by the two nurses from the ward whom we found standing at the door. A further member of staff stood outside. Our patient was lying in bed, a skinny, 50-something man who was staring at the ceiling and holding a vape cigarette in his mouth. I introduced myself and he mumbled back a greeting, asking my nationality (Bulgarian, as I clarified, hoping that this would break the ice). As there was no chair in the room, there was of course nowhere to sit. I felt it was too intimidating to be standing over him, especially as he hadn't even lifted his head from the pillow, so I sat down on the bed and started inquiring about his problems and views on ECT. I wasn't getting anywhere. His answers became less clear, and finally stopped having any relation to the questions. I couldn't get any information out of him at all. Did he have a thought disorder, or perhaps it was that vape between his lips that was making the words unclear? I asked him to remove it so that I could understand him. This didn't happen. His eyes were becoming more hostile and there was a threatening note in his voice. But he was still lying flat, head on the pillow. I kept my eyes on his arms, for any signs of the fists clenching.

The interview was not turning out to be productive. I felt that I hadn't done a good job and that I should give him more time, but it was clearly pointless to persist. I turned back to the three nurses, saying that perhaps I should finish now. They nodded their heads in full approval, and indeed rather too eager encouragement. I definitely got the impression they were happy with me to stop now. They looked tense. I was pleased that nothing more was expected of me and offered my hand to the patient, who shook it, and then I left the room.

On the way out I looked at Sam, who clearly wanted to share something with me.

'My heart was thumping,' she put her fist in front of her chest to demonstrate how strongly it had been beating. I inquired innocently as to what had disturbed her chest. Surely the situation had not been that tense?

'Didn't you hear? He said that he would smash your face in.'

So that's what Nigel had been mumbling towards the end of our talk. My heart wasn't thumping. I had felt no anxiety whatsoever, as I hadn't heard this. I must have looked very cool and brave. For a second I wondered whether to pretend that I had indeed been brave, but it was more fun to admit the truth.

We sat down with the staff nurse who provided further information. The previous night Nigel had pulled a bunch of hair from somebody's head and had bitten another member of staff who had tried to intervene. The situation was intolerable. Someone was going to be badly injured, and even if that was prevented, our patient was suffering from severe delusions and hallucinations, and two members of staff had to stay with him 24 hours a day, risking their own safety in the process. I gently suggested that ECT might prove highly appropriate and could indeed be the fastest way of improving his mental state. I was probing the mood, as many colleagues strongly object to the use of ECT in schizophrenia. But the nurse was nodding her head in approval again. She didn't want any more of her colleagues to be injured either, and she had to be there eight hours a day, not 20 minutes like me. It was a Friday, so we planned a session for Tuesday, to allow time for all the assessments to be completed. He clearly lacked capacity to consent for ECT and a Second Opinion Appointed Doctor had to be summoned from another hospital to assess Nigel and complete the form that allowed ECT to be given without his consent.

Everything was organised in time and on Tuesday morning I arrived, slightly late, to find a dozen people in the treatment room. Kara was presenting her action plan, which had every detail meticulously anticipated. Up to now, we had managed not to use force on anybody during ECT and were determined to avoid this if at all possible, using gentle encouragement instead. But Nigel was unpredictable even on a good day. If he became violent, two strong men were going to hold his arms, two more would restrain his legs, and a further one would hold his head. Once the needle went in the vein, the anaesthetist was going to give him the anaesthetic straight away and only after that give him oxygen through a mask. Kara was moving round the room, from the wheelchair to the bed and the floor, pointing to people as she explained the plan, making sure everybody understood their roles and knew their positions.

'Nothing can go wrong,' I announced hopefully, maintaining the air of coolness I had established during my first meeting with the patient. But inside I was wondering what to do if the situation escalated and we needed to restrain him. Nigel would never agree to have it voluntarily again, so I decided that if restraint was required, we would call off the treatment and try gentle persuasion on another day.

In the event, nothing did go wrong. Perhaps intimidated by the crowd around him, Nigel offered no resistance. In fact, he looked disinterested, lay in bed, accepted the needle and then fell asleep. Kara was explaining to him what was happening, although I don't know how much he understood. All was well, then, except his seizures: the anticonvulsants and benzodiazepines he was on prevented him from having a seizure on any of the three stimulations, each being 50% higher than the previous one and starting from the relatively high, emergency protocol dose. He was reported to have been more lucid for a few hours after the treatment but had then slipped back into his usual incoherent speech. There was no seizure at 922mC the next time, nearly the top of the machine range. We instructed his team to stop his Valproate and benzodiazepines without waiting for the planned tapering and changed the anaesthetic to Etomidate. These were setbacks, but he was settling down to having treatments without objections, which was the priority for now.

Having more or less wasted the first three sessions, we finally sorted out the seizures: 922mC with Etomidate. Some improvements were noted after five sessions: Nigel stopped lashing out at people, although he remained abusive. He was no longer lying in bed all the time. Quite the contrary, he was singing and dancing, and becoming grandiose. He thought that women were attracted to him and that he had royal blood. He was chatty and over-familiar with people, but one still felt uneasy being in the same room as him. He clearly remembered me and asked me to come closer to him, saying, 'I've seen you before.' Then he stretched out his hand to me - he had remembered my handshake from our first meeting. I still found it hard to understand his muttering, but it felt friendly. Or at least I thought it did. The electronic cigarette was still in his mouth and was only removed to make room for the oxygen mask. A student asked me why he was allowed a vape in the treatment room, which made me realise that nobody would volunteer to take it out of his mouth. After the seizure and rather quick awakening, we went through the same ritual of handshaking, after which he laughed. There was a change in his condition, no doubt about it, although he wasn't exactly healed. After just two good seizures, though, and with such a difficult case, this was not bad going.

After 10 ECTs and some more good seizures, Nigel's level of observation had fallen to checks every 15 minutes. Aggression had ceased, and there was no trace of his hostile demeanour. He was now coherent and easy to understand but looked disinterested and gave short answers. His understanding of his illness and of ECT remained poor, and he was still being treated on a section, although he seemed to accept the sessions as a welcome routine. Asked why he had ECT, as part of the routine capacity assessment, he usually replied that it improved his memory, easily convincing the assessor that he had no understanding of the treatment.

A medical student had just started a project with me on schizophrenia and ECT. He ended up doing all the assessments, very diligently, and I am relying on his accounts. After the initial severe aggression, Nigel had become more friendly and fully coherent, and had no bizarre behaviour or mannerisms. The scores on the Brief Psychiatric Rating Scale (BPRS) had fallen from an initial 118 points to 59, a 50% improvement. Pharmaceutical companies would consider a 30% or 40% average improvement in trials as evidence that a new antipsychotic is effective. No doubt there were also severe negative symptoms, such as lack of interests, apathy, and lack of emotional warmth, but I didn't expect these to improve. After a period of improvement, however, Nigel was becoming confused and disorientated. I wondered whether the intensive ECT course was responsible for the disorientation, rather than his illness. My plan had been to persist with two treatments per week until his improvement plateaued, i.e. until we reached the full effect. But his confusion was also confusing my interpretation of his condition. I advised that we move to weekly sessions, effectively progressing towards continuation ECT, which had by this time been entered into our protocol for schizophrenia. This would reduce his confusion, if it was a consequence of the ECT, rather than a feature of his psychiatric illness. I couldn't observe any change during the following weeks and so was none the wiser.

Nigel had qualified as a 'responder' to ECT by all possible criteria. Despite the vast improvement he had made, however, he was not well - far from it, in fact. He still lacked capacity to provide informed consent for treatment and had no insight into his illness. It was time to make longer-term plans. I did not think he would be able to comply with maintenance ECT if he was discharged from hospital. ECT had to be stopped before that, however, to see how well he could manage without it. When the frequency dropped to one session every two weeks, he got worse very quickly, again raising grave safety concerns. Our nurse Elaine took the brunt of it. While accompanying him in the corridor, she was cornered by him and had to defend herself on her own.

Fortunately, she made a good job of it, but the level of nursing observation of Nigel had to be increased back to one-to-one. He continued to deteriorate, with more episodes of disinhibition and aggression, despite ECT being intensified to once a week. This lasted for three months and we didn't stop ECT, only because we felt we had no alternatives likely to help. Nigel was already on depot (slow release) injection of antipsychotic, as well as more antipsychotics in tablet form. With hindsight, we should have given him two ECT sessions per week, but there is so little experience with ECT in schizophrenia, that we were still learning. A referral to forensic psychiatry was made, more out of desperation than anything. But after three months, Nigel's aggression gradually disappeared, he became co-operative once more, and his BPRS scores settled between 60 and 70 points. I was surprised by this delayed improvement and didn't trust it for a while. My medical student had finished his project long ago, so I was doing some of the ratings myself, still doubting that the improvement was real. The reports from the ward were also consistent and Nigel's demeanour remained friendly, week after week. His sessions could be spaced out to two-week intervals again, this time with no relapses. Plans could finally be made to discharge him to a rehabilitation unit, while still keeping the maintenance ECT. A re-start of Clozapine was also planned, but his neutrophil count was hovering around the lower range of the norm, so nobody felt brave enough to start it yet.

It is time to wrap this story up, as it is likely to continue for some time, with no definitive outcome. Nigel's depression has lifted, and in fact, he is now inappropriately cheerful, laughing loudly at any hint of a joke, finding everything funny. But the voices are still there. Although they tell him nice things, his face shows concern when he is asked about them. The conversations with him are still not productive, but there have been no acts of aggression for a long time. The pretty, young female nurse who last accompanied him to our unit through the hospital corridors, on her own, assured me that he is 'very friendly and no problem really' when I expressed concern about her safety. Somehow, he seems to appreciate that ECT is helping him ('It keeps my mind clear') and is happy to continue. We feel it is early to test whether the improvement will be maintained without ECT, but this will be the next step.

The 50% improvement in symptoms might seem a relatively moderate achievement but feels almost life-changing in such a severe case: it drastically lessened Nigel's aggression, saved injuries and anxieties among staff, and certainly improved Nigel's sense of well-being. And to go from close observation by two nurses, to discharge into a rehabilitation unit is no mean feat.

Nigel is not an exception. My student finished his audit on schizophrenia with this conclusion: *'Initial indication for treatment was completely resolved in seven out of eight cases. This is of particular significance, since in many cases ECT was prescribed in an emergency situation, such as life-threatening starvation or dehydration.'*

One thing still puzzles me: surely there are similar patients suffering from severe relapses of schizophrenia in our area, who would fit the referral criteria set in our new protocol? Why is it that no one else has been referred since we wrote that protocol?

17

A DEATH WISH

Psychiatrists see many people who self-harm. Thankfully, such actions mostly involve low risk. Sometimes they are a cry for help or a way of releasing inner tensions. But some people don't leave any chances of staying alive. Occasionally we meet people who should have died and even thought that they had died. When I was a junior doctor covering an A&E department in London, I assessed a person who had hanged himself from the banisters in his house. The rope had snapped, resulting in a fracture of a vertebra when he fell down the stairs. Did he deliberately choose a rotten rope, to give himself a chance of surviving? One item in his account clarified this question. He had heard that when people hang themselves, their bowels open. He felt that this would be a very unpleasant scene to find, and he didn't want to leave such a memory for his family. So he tied the legs of his trousers with strings, to prevent any mess dripping to the floor. This had been his main concern; the thought of survival hadn't entered his mind. I admitted him to the psychiatric ward. Other people show remarkable imagination when they are deprived of tools to kill themselves. One lady with a history of multiple self-harming attempts, whom I treated a few years ago, ended up in a police cell for her safety. She found a pencil on the floor, sharpened it with her teeth and stuck it through her neck, all the way through her throat. Luckily, she missed the large carotid artery.

The story I want to relate here is more recent. The background unfolded over the course of a morning. I had to read and re-read the short referral note from a local psychiatrist, with many exclamations and questions for my colleagues. They all seemed to have heard various bits of the story, which had been circulating round the hospital over the last few weeks. And with good reason. Few patients can have made a more dramatic entrance into our hospital than Ian who had arrived at A&E on a stretcher with a knife in his chest. Yes, a knife was actually stuck in his chest! It was still there as he was wheeled in, the handle protruding from his chest and the blade fully hidden in the flesh. And he had been taken first to another hospital, then transferred to the main one, a good half-hour away. All this time the knife had been sticking out of his chest. It was a suicide attempt and he had stabbed himself in the heart.

A few more minutes of digging through notes and computer pages defined more clearly the path that the knife had taken. It had entered the body right in the middle of the chest. 'Injured the right ventricle of the heart!' volunteered the anaesthetist with some respect in her voice. 'No, it says here the left ventricle,' I said. I had noticed another entry, although preferring to accept the anaesthetist's version of events, as it made more sense – you shouldn't be alive after a knife puncture to your left ventricle. Eventually we found a short account of the operation. It was the left ventricle and it was pierced through, not just scraped.

The anaesthetist and I discussed Ian with some awe. He had almost literally come back from the dead. But there were practical considerations, and the anaesthetist was already weighing them up. Until then I had just been admiring the man's audacity and thinking that ECT could indeed be a good option for somebody that desperate. Only then did I grasp the problem that was worrying the anaesthetist. If the ventricle was pierced, then during ECT, when blood pressure goes up, it might tear the wound open again. After all, we have to wait six months after an ordinary heart attack before giving ECT. And this looked riskier than a heart attack.

But there was more. Still looking through Ian's notes, the anaesthetist gave an exclamation, 'He was tasered!' The police had stopped Ian in his car. Alerted by his wife as to his intent to kill himself, they had given chase and cornered him. That's when Ian stabbed himself in the heart, right in front of them, before they could get him out of the locked car. He was still conscious, and the officers saw that his hands were still gripping tightly onto the handle of the knife. They feared that he was going to pull it out and bleed to death on the spot. They had read the situation correctly: Ian later told me that he was indeed about to pull out the blade, to allow the blood to pour out. So they tasered him. Ian remembered the pain and the immobility and was still conscious for a while after that. He blacked out on the way to the hospital due to blood loss. Saved by a taser?

How on earth hadn't his heart stopped, given that a taser uses an electrical current, with the metal blade providing direct electrical contact to the heart? Well actually, hearts are pretty resilient machines. Should I really worry about the electric stimulations from the ECT, then, if he had survived the taser? The thought was comforting but wrong.

I was impatient to see the man who had what it takes to stick a knife into his own heart. Perhaps his death wish had gone after returning from the dead. I went to the ward, accompanied by our anaesthetist and a junior doctor who had looked after Ian. It is a long walk through the corridors of the general hospital, full of people and moving trolleys, so there was time for the doctor to fill me in. Various details promised to make the treatment decision even less straightforward than first anticipated. The patient didn't seem to be depressed, I was told, nor was he psychotic. He was looking after himself; in the morning he was shaving and showering; his conversation was normal; his voice was confident, and he even smiled appropriately. Did he really need ECT? I had imagined a severely depressed person, tormented by delusions of guilt, who would easily recover by means of ECT. But this presentation would caution against this treatment. I was to change my mind some months later.

We were ushered into a small interview room by a nurse, as the hospital rooms each had several occupants, making confidential talk impossible. The man who joined us was well-built, strong and stocky, of average height, and looking quite fit for his 45 years. He sat down and engaged in discussion. He had already read a lot about ECT and felt he should try it. After so many antidepressants over the years, nothing had really made a change to the way he felt. So what was it that he did feel, what was making him suicidal? I tried to get some clear answers. The man started his story. Ever since he was 15 years old, he had had these intrusive thoughts of killing himself. There was no reason for them, as his life was going well. Some days the thoughts were very strong, other days, less so. Alcohol was nearly always a factor at times when he lost control, although not in terms of triggering the thoughts, as they didn't need any prompting. The so-called biological features of depression were missing: his sleep, appetite, and interests were not affected, his thinking was not slowed down and he certainly didn't experience any psychotic symptoms. He smiled at jokes, although he looked as if he was doing so out of politeness. So far, nothing to suggest he was a good candidate for ECT.

I was curious. I asked Ian to show me his chest and he lifted his T-shirt. A long scar ran from the top of his chest almost down to the navel. This was from the operation. It must have been substantial as they had apparently opened the entire rib cage, to gain access to the heart. Compared to that, the scar from the knife looked like a scratch. It was about 1.5 cm long, already pale and fully healed, three weeks after the stabbing. It looked very well positioned for a heart stabbing: between the third and fourth ribs, as I counted, on the left of the breast-bone. I inquired about the type of knife he had used. 'It was a combat knife.' He accompanied the short phrase by stretching his thumb and forefinger to a distance of about 12 or 15 cm, to show me the length of the blade.

Clearly, I hadn't learned the whole story yet. A combat knife? Plunged into the left ventricle? I had to get more of this story.

'So did you know that you needed to stick it between the ribs, between these two ribs exactly?'

'Yes, doc, I was a combat paramedic. I have treated people injured in combat.'

Ian had served in Afghanistan. Perhaps he wasn't frightened of being killed, or perhaps this was a natural choice for a person who didn't mind risk.

Ian was keen to start ECT. I explained that it would be wise to wait a few weeks, to allow time for his heart to heal and to reduce the chance of the wound tearing open during the session. Would he be safe if we waited? Ian was unable to reassure me on that point. He was still suicidal and didn't know when he might get the urge to kill himself again. We opted for an early follow-up with the cardiologist, who would be able to tell us how safe it would be to raise his systolic blood pressure to 220mm.

But did Ian really need ECT? He had felt suicidal for about 30 years. Such feelings were now almost part of his personality - how was this going to change? The thoughts were intrusive, and while he didn't like them, they were too powerful for him to resist. He admitted to feeling depressed, despite his relatively trim appearance, and he had horribly low self-esteem. He felt guilty for letting down his children, but this was an understandable and rational reaction after the suicide attempt, and surely not a delusion of guilt. And if his depression did lift, what were the chances of this change enduring? All in all, not much to go by while assessing his suitability for ECT, but do I really know which person or what symptom will respond? 'He wants ECT, he will probably kill himself without it, and there is some chance it will work,' I mused to myself. And in fact, we had seen people with similar isolated suicidal ideation who did not look depressed outwardly but who were effectively hiding their feelings inside.

The decision was not that complicated after all: it would be more difficult to refuse treatment and tell Ian there was nothing we could do for him. And so I agreed to treat him. The other three or four people in the room nodded in approval. I knew that even if Ian managed to shed his death wish with this round of ECT, the problem would not necessarily be solved, as it would probably come back sooner or later. But that was a discussion for another day. The question was whether ECT would relieve him of his suicidal thoughts in the first instance. I would know this only many weeks from now, when I came back to write the outcome, I thought, while writing this introduction that evening.

My patience was finally rewarded. We started treating Ian two months later and to my surprise, the heart surgeon's main worry was not the scar in the heart, but the scar in the breast-bone. It had been cut through during the operation and the bone needed time to heal. The surgeon recommended waiting three months to prevent it from splitting open during a strong muscular contraction. Ian didn't want to wait that long. We settled for an alternative: full muscle paralysis. Our anaesthetists opted for Rocuronium and reversal of its action with Sugammadex. Rocuronium is used for general surgery procedures, as it keeps the muscles paralysed for much longer than Suxamethonium. Sugammadex is an antidote to stop its action. As we needed to reverse the paralysis after about five minutes, Ian needed a full dose, costing a silly amount of money, but that was not an issue. A nerve stimulator was used to determine when his muscles stopped working, by delivering a small electric current over the forearm and observing whether this provoked a muscular contraction. When the muscle stopped twitching, we would know that he was sufficiently paralysed. We started titration with 80mC, predicting that he would have a seizure, so the procedure wouldn't be wasted. It would only be a modest seizure, to avoid causing damage and after which we could reassess the plan. Ian did have a seizure and not only according to the

EEG. His muscles twitched visibly despite the anaesthetist's assurances that he would be fully paralysed. My face twitched in a grimace as well; this looked uncomfortable. Perhaps it is not the same thing to be immobile during surgery as to have an epileptic seizure which brings every last bit of muscle strength into action. Anyway, Ian's chest thankfully remained intact, his heart ticked rhythmically and his blood pressure gave no cause for concern.

After his second session had finished and he had been moved into the recovery room, I heard wailing sounds. I rushed in, panicking that Ian's breathing might have been affected by the antidote to the muscle paralysis having worn off for some reason. The noise was indeed coming from Ian's mouth but it wasn't caused by breathing problems. He was sitting in bed, awake, crying uncontrollably and repeating, 'I can't go on like this'. He was holding his head in his hands, eyes wide open, staring in despair in front of him. He suddenly reminded me of a painting that I show to medical students at the start of my lecture on depression. I have an opening line:

'A person with severe depression can feel worse than anyone else. This is because what gets damaged in this illness is this part or function of the brain that controls our emotions. When that mechanism is broken, the patient may feel that he or she is in the worst possible situation. Without any control, the mood slides down and might reach the absolute bottom, the worst possible mood one can feel. The patient may experience the ultimate suffering.'

I support this point with a slide of *'The Scream'* by Edvard Munch. A peaceful landscape at sunset, contrasting with a terrified man holding his head and screaming. Yes, our patient was experiencing the Ultimate

Suffering! He was genuinely depressed. During the twilight state of awakening after ECT, his mood went out of control and dipped down to the bottom of the abyss. I had just changed my mind about his prospects and was feeling hopeful. This kind of depression was not just treatable but suggested a good prospect for ECT.

'Ian, we will get you better,' I told him. 'Just give this treatment a chance, and don't do anything silly.' Of course, I asked Jess to repeat this instruction before Ian went home, in case it slipped his mind. Jess used many more words than I did - she is good at this.

I started writing this as a story about giving ECT to a suicidal person with no obvious depression. The story had already changed: we were treating a depressed person. But after the third treatment the story changed again, this time for the worse. Just after the seizure I noticed a worrying image on the ECG monitor. The electrical activity of the heart had changed from the almost normal complexes - I say 'almost normal', as Ian did have negative T-waves, indicating some damage to the heart muscle after his stabbing and operation - into huge, broad and distorted shapes, that followed at a rate of about 110 per minute. Was this the dreaded ventricular tachycardia, the irregular heart rhythm that can result in death? His pulse was full, the ECG shapes were regular with some intervals in between, so I was hoping that these only indicated some change in electrical conduction caused by the strain. The face of the anaesthetist was stern, however. 'Do you get these in ECT?' she asked me, hoping for reassurance.

'Well, we get all sort of things, but no … not this.' After two minutes the ECG changed so suddenly, that I missed the exact point of change. It came back to almost normal. Almost normal, as a prominent depression of the

ST interval was added, that usually indicates ischaemia. We occasionally see such changes after seizures. They should normalise within a minute, so I relaxed. Another two minutes and the ST depression disappeared as quickly as the previous nasty pattern. There had been no drop in blood pressure or oxygen levels. There were no more extra beats and no further issues.

The real worry was what to do next. After a discussion with Ian's heart surgeon, the opinion was that this was indeed ventricular tachycardia. I admit that I had known it in my own heart but was casting round for other explanations, or should I say excuses, to justify giving Ian more ECT. The surgeon suggested that the scar left by the stabbing had possibly damaged the blood supply to part of the heart as well, resulting in further scarring. A literature search returned a very clear statement: 'The most common cause of monomorphic ventricular tachycardia is scarring of the heart muscle from a previous myocardial infarction. This scar cannot conduct electrical activity, so there is a potential circuit around the scar that results in the tachycardia'. Everything fitted together. Ian did have a scar, and this resulted in the monomorphic ECG complexes that I had described to the surgeon.

Ventricular tachycardia can result in swift death and the scar was not going to heal with time; it was going to remain a scar, so the problem was not going to disappear even if we waited a few months. I had to give Ian this news, knowing it meant that he might kill himself. What a situation! Damn! Whatever we did, no matter what we did, it might result in his death. My only slight hope was that the cardiologists could find a way out in the future, unlikely though that may be.

One year later

I am picking up this story after 12 months. I had been checking Ian's computer records for any developments, wondering whether the scar in his heart would heal up against all probability, so that the cardiologists would give us the green light. But with the passing of time, it was also becoming clear that Ian didn't need more ECTs. He was getting on with his life and was holding down a job. He had finally had an exercise ECG to check how his heart reacted to exertion, and that had resulted in an episode of ventricular fibrillation, I presume a similar picture to what I had seen. This excluded any thoughts of further ECTs. Ian wrote me a letter about this. Despite the setback, I felt the letter sounded positive. Perhaps the close encounter with death had changed his outlook on life. Or perhaps it was the Lithium that he had started. Or both. This wasn't due to ECT - after all, he had only had three sessions. He was alive, that was the important point. In his letter, he wrote that he was honoured to be included in my book. No, Ian, I am honoured.

18

CHARCOT-MARIE-TOOTH DISEASE

Olivia was trying to grab my attention. I was updating records on the laptop, sitting at my desk that is helpfully positioned in the treatment room to give me the best view of events.

'This new referral... I went to see her on the ward yesterday. She looked very poorly, extremely slow, I could hardly wait for her answers. And no facial communication. She has some neurological problem... Charcot something.'

Olivia now had my full attention.

'Do you mean Charcot-Marie-Tooth?' I asked without much hope, not dreaming for a moment that anyone would bother memorising the full title.

'Yes, that's it!'

Olivia is good! How did she remember it?

My excitement was provoked by the mutation that normally causes Charcot-Marie-Tooth disease: a large duplication of genetic material on chromosome 17. In my other life at Cardiff University, I conduct research in genetics and my main interest is on deletions or duplications of large stretches of chromosomes, called copy number variations (CNVs). A number of them can cause psychiatric disorders, so these genetic changes are of great interest to psychiatric geneticists. Somewhat disappointingly for me, my genetic research has been confined either to the laboratory or to the computer, and I have only interviewed a small number of people who carry such CNVs. The CNVs involved in neuropsychiatric disorders are rare: only 1% of the general population carry one of them and this proportion rises to 2%-3% among those with severe psychiatric disorders.

The particular CNV involved in Charcot-Marie-Tooth (CMT) is found in about one in every 3,000 people. It is a duplication of a large section on chromosome 17 which affects a gene (PMP22) involved in the insulation of peripheral nerves (known as myelination), enabling the lightning-fast conduction of nerve impulses along the nerves. Carrying this duplication, that results in three copies of the gene instead of the usual two, leads to a neurological disorder presenting with weakness and atrophy of the muscles. It begins in adolescence, starting in the lower legs and may later affect the hands and cause sensory loss. We had conducted studies on thousands of psychiatric patients and healthy controls and had shown that this particular CNV does not affect cognitive abilities and does not lead to psychosis, although it increases the risk of depression, possibly due to the associated medical problems. I had not seen a patient with this CNV yet, let alone one who also has severe depression.

I waited impatiently for the clinic to finish so that I could go and see our new patient. I doubted that she had this specific genetic mutation, as there are several other causes that can produce a similar clinical picture, although the duplication is the most common one. At first, Angela did not appear to be somebody who would be able to tell me which genetic mutation she was carrying. In fact, she did not appear able to answer even much simpler questions. As Olivia had noted, she was very slow, kept staring at us and moving backwards, as if frightened of something which wasn't there. She didn't complain of depression and didn't think that she needed ECT. I was keen to do a basic neurological examination. Angela's fingers were quite strong, and she squeezed mine quite well when I prompted her to do so. But when I asked her to pull my arms towards her, the pull was feeble. As she was standing, she needed the support of her legs in order to pull me, and that wasn't going well.

'I have a problem here.' She slowly touched her knees and then tried to glide her fingers further down towards the calf muscles, clearly finding it easier to point than to express herself with words. She was wearing orthopaedic shoes, as such patients develop deformities of the feet due to the poor sensation typical of the condition.

'No, my hands are okay,' was the answer to my next question.

I couldn't hold back my most pressing question any longer.

'Do you know exactly which type of Charcot-Marie-Tooth you have? There are a few types, like 1 and 2.'

'It is type 1A,' came the surprisingly quick and specific answer. And then she slowly related to me how she had had the disease from an early age, receiving a genetic diagnosis in 1992.

'Did they say it was a duplication?'

'Yes.'

Perhaps she didn't give me the correct year of diagnosis, as the test was only developed in 1994, but it was now clear that we were talking about the same genetic condition. The illness was described more than a hundred years earlier, in 1886, by the iconic Professor Charcot in Paris, whose demonstrations in the Salpêtrière Hospital drew captivated audiences and are preserved for posterity on paintings familiar to medical students.[15] The other two words that complete the long name of this disease are those of Charcot's pupil Pierre Marie and of English neurologist Howard Tooth who had written a separate paper on the condition in the same year.

Angela was adept at describing her neurological illness but not her depression. As Olivia had remarked, she didn't seem to realise that she was depressed. The notes indicated that the depression had started within the last two years, after some stressful events - perhaps also due to the difficulties imposed by her impaired mobility, I imagined. Now, she was losing weight, her mind and body were slowing down, she was becoming paranoid, and the medications were not touching the problem. ECT was the obvious choice, as she had clear psychomotor retardation.

Our anaesthetist spotted the problem first, after we returned to the unit: 'We can't use Suxamethonium'. This muscle relaxant could, theoretically at least, lead to malignant hyperthermia.[16] It would also reduce the strength of the already weak muscles, which could cause breathing problems after the seizure. We started researching ways round the problem. The risk of hyperthermia sounded more theoretical than real to me. Many such patients are reported to have had no complications after anaesthesia. In fact, these patients have more than their fair share of operations, done mostly on their feet, which suffer from the reduced sensation and

---

[15] *A Clinical Lesson at the Salpêtrière*, 1887, by André Brouillet.

[16] Malignant hyperthermia is a reaction to some drugs used during anaesthesia. Symptoms include high temperature, muscle rigidity and a fast heart rate.

strength. The anaesthetist suggested we use a non-depolarising muscle relaxant (Rocuronium), which should avoid the risk of hyperthermia, and that we terminate the paralysis with Sugammadex, which reverses the paralysis by binding to the Rocuronium.

I couldn't find any reports at all on ECT in patients with Charcot-Marie-Tooth until the next day when Olivia printed out a short paper for me, which the authors claimed to be the only report of ECT given to a CMT patient. They had used Rocuronium. I began to wonder whether our patient even needed a muscle relaxant (I would find out later that this was a bad idea). The purpose of the muscle relaxant is to prevent people injuring themselves during the severe muscular contractions of a seizure. I could not see how Angela could mobilise enough muscular strength to cause herself any injury, however. This was only a thought-provoking point for the staff and two students: of course we would use a muscle relaxant. We decided to go for a low dose of Rocuronium and lower it as much as possible for the subsequent sessions. The first treatment was to take place in an operating theatre, as is common with high-risk patients, just in case of problems. This was a very sensible precaution, as we didn't know how Angela's breathing would be affected.

A couple of days later everything was set, and we assembled in one of the pre-operative rooms, just after 8 am, to avoid interfering with the theatre list lined up for later that day. Angela lay down with no fuss, although she didn't quite understand what was happening. She had been placed on a section of the Mental Health Act the day before, as she had no capacity to consent. We set the machine at 80mC charge, our standard first dose for middle-aged patients. As we were getting ready, needle tucked into a vein and the anaesthetist aiming a syringe with Thiopental anaesthetic at it, Olivia started reading the safety checklist. One of the items refers to teeth problems.

Angela's teeth had been examined the previous day, but I was slightly perturbed when we asked her to remove her dentures, which exposed a sole, rather long incisor. It protruded ominously, and the pressure of the clenching jaws during the fit was clearly going to concentrate on that one particular spot in her mouth. For a few seconds we wondered what to do and proceeded with placing the soft mouthguard, hoping that it would soften and re-distribute the pressure. All patients get a mouthguard in order to prevent any damage to the teeth or tongue as teeth clench during the electrical stimulation, even in well-paralysed patients. The single tooth seemed to rest snugly over it, not in any immediate danger.

Angela had a decent seizure with the first stimulation. The muscle relaxant dose was indeed low, due to our cautious approach, but still I was surprised how much muscle force she managed to muster. The legs, as expected, didn't move much, but the arms and fists suddenly looked full of strength. The clenched jaws and mouthguard portrayed one of the stigmatising stereotypes so beloved of movie makers and the anti-ECT movement. Angela's face showed the typical reaction of all facial muscles contracting, despite her weakness, and she grimaced strongly, as if in disgust at what was being done to her. There were no complications: she didn't stop breathing, her oxygen level didn't drop, and her heart rate remained regular. This was a full success. The fit was clearly above seizure threshold level, so I advised that the dose only be increased by 50% next session, hopefully just enough to bring the EEG trace into a better organized pattern. Our concerns about breathing problems had been unfounded and we were going to increase the dose of the muscle relaxant at the next session. Job done.

I offered to stay in the theatre recovery room, while Olivia and the junior doctor went back to the ECT unit to treat the next patient. I was waiting with the anaesthetist and the recovery nurse for the patient to wake up, which was taking slightly longer than usual, perhaps not surprisingly, as she struggled to talk even when fully awake. After a couple of minutes, the nurse removed the mouthguard and frowned when he saw blood on it. He opened the mouth to inspect and there we saw the long incisor looking even longer and pointing in a slightly different direction than before. It was completely loose and came off without resistance. It had taken all the pressure of the jaws and, despite the mouthguard, had broken.[17]

We do warn patients that dentures or loose teeth might be damaged during ECT and indeed this is probably the most frequent side effect of the procedure. But this felt preventable. The ECT Handbook gives good advice on dental problems. I re-read the relevant chapter that evening, noticing the advice for custom-made bite guards, and getting a dentist involved if need be. In the concern around Angela's CMT disease and the dangers of muscle relaxants, we had over-prepared for life-threatening anaesthetic complications and had not paid enough attention to the more mundane risk of tooth

---

[17] That a patient suffering with a disease called Charcot-Marie-Tooth should lose a tooth, is a strange coincidence. The name of the neurologist Henry Tooth does not imply any dental problems.

damage. In fact, we had possibly made it worse, as the lower dose of muscle relaxant might have contributed to the fracture. On the other hand, the tooth would have been put through the same pressure at each session, so it might well have come out eventually, even with the best of preparations. Still I felt guilty and annoyed with myself and was only reassured somewhat when I learned that Angela would get free new dentures, as a hospitalised patient. And I would surely sit down with her and her family and explain the dilemma we had been facing and what happened that day. If she made a full recovery, all would be forgiven, I told myself. The hospital dentist removed the rest of the tooth later that day.

Things settled down over the next few sessions. The remaining teeth still made precarious contact with one another when the dentures were not in place, but they were holding up. The arm muscles were not contracting so strongly that they would cause any injuries, but strongly enough to tell us that the seizures were good - so good indeed, that we only needed to stimulate her with 103mC for the first few sessions. The small dose of Rocuronium was not causing any concerns, and in fact she never stopped breathing spontaneously. Our initial concern had been quite unfounded, but it is always better to err on the side of caution. After a couple of weeks, one anaesthetist decided to use the standard Suxamethonium for muscle relaxation. All went well and this became Angela's standard treatment.

The CMT1A disease, such an initial concern, was becoming almost irrelevant in terms of her management. We could get back to the real business: treating her depression. This was progressing slowly. After three sessions, Angela was still slow in replying to simple questions. When asked what side effects she should expect from ECT, she paused a few seconds, then slowly moved her finger in the direction of her mouth ('dental problems' was certainly one correct answer). But there was some reactivity of mood and expression on her face, that hadn't been there at the start. She told us that ECT was helping her, although I wasn't sure if this was her genuine self-assessment, or whether she was trying to say what was expected from her.

The changes continued at a worryingly slow rate, although each week she scored slightly better on the depression scale. It took 14 sessions before the scores dropped into the remission range, despite us keeping her seizures strong. Her walking had improved from a hesitant waddle to a confident quick pace. There was a smile on her face. But she still wasn't well. She would still take a while to answer any question that required consideration. And sometimes her gaze would drift to one side during the conversation, or she would turn around to look behind her. While young, she had suffered a psychotic episode during which she had heard voices. She had been well for a few decades after that, without medication, but was she maybe hearing something again? Or was it perhaps post-ECT confusion and she would regain her speed once treatment stopped? I spaced out her sessions, but this didn't improve the problems. Even worse, she became more hesitant and her depression ratings jumped up. This wasn't confusion from ECT, it was still her unresolved retardation and depression.

Nineteen ECTs had now been given and I was running out of ideas. Angela was described as being very well one day, but not so good the next, and was hesitant and slow each time I saw her. She had improved a great deal; her presentation was so much better than it had been at the start. The HAM-D scores suggested that she wasn't even depressed, but we knew that this was deceptive: she was not well. This was not a presentation of Charcot-Marie-Tooth disease, which shouldn't really affect the brain, and in any case, she had been back to normal for a few days at a time. Spacing out ECTs, or alternatively, giving them twice a week, was not helping. I kept re-examining the chart with ECT sessions but couldn't see anything that could explain the lack of progress. Perhaps we should stop treatment, observe, and then start again afresh if she deteriorated, was my feeble advice…

I am picking up this story again, writing exactly one week later. I could re-write the last paragraph, but I am tempted to leave it, so that you can follow how both Angela and my advice changed in just seven days. Christmas had just been and gone but I did not put on my Santa hat in the unit, as I didn't expect any joyful transformations among the three patients who had been booked between Christmas and the New Year. Wrong! I was in for a happy surprise. Angela looked transformed. She was smiling, talking at a normal pace, quite fast in fact, responding quickly and sharply to whichever question I put to her. And she was looking around with interest and asking questions of her own. This was a totally normal conversation and I was wondering why I had ever doubted that she could be so well. She was out of her depression after 20 ECTs. She still didn't know what had improved in her and admitted that she didn't remember how unwell she had been. It sounded as if she had been in a different world, but her memory of it had faded like a dream, something I have noted in other patients whose realities change dramatically after treatment.

I know that more problems may lie ahead, but I can relax. We now know that Angela can achieve full remission with ECT, and that the depression and her neurological condition have not left any permanent damage. Some combination of medications, ECT and psychotherapy will eventually be worked out to keep her well. And if the depression comes back, she can always have a few more ECTs twice a week.

19

HYPOXIA[18]

'So why is he alive?' asked Olivia with some incredulity in her voice, after I summarised the story of our new patient. I don't think she was questioning the sincerity of his suicide attempt. She was just trying to understand how he had escaped with a whole skin after plunging into a lake weighted with bricks. He should not be alive, indeed.

I had gone to see Colin on the ward after receiving an e-mail requesting a second opinion. The information was minimal, and I couldn't glean too much more from the computer records, as he had been admitted to us from another hospital. The man was in his 60s, unshaven, unkempt, and clearly troubled as to why the nurse had called him to see me without warning. I took the main bits of the history, which was not too difficult, as it had all started only 18 months ago, and his answers were to the point. Colin had had a fairly successful life, had held a good managerial job, and was married with children. And then a health problem came out of the blue: an operation ended in complications, and suddenly life could no longer be taken for granted. Colin became depressed and wanted to end it all. There was nothing to look forward to and nothing else to think about but killing himself. He had tried this three times, most lately by drowning.

---

[18] Low level of oxygen in the body.

I wanted to hear some details of his drowning attempt, to get a feel for how determined he was to kill himself. After all, what do you have to do in order to drown? If you can swim even a little, it makes things difficult, as you need to make sure you can't swim back to the shore – a natural instinct that should kick in. Some people jump from a height, some make use of the coldness of the water. I was leaning forward in my chair as Colin gave me the details. There was a lake near where he worked. However this was summer: he wouldn't freeze and he could swim. He took several bricks, so that they would weigh his body down in the water.

'But how did you tie them to yourself?' I continued, insisting on all the details. Colin described how he had put them in two plastic bags, then tied the two bags together and put them round his neck, before jumping into the water. When he was in the water, his body floated up, while his head was pulled under the water by the weight of the bricks. This led to the plastic bags sliding off his neck and down to the bottom, so he floated back to the surface. There was obvious disappointment in his voice when he narrated what he felt was a personal failure. Well, I can hardly think of a surer way of drowning oneself than tying a few bricks or stones to yourself. He had my full respect. This was a determined pursuit of death: his illness was serious. In addition, I noticed that Colin was taking quite a long time to answer my questions. He was not hesitating as to what to say - he was just finding it difficult to express himself, to find the words, to make sense of what had been going on. This was not the senior manager of a couple of years back; no way would he be able to chair a meeting in this state. Colin had psychomotor retardation.

I should have been pleased at this point, as retardation is a clear positive prognostic sign for response to ECT. But things are seldom that simple. My colleagues in England had also spotted the signs and he had already had two courses of ECT in two different hospitals before coming to us. I knew of both centres and had no doubt that he had received proper treatment. The first course had lasted a full 12 sessions. Colin did get better, but not completely well, and then he stopped. After two weeks he was depressed again. Two months later he was so poorly that he had the second course, at a different hospital. This time he had eight sessions. Why only eight, he couldn't tell me, but he did remember feeling better again and then becoming depressed once more soon after.

I was picking up the positive sides of this story and presenting them back to him. 1) He had a type of depression that should respond to ECT; 2) ECT had clearly worked: he got better twice and relapsed twice soon after it was stopped. So we could expect him to get better again. On the negative side, he clearly didn't respond that easily and also relapsed very quickly. So if he did have another course, it would have to be a long one, and he would need 'booster sessions' to prevent relapse. I thought to myself that he would in fact need quite a few 'booster sessions' and at quite frequent intervals, and that indeed, he needed to stay well for most of this time, if his illness was to take a good trajectory. The question was whether he would even reach full remission, as he seemed to have failed to do this on two occasions. I didn't want to talk about it right now - it would be easier to discuss the future when he was well. Ah yes, and he would probably need Lithium and a stronger antidepressant.

'When can I start?'

I realised that I was preaching to the converted.

And so we started. Seizure threshold was rather high and increased further, so that by the fourth session, already at 368mC, Colin had a missed seizure, despite receiving twice the electric charge of the seizure threshold established on the first day. I was building a hypothesis that he hadn't reached remission during his previous courses because he had always ended up having poor seizures. I still had not received the details of those previous sessions, so I had no proof that this had been the case. I wanted to avoid a scenario where we increased the dose each time he had a bad seizure but still didn't produce a good one, as his seizure threshold would also have increased in the meantime. I was worried that we would be chasing good seizures and be stranded one step behind each time. And with poor seizures, he would not reach remission again. In my experience, it is always better to do something more pro-active and to stay ahead of the developments. There was an obvious solution: change the anaesthetic to Etomidate which always improves seizure quality and duration. So the next time we switched to it, and Colin had a great seizure, 42 seconds. There were a couple of extra beats on the monitor, and his oxygen saturation dropped to 69% for a couple of seconds, before quickly increasing back to 100%. Thirty minutes later Colin was orientated and told me that he felt fine.

His weight was a bit over what we would promote as ideal, and as is the case with such middle-aged men, his abdomen was exerting some pressure on his lungs when he lay down. Such people can suffer from sleep apnoea or, in our clinic, tend to drop the oxygen saturation in the blood after seizures. It doesn't help if he has nearly a minute of strong muscular contractions while his paralysed muscles cannot open his lungs to take in oxygen, as had just happened. Next time we would ensure he was even better pre-oxygenated, and that ventilation was started before the seizure was finished, I reassured myself.

Next time came and the plan failed dismally. After the anaesthetic, Colin's fasciculations (the fine muscle twitches, caused by the muscle relaxant) took too long to end, perhaps three minutes. The trouble is, we didn't want to shock him before he finished fasciculating, as his muscles wouldn't be sufficiently relaxed and he would use up too much oxygen. The anaesthetist had already stopped using the bag that forced air into his lungs and was waiting for us to proceed. As we waited, I noticed that his oxygen level had dropped from 100% to 96%. For you and me, this would be normal. But for Colin, this meant he was not over-oxygenated, as I wanted him to be. During the next two to three seconds I reasoned that a further delay to allow more ventilation would require more anaesthetic, more muscle relaxant, and the outcome would be even less predictable. I nodded to the junior doctor and to the nurse to apply the shock. Another very strong jump (not enough muscle relaxant or we hadn't waited long enough?) and 42 seconds of strong contractions ensued. His colour was already changing during the seizure, and he was becoming more purple, especially his ears. The oxygen was now down to 60% and everybody was getting into a state of high anxiety. I looked again at the monitor and noticed the number 37. This was the pulse rate. Thankfully, the seizure was over, and the ventilation bag was being squeezed regularly by the anaesthetist, pumping 100% of oxygen into Colin's lungs. A few seconds later the pulse rate was already picking up and so was the oxygen level in his blood - thankfully the crisis was averted as always. He had suffered a bradycardia (an overly slow heart rate), probably precipitated by the low oxygen level. Ironic, perhaps, that we had had to panic over the lungs Colin had done his best to deprive of oxygen when he had tried to drown himself.

We needed a plan. In choosing the right anaesthetic, we had created a new problem. If we switched back to Thiopental, Colin would have poorer seizures and might not get better. With Etomidate, we were not only risking his health, but surely making his memory problems worse, as the neurons are deprived of the normal levels of oxygen for a few more seconds each time. I had to reduce the electric charge, make sure he got more oxygen, and possibly increase the dose of the muscle relaxant, in the hope this would make him consume less oxygen during the seizure. But this would also reduce his spontaneous breathing after the seizure, so more muscle relaxant could cause more harm than good. This needed a good discussion with the anaesthetists, but we should be able to sort it out definitively. By the way, after five sessions his mood was unchanged. I wasn't expecting miracles.

I had been thinking about these options over the course of a few late evenings. The records from Colin's previous ECT course had arrived in the meantime. My colleagues had faced similar problems: strong muscular contractions, high seizure threshold, cardiac extra beats and, a new one, atrial fibrillation (highly irregular heart rate). That Friday I discussed the problem with the anaesthetist. Perhaps we could give Colin glycopyrrolate, an anticholinergic that would help ensure his heart rate didn't slow down. Or maybe we could give him more muscle relaxant, wait longer for it to work, and ventilate him throughout the procedures. And when everything was ready, something in me clicked. Did we really need to push our luck? Colin might respond without achieving great seizures. Why not go back to our original anaesthetic Thiopental and just increase the electric charge? We were still below the half-way point of the machine power, and at worst he would only miss a couple of good seizures. But this way, Colin would be safe. Destiny had saved his life in the lake. Perhaps he had several lives, but did we really want to test that? His lungs had already been tested once under treatment. We quickly switched back to Thiopental and made a modest increase in the electric charge.

With the drama and tension reduced, everything was going smoothly. With the luxury of extra time, we were able to see that the muscle twitches were going on for an unusually long time after the muscle relaxant was released into the vein, so perhaps he must have been given the shocks before being sufficiently paralysed. The EEG showed a good seizure (although much shorter, 17 seconds), there were very gentle visible muscle contractions, a stable oxygen level and only rare extra systoles, that I described to the two junior doctors as completely acceptable, while almost patting myself on my shoulder for the shrewd decision.

Why are things always more complicated than they seem? Ten minutes later the recovery nurse opened the door that connects the treatment and recovery rooms, to tell me that Colin was in atrial fibrillation, or AF, as she said. This was the correct diagnosis. He had suffered with this occasionally over the last year and during his previous ECT course, and was on anticoagulant medication to reduce the formation of blood clots, but not on any medication to slow down the pulse rate or improve the heart rhythm. We do give ECT to patients with established AF, but newly developed AF needs attention. It can run at a fast frequency, placing strain on the heart muscle, so he needed care and observation, and possibly treatment to get into a normal rhythm, or at least to slow down the rate to below 100 per minute. We left it to the medics to sort out and hoped to see him again in a regular rhythm on Monday.

On Monday Colin was back, unperturbed by what had happened to him, and not even keen to talk about it. I guess if you are constantly thinking that you should die, a few palpitations might not cause the usual distress. I didn't want to trouble him with such questions and just felt for his pulse. It was regular, about 70 per minute. The cardiologist had prescribed Bisoprolol but I was a bit surprised that 1.25mg was enough to restore his sinus rhythm. Colin didn't suffer any more AF, but this episode had left me even more fearful of changing to Etomidate again. I resorted to increasing the electric charge instead.

Over the next few weeks we continued to struggle with seizure quality, managing only between 11 and 17 seconds of visual seizures, with varying quality of EEG traces. I reassured myself that with poorer seizures Colin could still get better, it would merely take more sessions. And his depression scores seemed to be nudging down to 11 or 12. The conversations with him were easier, he was smiling broadly and pleasantly when he greeted me, but the speed of his responses was still not what I expected from him. He was still hesitating and searching for words, just as at the start, although this was now much more subtle. And if I had any doubts as to whether he was well, these were easily crushed: he was still thinking that he ought to die and even attempted to kill himself while on the ward, although the effort was not as determined as before.

I had been too cautious with the ECT parameters. Colin had already had 19 sessions and frankly was not responding well. There was no point giving him this type of ECT; he was only experiencing the side effects. So we tried Etomidate again. The electric charge was reduced from 748mC to 403mC, much more cautious than usual but fully justified after the previous experience. He had a very good seizure which lasted for 29 seconds, a perfect duration from my point of view. The anaesthetist was taking no chances with the oxygen, which stayed above 90% throughout. But the pulse rate was gradually slowing, still with perfect narrow complexes and very regular, but dropping down one beat or two in speed at each new change on the monitor. When it showed 45, the anaesthetist jumped into action with a syringe of glycopyrrolate. The heart rate dropped further to 40, before picking up gradually. After another 30 seconds, the tension was all over. Oxygen and blood pressure were never a problem. Colin took 45 minutes to regain his orientation, a longish time.

It was time for a multidisciplinary team meeting. We had few options left and needed to share the risks with Colin and his wife, in order to allow them to decide how to proceed. There was no point continuing with Thiopental as an anaesthetic, as Colin was not going to reach remission with this. We could only achieve remission with Etomidate. Perhaps we were going to reduce or even abolish the risk of bradycardia if we pre-medicated him with glycopyrrolate, but if he needed another 12 or 20 sessions, he would be at risk another 12 to 20 times. My other concern was his questionable improvement. Years ago, I might have suggested that we continue with stronger seizures. But I am more realistic these days: even if we managed to get Colin into full remission, his condition was very resistant to ECT and he would probably relapse. He was likely to need a long continuation treatment, with short intervals between sessions. If I was certain that this would keep him well, I would go along with it, despite the risk. But I was not certain at all, in fact I doubted whether he would get well even with Etomidate.

These are the lines I've been thinking along, but I am now saying it all aloud to Colin and his wife, his consultant nodding in agreement. And as I am going through the arguments, I am convincing even myself that it is better to stop and to find different solutions. We should continue with CBT, institute changes to his antidepressants, and make a referral to a sleep clinic, as his sleep apnoea might be one reason for his poor response to treatment. And we would review him in a couple of months and find out whether he had actually benefited from ECT. All this might be correct, but I am clutching at straws. Let's face it: this is an ECT failure and I am not sure of the reasons. Is Colin's depression of a type that is not responsive to ECT? Did he need stronger seizures? He belongs to that one third of patients who do not respond to this therapy. Perhaps I have to accept that we might not find an explanation every time this happens. Perhaps we could find something positive to instil in him at least, so he doesn't decide to tie up those plastic bags more tightly at some point…

I was apprehensive prior to the three-month follow-up meeting. I expected bad news and was wondering what to suggest that didn't involve more ECTs. But Colin looked a bit better, if anything. His wife confirmed that impression and so did his HAM-D score, which Sam had assessed earlier: it was 10. Colin had been discharged from hospital and was making small but reasonable progress towards getting used to life in the outside world. The retardation had gone, and our conversation was progressing at a normal pace. He had even started wondering whether he might be able to go back to work. Was this progress due to the ECT or the change in medication that had been discussed at the last meeting? He was now on Lithium, stronger antidepressants, and an antipsychotic that was less sedative. Nobody was in a mood to argue, so we settled that the improvement was due to all these factors.

With the prospect of going back to work now on the table, the conversation shifted to memory problems. I wasn't surprised that these had developed. Hypoxia, high electric charge, and long recovery times were all factors that I had expected would make Colin's memory worse. He gave an example of forgetting the names of some business contacts and was wondering whether the memories would come back.

'He has forgotten some things going back over several years,' his wife added. 'He doesn't remember what happened during the first hospital stay. I thought ECT was going to affect memories just over a few months, but these things happened a long time before his first course.'

'Yes, forgetting events during the ECT course and a few months before it should be expected.' I was quoting our standard warning. 'But occasionally it can go back over several years.' I had seen a few people telling me that and was now wondering how common this problem was. 'But have you forgotten important things, that can impact on your functioning?'

'Well, I wonder why he needs to remember what happened during that hospital stay?' This helpful suggestion was made by his wife and came rather unexpectedly. It seemed that nothing vital had been forgotten, so why did they look so worried? I remembered a patient telling me that her memories were extremely important to her. For example, she had forgotten a holiday that had taken place three years earlier, and the memories could not be revived even after she was shown the photos. She stopped treatment rather early. Another patient felt he had forgotten many personal events from the previous five years, including giving a speech at a funeral, but still decided to continue, as ECT had kept his depression at bay and he was terrified of it coming back.

'Are you worried that you will develop dementia?' I had grasped the main source of concern. They nodded, and I felt in more familiar territory. 'ECT doesn't cause dementia. Neurons are not destroyed. You can forget facts, events, but not any skills or abilities. Your brain can still solve problems and you will remember new material in the future.'

Colin had just completed the battery of cognitive tests at the three-month follow-up assessment, so I turned the laptop towards him and showed him the results of his tests. The time on the Trail Making Test had actually halved compared to the pre-ECT score. The complicated Complex Figure had improved too. He had remembered six digits backwards. The only test that was not performed well was the memory one: remembering names and objects shown on a computer screen. Well, we didn't have a baseline, they observed, we were comparing his performance to that prior to the ECT, but he had already received another 20 sessions in the past. And of course, his depression was much better, no doubt contributing to an improved performance. This was all true, but still, dementia was not on the cards, that was clear.

'So why do depressed people forget more?' was the next question. 'Are there particular types of memories that are more affected by ECT?' This felt like an exam, and the danger of being failed by my examiners was real.

'Difficult to tell, and probably there is not that much good research.' I reflected on my knowledge of the subject, and a previous not very successful attempt to find definitive articles. 'It is the autobiographical memories that are most likely to go: events that the person has experienced, telephone numbers, what you did on a particular day. You don't forget skills, such as riding a bicycle or playing the piano. The emotional memories are less likely to go, too.' Here I suddenly got going again. 'If you experience fear, or pain, or happiness, you are more likely to remember the event anyway. We can't possibly remember everything that happens around us, what we see or hear, it is just too much. The brain has to decide what is important and will forget everything else. If an animal feels pain or fear, this is important for its survival and it will remember to avoid that situation.' Colin was nodding in understanding.

'So perhaps if you are depressed, your emotions are blunted, so you can't remember things, as the emotions are not involved so much?' I was on the edge of my chair: this sounded such a great explanation. I am sure there are papers on that subject and readers will correct me, but I will not spoil my joy by searching the literature to find out who said this first.

We agreed that there was no need to have more ECTs now, as Colin was on the right track, and there had been so many complications and side effects. And then I was surprised again. They asked whether he could have ECT in the future, if things got worse. 'Yes, of course we will consider it,' I replied. We would indeed, but I so much hope it doesn't come to that. We shook hands at the door and I muttered something in response to his thanks, unsure of how much I had helped.

20

DELIRIUM

There was nothing unusual about James's illness, so I wasn't planning to write his story. But what happened today was so dramatic, that I sat down in the evening to write it down, before my memory of the details faded away.

James was suffering from episodes of depression as part of his bipolar affective disorder. He hadn't had manic episodes for years, and he was not psychotic. Just a straightforward severe depression with a HAM-D score of 29. Or should I say almost straightforward, as he had been thinking of hanging himself and found it difficult to resist that urge. This was the main reason for his referral for ECT. He was just under 60 years old and looked quite fit. I had been away, so hadn't met him until this morning when he walked through the door of the treatment room and acknowledged the introductions to each person present. James had been on Carbamazepine until two weeks earlier, as a mood stabiliser. This was stopped because of the ECT, as it is an anti-convulsant and so would prevent effective seizures during treatment, but as usually happens, its effect had not disappeared. For his first treatment he had been stimulated three times and had had something reminiscent of a seizure at 184mC at the third attempt. For his second session this dose had been doubled, but he still only had a poor seizure of 13 seconds, both visible and on the EEG. Normally after such developments, I would switch to Etomidate for our anaesthetic to lengthen seizure duration and improve quality, but as already intimated, I had been away. I prefer to initiate anaesthetic changes myself, therefore the doctor who administered the treatment had instead increased the electric dose to 461mC, following the protocol. The resulting seizure had been even poorer, just 12 seconds duration of muscular contractions and 15 seconds of poor EEG activity. Today I was in the unit and it was time to switch to Etomidate. Just to be on the safe side, I reduced the electric charge. I would normally keep the same charge after a very poor seizure, but 12 seconds wasn't insignificant, and I had not witnessed the previous seizures myself, so I decided I had better be cautious.

ECT at 368mC, Etomidate anaesthesia. The usual myoclonic jerks, a common side effect from Etomidate, but nothing exceptional. Jane, the anaesthetist, is satisfied that our patient is asleep and injects the muscle relaxant. For nearly a minute James continues to have some myoclonic movements, some of them now probably caused by the muscle relaxant, but they can be hard to distinguish. An arm shoots up, but this is not a voluntary movement, we agree. He is ready. Mouthguard in, the SHO is ready to start, but the anaesthetist is not sure whether James is properly relaxed yet. Kara remembers that he had been slow to fasciculate the previous time, but we have not yet seen how he reacts to Etomidate, so nobody knows for sure. I give the nod to start and the anaesthetist agrees. The muscular contractions during the electric stimulation are quite strong, arms and legs stretch and freeze for a few seconds, tense and shaking. We wince and agree to wait longer next time for the muscle relaxant to take full effect or to increase its dose. James relaxes his limbs a bit and they slide into the usual rhythmic, symmetrical contractions. The seizure lasts for 35 seconds and has a clear EEG endpoint at 41 seconds. EEG is great and Kara comments, 'He will get well now'. She had been worried about his response to the question on suicidal ideation the last time she completed the HAM-D. Everybody is happy.

I linger at the bedside for a bit, watching the cardiac monitor, as this is the first strong seizure James has had so far. Not a single extra beat. Pulse rate stays at about 140, regular, then gradually slips down to 120. A bit fast, but nothing unusual; time to go to the desk and make notes. But I don't go to the desk. Something has still not settled. The anaesthetist looks focused and keeps James's chin up, while squeezing the breathing bag to give him oxygen. I notice the source of the concern: oxygen level on the monitor is 90%. 'He is a smoker,' Jane explains. Nothing strange, really: it is common for oxygen to drop slightly after a seizure, and James's level is expected to drop even further, as he is a smoker, and has gone through excessive physical activity for half a minute without breathing. He will be fine. But I don't go away, and we continue to watch his movements, his pulse and his colour. Yes, his colour is not right, he looks purple, as if his oxygen level is much lower than the monitor suggests. He starts breathing on his own, and we lift him up slightly in bed, to facilitate this. He breathes heavily but after another minute his skin colour goes back to a pinkish normal, and the monitor shows 98%. No problem, as always.

But still I stay by the bed and still the anaesthetist is focused on him, as if we both sense something is not right. Then James's eyes open and he looks round. This is strange: after only five minutes he should be deeply asleep after such a strong seizure. He should take perhaps 10 minutes to open his eyes. The eyes close, then his arm goes towards his mouth, to push away the oxygen mask: he doesn't look comfortable. Then he twists his body to one side. His pulse rate is static at 135 per minute, regular. It should be well below 100 by now. He is breathing well, he is not moving, why is his pulse rate so fast, and what is going on? He must be feeling anxious, I can't see any other explanation. 'Looks like he is one of those people who get agitated after the seizure.' The words come from my mouth, but I didn't know how prophetic they were going to be.

James continues to struggle with the oxygen mask, then sits up in bed, and twists to the side again. He's looking around with his eyes wide open, but not focused on anything. He is confused. We begin to worry, as he might fall out of bed or hurt himself on the safety rails designed to prevent accidental rolling out of bed. Then he turns around and kneels on the bed, facing its head. He starts growling and shouting something incomprehensible. Then he concentrates on the pillow and starts delivering punches into it in quick succession, shouting at the same time.

We have a problem. We get hold of his shoulders, trying to keep him safe, repeating to him that everything is fine and that he is doing all right, while trying not to fight with him, as this will only scare him further. But this doesn't help; he is getting more frightened now that he sees real people fighting with him, more agitated, lashing his arms around chaotically, shouting and bellowing as if he is being slaughtered. At this point I notice that he is quite a strong chap and that we are making very little difference to his movements. Kara loses no time and shouts for somebody to call the hospital crash team.

It is reassuring to see how quickly the team appears, perhaps 15-20 seconds after the SHO presses the alarm button on the identity card hanging around her neck. The tempo rises, there are people glued to each of James's limbs, others holding onto his head or to parts of limbs. He is overpowered, but still continues to growl and to wriggle with every possible muscle. I give up trying to reduce the intensity of the struggle, as his confused mind must now be gripped by utter terror, maybe imagining being attacked by nightmare enemies, or animals, or whatever images his brain is producing. 'Midazolam!' we shout, as we are now able to give him intravenous medication. At once 1.5 mg of this benzodiazepine goes in, but there is no obvious effect. And then his venflon is ripped out, despite the four hands trying to keep it in place. A new struggle now starts in an effort to secure access to a new vein. The anaesthetist is calm and decisive, but her fingers are shaking, as she can't do much about the adrenaline rushing in her blood. It doesn't help that she can't squeeze herself between the five people on that side of the patient. It doesn't help that despite all the well-intentioned hands clutching at his arm, wrist and fingers, he still manages to wriggle them enough to make the needle pop out of the vein again. 'Too many people,' the anaesthetist rationalises. She tries his foot, which has less room to wriggle, being held down by a few people. I get hold of the other foot, which is causing enough havoc to disrupt the procedure. Sounds easy enough, but I am again surprised how difficult it is to hold onto it. At one point my fingers are squeezed against the metal bar on the side – quite painful. I can only admire the strength of a delirious person, and I just hold onto that foot for dear life, while two more people are taking care of the upper sections of that same leg. The venflon is in and all care is taken to prevent it being ripped out again, so it is strapped in a bandage, with a little hole cut to make an opening for the syringe. This simple procedure is taking longer, as the hand holding the scissors is also shaking. Another 1.5 mg Midazolam goes in.

No effect. James is still shouting and fighting his lost battle with the whole army of nurses and demons, while the anaesthetist and I are beginning to worry that he might exhaust himself and put his cardiovascular system at risk. We discuss what to do next. She is reluctant to use an anaesthetic and I agree. Intramuscular Haloperidol (an antipsychotic) looks like the best option and is also what they use for delirium on the medical wards, so we prepare to give him 5mg. But by that time, James has slowed down. The anaesthetist positions herself next to him, face to face, and explains to him very loudly that he is in hospital and safe. He gets a bit of that message, after a few repeats. Then we gradually release his limbs and he quickly relaxes. The whole event has lasted 35 minutes. At 40 minutes he is calm and at 60 minutes he is talking coherently.

'No, next time we go back to Thiopental', I answer the SHO's question regarding the plan for the next session, although I noticed the cheeky smile on her face when she asked.

Before the next session I had a chat with James. He was his usual gentle self, kind and polite. He was still depressed, rather disappointingly after such a strong seizure. He didn't have any memory of the events - not surprisingly, as he was not conscious. I didn't want to give him too much detail for fear of upsetting him but explained that he had been very agitated and disorientated. Post-ictal confusion – the altered state of consciousness just after a seizure – is a usual response to the seizure, and patients gradually regain their orientation. Post-ictal delirium is rare. James, however, was more concerned about figuring out why he was depressed. 'I was a very fit man, doctor. I was never unhappy, I did all the right things. I was strong, exercised a lot. I was a very good boxer…'

I tried not to show any reaction. I was glad that it was the pillow that took his punches!

James continued ECT on the previous dose of electric charge and with Thiopental. There was no further hint of delirium, but his seizures were poor and his depression didn't lift. After another three lame seizures of around 15-second duration, I increased the electric charge, from 461 to 553mC, around 15% increase, following our protocol for dose change after poor seizures. The anaesthetist commented that it wouldn't matter if he was on Etomidate or Thiopental, as it could be the seizure itself that might have caused the delirium. I fully agreed, but many people tend to blame Etomidate for increased confusion and agitation, so we can't be certain what caused the delirium.

We were watching carefully for any untoward signs. The seizure was 23 seconds and the quality was good. The anaesthetist injected 0.5mg Midazolam, just in case. James remained settled and his pulse rate quickly came down to 80. Clearly there were no signs of delirium and he was wheeled out into the recovery room, where he lay quietly. After eight minutes, a recovery nurse rushed into the treatment room, asking for help. I put my head through the door and saw James waving his arms in the air, trying to stand up in bed, with the nurses trying to keep him safe. 'Midazolam!' The anaesthetist hadn't seen the previous episode and was not running fast enough. 'Quick, before we lose the venflon!' I urged her. Somehow, she got one milligram in the vein, before the venflon flew up into the air and the floor was sprinkled with blood from the orifice left on his wrist. The crash team were quick as usual and James had one member of staff on every limb. The story was unfolding with annoying predictability: the anaesthetist begging for some access to a limb, James shouting as if he was being murdered, nurses hanging on to parts of his body, and me standing one step back, trying to instil some calm into people, knowing what the outcome was going to be. The outcome came sooner than the previous time, the whole episode lasting only 18 minutes after the seizure, perhaps because the seizure wasn't as strong as before, or because James had Midazolam straight away. At any rate, we couldn't blame the Etomidate any longer. It was now clear that it was the good seizure quality that caused the delirium, and Etomidate just boosted the seizure quality. One question answered.

What should we do next? We had little option but to continue with ECT, as James was a suicide risk and medication had not worked. If we stuck to lower electric doses, we would easily avoid delirium. However, after seven sessions his depression was not showing any signs of improvement, so perhaps he did need stronger seizures – yet, stronger seizures caused delirium in his case. A bit of a Catch-22 situation. We could give him more Midazolam next time. This had worked well with a couple of previous patients. But these had been elderly and frail people who were getting agitated for a few minutes after their seizures. They had just needed two nurses to hold their arms to prevent them from falling over and injuring themselves. Nobody had yet required restraint; nobody had fought with imaginary enemies. We couldn't risk another fight with James. Was the margin between therapeutic and sub-therapeutic seizures really so narrow with James, that the therapeutic seizure resulted in delirium? This seemed unlikely. Our handbook states that if there is delirium, we should re-examine the need for ECT or consider the possibility for right unilateral treatment (both electrodes placed on the same side of the head). After deliberating this for a while, I settled for a lower electric dose, that we knew didn't cause delirium, arguing that it might take a few more sessions than usual, but would surely produce decent seizures with some therapeutic effect. James would receive one milligram of Midazolam routinely, we would have the crash team on site, and we would secure the venflon with a bandage. No problem. The real problem was to get him well.

James recovered the following week, assuring me that he 'had not felt that good for many years'. He was so well, that people recalled that his diagnosis was manic-depression and started worrying about him developing a manic episode if he received more ECTs. Having to balance the twin concerns of delirium and mania made the next treatment decision an easy one: we would stop the ECT.

I wish the story had ended there. But here I am, six weeks later, sitting down to continue writing. James was a proper manic-depressive. His mood would swing from one end of the scale to the other, with nothing to stop it in the middle or slow its progress. For a while, I kept meeting a smiling James once a week and postponing the ECT, pleased with his exceptional progress. But on the fourth weekly appointment, he had slipped back into his dark mood and suicidal ideas. I reassured him that we knew that ECT would help him again and noticed that this obvious statement didn't sound too convincing to him.

After two more poor seizures, he was not getting any better and we started thinking about Etomidate once more to help boost seizure quality. Events so far were compatible with the explanation that only the strong seizures were therapeutic for him. The 'combat' team gathered again, we introduced the boys to James and explained that they might have to hold him down for half an hour. 'No problem,' he reassured us. I reduced the electric charge and we proceeded. He had 2mg of Midazolam after another excellent seizure. James was peacefully asleep, but we didn't wave the strong boys away. At the seventh minute his arms started moving slightly, his eyes opened and everybody took hold of their pre-assigned limb: the heaviest man on his legs, one man on each arm, and the anaesthetist in charge of his head, or rather making sure his airways were open. It is so much better when you are prepared for it! We just counted the minutes, looking at the monitor that showed a pulse rate between 150 and 170, with a 100% oxygen saturation when the oximeter was allowed to stay in place, explaining to him in a loud voice what was going on, and giving him first 20 mg of Propofol anaesthetic and later another milligram of Midazolam through the tightly bandaged venflon. At 22 minutes he nodded that he was awake and understood what was going on. The boys released their grip and their faces beamed with satisfaction, seeing that James was not trying to get up. A good job done, everybody!

A good job, but could we do this time and time again? I sat down with Kara to chat about the long-term plan. It is Kara who really runs the unit. She has to answer to the hospital managers, to organise the salaries, the equipment, the training, and so on. And if something goes wrong, she will be called first to explain and to write the report. She has a clear mind and corrects me when I go off-piste with some crazy plan or when I want to treat somebody who is physically unwell. I knew that she considered James's treatment too risky and that she would want me to reduce the electric charge or to stop his treatment. I was wrong. 'Yes, we will continue like this. I am not having him kill himself!' Kara stated as a matter of course. Decision made, entirely in the patient's interest. Kara had my respect, although I forgot to express it at the time.

Why did I think this was the end of the story? After two episodes of delirium, I expected James to be well. This was on Thursday. I told him to come back one week later. The next day, Friday, I received a worrying WhatsApp message, written in the usual cryptic style: 'Delirium not well, can I tell him to come on Monday?' What was going on? Why did he reach remission during the first course and keep it for a month, while now he can only stay well for 24 hours?! The seizures were good, after all he was experiencing delirium after each one! His prognosis suddenly became very bad. Just as well we didn't switch to right unilateral ECT, as I would have blamed that for his lack of response and got into a real muddle.

On Monday we had Rob as our anaesthetist. Rob works in cardiac surgery and has seen a lot of deliriums: they are common after cardiac operations. He suggested we keep James asleep with an anaesthetic, Propofol, after the fit, until the delirium was over. So when James moved his arms at 7min 30sec, he gave him a dose of Propofol, about 40mg. Then he continued giving him 20mg every two minutes. He was casual and confident, as if injecting water. The strong boys noticed that he was in control and gradually stepped away from James's limbs. A total of 170mg of Propofol were given over 10 minutes. And then at 18 minutes, James looked at Kara with more focused eyes and confirmed that he knew where he was. It was all over. Propofol can be dangerous, it can stop breathing if given in high doses, but when administered by a consultant anaesthetist, who has the full anaesthetic equipment at hand, you feel that things are under control.

Delirium was now sorted, but James kept me worried. He was not responding. I was convinced that after only a month's break, ECT should work straight away. And when it didn't, I admitted that I was out of ideas. The only hope I could give James was that he responded once, so he should respond again, like most of our patients over the years. Despite his deep depression and suicidal feelings, he appeared more optimistic than me and declared that he would continue with ECT. Luckily, he was not complaining of side effects and he didn't share my concern. Finally after eight sessions, he was well again, that is, he was well for four consecutive days, rather than for just a few hours after an ECT. I admit that this was a huge relief. His long-term prognosis was still quite bleak, with these very short periods of well-being. He could easily be one of that small number of people who reached remission but managed to keep well only while having ECT once a week. They all gave up eventually, apart from the lady described in this book who managed to space out her treatments after a few years. But at least we knew that we could offer something to make him better, and he didn't seem troubled by the memory problems that had crept in. He had forgotten some events spanning quite a few years back. I asked him whether these had impacted on his functioning. He thought carefully but the closest to a problem was a worry that he experienced when he started work again. He thought that he had forgotten how to tile a wall, but the knowledge came back quickly once he had started. Also the limited number of items on a shopping list that he could retain (three) had not caused conflicts.

As for the delirium and the need to call the strong boys, this had become a bit of a routine which had to be adhered to by everybody, regardless of their rank and experience and, on the positive side, gave us an opportunity to exchange ideas and to teach students.

'Just don't change anything, okay?' Kara would instruct every anaesthetist, leaving no room for objections. And it worked each time: 10mg Propofol per minute for 20 minutes. There was no more fighting…

I have decided that this is the last time I will add a follow-up to this story, whatever happens. It is now one and a half years since James started his maintenance treatment. Things are going well. The interval between sessions was extended very gradually and is now three weeks. We are planning to stop ECT soon. James still has some bad days when his dark moods suddenly return, and he feels the urge to kill himself. But he knows that his mood will settle again the next morning or in a couple of days, so he waits and goes out to walk his dog. A few months ago, one anaesthetist dared to change the routine when Kara was not around and decided to keep him asleep with inhalation of another anaesthetic, Sevoflurane, instead of intravenous Propofol. Now the steady level of anaesthesia provided by the flow through the mask seems to be working even better. James is asleep for 20-25 minutes and then wakes up relaxed and in a good mood. We still call the strong boys for the morning, but they only hang around and chat at the back of the room. The new medical students look on slightly bemused, not sure what all the fuss is about.

21

CHILDREN

Children are very much the exception in ECT, so much so that the day I received an urgent referral for a 17-year old, I had to refresh my memory with a quick look at our treatment guidelines for young people. Of course, 17 is not a child as such, but persons under 18 count as children when it comes to ECT legislation. We had not treated a young person with ECT since I had started work in our unit, simply because nobody had been referred during all these years. Indeed, only two under-18s on average have ECT in the UK each year.

It makes sense that ECT in youngsters might be harmful; the brain is still developing, and the electric current, or the seizures, could interfere with neurons making the right connections. But surely, so will severe untreated mental illness. Apart from the different legal requirements for the involvement of a Second Opinion Appointed Doctor, I couldn't find much difference in the guidelines that I could take into account in terms of actual treatment. The seizure threshold would be expected to be low, so we should start with a very low electrical charge, but beyond that I couldn't find any clear differences.

The case was an emergency. Amelia had stopped eating about a month ago. She did not suffer from anorexia - she had done this in response to the voices she heard. This had happened a few times before, but this time it was dangerous. She had a nasogastric tube inserted but tried to pull it out all the time. To prevent this, two nurses were constantly with her, one on each side of her bed, each one tasked with grabbing her arm if she tried to reach her face and pull out the tube. Day and night. And it wasn't just the tube they were concerned about. Amelia would also try to bang her head against the wall and furniture, and even on the hard edges of furniture.

Amelia had started self-harming at the age of eight. From the age of 13 she had started hearing voices. Since then, she had been in hospital for most of the time and had not attended school again. Medication seemed to have done little to improve her condition. She could see angels who smashed their heads into the walls every time she ate something, and who kept shouting at her, 'Look what you have done to us! Stop eating!' After four years of illness, action had to be taken. ECT now seemed the lesser evil.

Our nurse, Danielle, had gone to perform Amelia's cognitive assessments but hadn't managed to complete much. Amelia was lying in bed looking at the ceiling. She wasn't allowed to use a pen to draw the Complex Figure or to connect the numbers and letters on the Trail Making Test, in case she stabbed it into her skin. Until Danielle's account, I hadn't known about the nurses keeping an eye on her arms day and night. If she hadn't been under 18, ECT would have been given much earlier…

The first time I met Amelia was on a Monday morning when she arrived from the specialised child psychiatry unit to have her first treatment. Even as she was being transported, events were unfolding, each one worthy of some gossip among the nurses, and at a rate that made me take notes, so that I wouldn't forget the details. The girl had asked to be covered with a blanket while being transferred from the ambulance to our unit.

Not due to the cold weather - the blanket had to be put over her head, so that she wouldn't see anything around her. Agoraphobia, I was told. And before she left the secure unit, she managed to pierce her thigh with a fork.

I tried to get things clear with the staff who accompanied our new patient.

'What was a fork doing in the room of a girl who is being fed through a nasogastric tube?' I asked. 'And did you not know that she had done the same thing in the past?' I muttered under my breath.

'It was just there.' The nurse looked bemused herself, noticing the irony of the situation.

My first surprise was that Amelia did look like a child. I had more or less assumed that a 17-year-old would be a young adult and that we were to treat her as a child only because of the administrative implications. But no, she looked like a fragile, helpless and frightened child. Her eyes were sad, and her voice so quiet that I had to lean close to hear her words. She told me how she had started hearing voices four years earlier and how she had been in hospital for most of this time. She said that she was feeling depressed and wanted to die. The voices were disturbing her, she could hear them all the time now, even during our conversation. They were coming from inside her, she explained, and were not the voices of real people. They were telling her not to eat. There was a large wound on her forehead, about a week old and now that the scar had peeled off, it revealed the thin, pink skin underneath. 'Did you bang your head?' She nodded.

The notes added other episodes of her punching her face, pulling her hair and cutting herself. She was sitting in a wheelchair, explaining that she had been lying in bed for a month and so she would feel weak and wobbly on her feet if she tried to walk. Her lips were dry, but the fluid intake had been assessed as appropriate by a dietitian, and her blood pressure and pulse rate were normal. She was not dehydrated but was becoming very weak from immobilisation. Her movements and speech were slow, suggesting some element of psychomotor retardation (a good sign, I noted). And she said that she was hoping to get better, probably another good sign. Yes, she herself did want to have ECT, although the treatment had been legally authorised by a Second Opinion Appointed Doctor.

I had planned to start at 46mC electric charge and bilateral treatment. This is our protocol for people below the age of 30. I am sure most clinics would start at an even lower dose, as she was technically a child. I was resisting that, due to the element of urgency. In the end I got cold feet (what if something did go wrong with a child in our care…?) and lowered the starting dose by one step, to 35mC. We also decided to use Glycopyrrolate, to avoid possible slowing down of the heart rate, and to have an ampule of Diazepam ready, in case her seizure was prolonged, as can happen with young people. In the event, there was no seizure at 35mC but a very good one at the next stimulation at 80mC, with no complications. I decided not to increase the dose at the next treatment, as the EEG traces seemed perfect.

On the evening of that day I wrote up my notes, concluding, 'I don't know how much to hope for here. Eating and drinking will probably get better, but would she be able to leave the hospital and start some semblance of a normal life? I am very doubtful at this point'.

At the second ECT, another sign gave me more hope. This wasn't due to the fact that Amelia was less anxious when travelling in the car, as the nurses reported. It was because she was crying when she lay down in bed, before the treatment. This was an emotion more typical of depression than of schizophrenia, a differential diagnosis that had to be considered in the light of her persistent hallucinations. And at least it showed that her emotions weren't blunted, as can happen in some cases of chronic psychosis, where it indicates a 'negative symptom', i.e. an emotional ability or drive that has been lost in the course of a psychosis and is unlikely to come back. If we were indeed dealing with an illness that was closer to depression, we were in with a chance, even after four years and even with this early onset.

I wanted to pick up on any hint of improvement, so I went towards the entrance of the hospital to meet Amelia on the morning of the third session. A whole group of people appeared at the other end of the corridor: Amelia in a wheelchair, surrounded and followed by five young women.

'She is on four-to-one monitoring,' Kara explained.

'Why?' I didn't get it and resorted to flippancy. 'She is a frail girl, surely it's enough to have one person for each arm, she only has two arms, doesn't she?'

'Yes, but one needs to hold her legs if she starts fighting. And a fourth one is needed to supervise everything and intervene if something goes wrong.'

Kara has worked in secure units and knows the restraint protocols for psychiatric patients. She found nothing unusual in the arrangements. There was no time to ask why there was a fifth person here today, as they were now close to us. 'Why don't they just use straps on her hands?' whispered the young SHO who had also accompanied us in the corridor. She had probably seen things done less kindly in her country of origin. I had also seen things done differently 30 years ago, during my work in a hospital in Bulgaria, where two members of staff covered the night shift for the whole acute ward. One or two difficult patients usually had their arms tied with special straps to the sides of their beds during the night.

Amelia had eaten something the day before, which was greeted with joy by the team. Not really a sure sign of improvement yet, though. Voices were still constant and terrifying, angels were still appearing before her, and her legs were shaking with anxiety. But there was no blanket over her head, and Amelia was hopeful that ECT would work on her depression. And then she surprised me with another positive sign. I had popped out of the waiting room and when I came back, saw that the wheelchair was empty. Amelia had got out of it and had swapped it for one of the armchairs. Then she just walked on her own to the treatment room. There was no crying, even after the first needle missed the vein. Was this a good sign?

The two medical students in the room were asking me about the diagnosis.

'Well,' I hesitated, and stepped away from the treatment area, so that Amelia couldn't hear us. 'It could be psychotic depression, and she has all the symptoms you can think of to support this diagnosis. But these constant voices worry me, as they would be more typical of schizophrenia. And I can't describe those angels that keep banging their heads on the wall and shouting at her, as depressive delusions. Nor can I explain why the voices sometimes say nice things to her - this is not congruent with depression. But she doesn't present as schizophrenic and her emotions are well preserved. She is also anorexic at the moment, but doesn't have the typical body image problems, so I don't want to call this anorexia. I think she is suffering from severe depression, and the very early onset is causing some atypical features. Patients don't always fit neatly into our diagnoses, it is all a continuum really.'

'Can't she be diagnosed with schizoaffective disorder?' insisted the student. She was a good student and this was the diagnosis that would best fit our classification systems, if we followed the rules. But I had become a bit cynical about our diagnoses over the years. In any case, new genetic studies indicated that there was a huge overlap between the common psychiatric disorders.

'You are right, this is what it could be called, but it still implies symptoms of schizophrenia, and I do not accept this. But there is a continuum between our diagnoses, and she has lots of symptoms of different disorders,' I wriggled out of anything more definite.

What was more relevant in my mind was that this was a chronic, severe, psychotic disorder and that it had started at an early age. Amelia had not been able to go to school for four years, hadn't interacted with peers, and hadn't had enough stimulation, having spent most of this time in hospital and much of it in bed. It was a bad mixture and she had a lot of catching up to do, if she recovered.

More good news was evident after seven sessions. Danielle entered the office with excitement on her face: Amelia had walked on her own from the taxi, through the long corridors of the hospital, all the way to our unit. And she hadn't needed the nasogastric tube over the long bank holiday weekend. We sat down for another chat. There was some spontaneity about her, she looked more like an independent human being, was not clutching the hands of the nurses and responded more quickly to questions, with a voice that sounded slightly louder and clearer. The fear in her face had almost gone.

But some things hadn't changed: she told me that the voices were still there, every minute of her life. The staff reported that she had thrown herself on the floor after a family visit, had tried to harm herself and stated that the voices were horrible. I always believe people when they say they hear voices, even if they don't look as if they do. But here I found myself wondering whether these were in fact psychotic experiences, or Amelia's way of describing her own thoughts or fears. The voices were now more controllable but got nasty if she started eating. She would now allow herself to be spoon-fed by the nurses but was still unable to feed herself. A great step forward from the nasogastric tube, but I still couldn't see how the voices would disappear or how Amelia would cope with life without an army of nurses rushing around her, let alone how she would develop any of the usual interests that her peers normally have. The nurses were happy to tell me that Amelia was more interested in doing things now, but the list of activities was not encouraging: colouring books headed the list and the outside world was still being ignored. Amelia was still frozen in her own universe and it would take a lot of work to get her back on track.

I didn't think ECT would do much more to improve her mood and interests, but it was her best chance to prepare to face the hostile world outside. She was used to being in a safe place, with nurses to turn to all the time. She was frightened of going out and this fear was probably getting stronger every year, as more time passed with her being cut off from that world. It would be a monumental feat for her to live an independent life.

Perhaps we should aim for more modest goals: eating with no prompting and no close observation in supportive accommodation or at home, and finding enjoyment in life, instead of hitting her head on the edge of the cupboard. ECT should continue twice a week until there was no more improvement, then should be spaced out over a few months but not stopped completely, I suggested to her and her team. The agreement was unusually unanimous: everybody was aware of the enormity of the task.

There were some improvements each week. One week we learned that Amelia had started feeding herself – a real break-through. Another week, she had been out in the garden. The observation level was reduced to one-to-one. After 14 sessions, however, it looked as if the improvement had peaked. She was still hearing voices all the time, self-harming continued, and she seemed content to stay in hospital. I agreed that we could move to weekly sessions. After the first break of one week, things seemed to have progressed further: Amelia had been eating with the other patients and there were plans to attend the hospital school again; the nurses sounded really pleased. Most encouraging of all, she was paying less attention to the voices. 'Something clicked in my mind, I was able to enjoy the moment.' Perhaps this statement was more to do with her having psychotherapy, than ECT. But hey, she was now able to have psychotherapy, and this was because of ECT!

The next few months were not encouraging. The interval between ECTs was increased to two weeks and then again quickly to three weeks. The team felt that it was time to stop it, assuming that it had already played its role. Amelia's mood slipped down, and for a few days she started refusing to eat again. However, she still kept saying that ECT was helping her and insisted on continuing. And somehow, she started improving again, looking better and more motivated each time she came. When the interval reaches three weeks, time seems to pass faster (for me at least), so when she completed her second 'course', for a total of 24 sessions, it was already seven months since she had first appeared at the door, in a wheelchair, covered with a blanket. She was now talking about discharge to a general ward and another hospital, away from our area. I was sure that she needed to continue with ECT and was worried about her relapsing. But the anxieties about giving ECT to children were too strong and, I suspect, played a part in the decision. During this time, I was contacted twice by journalists asking me to comment on the inappropriate use of ECT in children in the UK. They didn't know I was treating one - it was a coincidence. In preparing my response, I obtained the figures that only two children per year had been treated in the UK over the last few years. Neither of these had been below 16 years old. It seems that UK psychiatrists are not that keen to unleash electric currents onto those who are most vulnerable. I argued this in a more measured fashion. The figures raised a different question in my mind that totally contradicted what the journalists were worried about: why are so few children treated with ECT? There must be some very ill young people in the UK. Are they missing out on this treatment because of its controversial reputation?

Five months after the last ECT I made contact with the hospital where Amelia had been transferred to. Her new doctor gave me an account that I didn't expect. Amelia had continued to improve without ECT. She had received dialectical behaviour therapy and had engaged well with it. She had appealed against her section, had won the appeal, and now they were making preparations to discharge her. I was perplexed. 'But is she really well?' I worried. 'Even when her depression improved here, she still looked so frightened and weak.' No, the improvement was genuine; she had made good plans for the future, was the reassuring reply.

I contacted Amelia and we spoke on the phone. What I heard made me really happy. She was not only doing well and looking forward to the future but felt that she should do something for us. I was exploring cautiously what she was talking about. She was offering to talk to patients about ECT and even to talk to the press. Anything, to help spread the message.

'So you think ECT helped you?'

She had no hesitation. 'A year ago, I was stuck in bed, I couldn't dream that I would get well. And now I am going home!' Her voice had been firm and confident throughout the chat. Mine was getting wobbly. This girl had achieved something remarkable. She had lifted herself out of a seemingly chronic illness, finding mental strength where none seemed to be left. And already she felt that she should help others. I was humbled. Yes, I don't think it was the ECT that brought her all the way there, it was her own will and inner strength and the great care she received in the hospital. But - perhaps I am biased - I will not discount the contribution of ECT completely.

22

BECOMING A PSYCHIATRIST

I was always expected to become a psychiatrist. My father was one of the best-known psychiatrists in Bulgaria. Towards the end of his career he was the Head of the Department of Psychiatry at the university in the capital, Sofia. His colleagues, who occasionally came to our home for dinner, assumed that I would follow in his footsteps. I was not very interested in their medical conversations but enjoyed the anecdotes about their lives as students.

When I was a child, my father would sometimes take my mother and me on long, leisurely journeys around the country. These were holidays, but he was also following up patients whom he had looked after as a young doctor. A trip to the seaside, normally a day's drive even in our small car, could take up to week, as he would stop to enjoy the natural scenery or leave the main road to get to a small village and knock on a door where a former patient lived. I still remember one of the more exotic visits, about 50 years ago. We went to an old asylum with large grounds in the countryside. It was the largest in the country, remote from towns and villages and set within a beautiful river canyon. Over a thousand chronic patients were kept there, mostly schizophrenic, out of public sight. I was slightly surprised that I was allowed to walk in the alleys of the park, unsupervised, surrounded by these enigmatic figures, some with strange gaits, some looking distinctly odd. I must have been only nine or ten years old. Perhaps my father wanted to show me that his patients meant no harm.

The head of the hospital, who was a good friend of my father, lived there in a rather grand house, built in the pre-communist era, that stood within the grounds of the hospital. He had a daughter my age, a pretty and playful girl, and we made friends. On the first or second morning of our stay she said, 'Let's go and see the White Lion - he lives on the hill up there.'

My father had told me about the White Lion before the journey, so I knew what she was talking about. The White Lion was a patient, a long-standing schizophrenic patient, perhaps the best-known in the country. He had chosen the name himself. He had been a very intelligent young man, an engineer, who had fallen prey to a strange illness that made him imagine fantastic plots. He had developed the most elaborate delusional system, with him assuming the role of a king, or perhaps even ruler of the universe. There was even a little book written about him that my father had shown me. It featured elaborate drawings and three separate alphabets that he had developed for different purposes, complicated and bizarre, and of course never used even by their creator.

I wasn't sure if I should go there without any adult protection - what if he were to attack us? My father nodded in approval, however, so off we went. The girl led us on a path that meandered through meadows and trees and finally opened onto a small hill. The place was cordoned off by strings, threaded through with shiny wrappings and dangling bells. They were flapping in the gentle breeze. There were some odd objects scattered on the lawn, including the scull of some large domestic animal. There was an eerie feel to the place. On the upper side of the lawn was the White Lion, sitting in a tattered chair, his throne. He spent his days there; this was his kingdom. The hospital had allowed him full freedom to enjoy his delusions. I was still on edge, but I relaxed after he greeted us kindly, with an air of magnanimity. We only exchanged a few words; he wasn't that interested in us and I didn't know what to say or ask, and then we went back.

You might think that this was the formative experience that made me embrace psychiatry as my destiny. Well, nothing of the kind. I became more interested in maths and would probably have become an engineer, if my mother hadn't put all her persuasion skills into guiding me into medicine some years later.

As a medical student, I was put under further pressure to choose psychiatry, especially as I was studying at the medical school where my father was teaching. I was, of course, not going to follow in his footsteps. Cardiology looked so much more exciting and I was following a charismatic lecturer who was tutoring me towards that goal. One summer I picked up one of the thinner textbooks on psychiatry from my father's library, to explore that world, just in case. It was in German. The language is hard even in everyday talk, but this felt very difficult. I took the book for my summer holiday reading at the seaside. In two weeks I managed fewer than 10 pages. This stuff wasn't for me. There were better things to do both on the beach and in medicine.

Making a choice

I will now tell you how medical students in communist Bulgaria used to choose their post-university placements. After graduating, we were required to work for three years outside Sofia, to help fill the gaps in the provincial hospitals. Some people had already negotiated their placements - I never figured out how they did it. The rest of us were gathered in one of the lecture halls, seated on one side of the amphitheatre-shaped hall. On the other side were seated quite a number of hospital heads, who wanted to pick up good juniors for their departments. We would stand up one by one and the senior doctors would ask each student if they would like to come to their hospital. I think that most students had already made their contacts and the offers were predictable. We had already filled in our preferences. I can't believe now how naïve I was in those days, but I had put as my first choice to work in a town in the south of the country, that had recently become a ski resort: Bansko. It had installed its first fast three-seater lift a couple of years earlier and I wanted to combine my work with some skiing. I am still looking for such a job. I was scanning the senior colleagues desperately to see if the head of the Bansko general hospital was in the audience. I had done no research on this, had made no attempt to contact them in advance, and indeed I have a suspicion that they don't have a general hospital, even to this present day. So when my turn came to stand up, I was unprepared. I noticed the large figure of the head of psychiatry at one of our general hospitals. I knew she had spoken with my father, asking whether I would like to work with her in her town. She raised her hand and asked me if I would like to come to the psychiatric ward in her hospital. Had there been a collusion between her and my father? I scanned the other white-haired doctors. I wasn't looking for the Bansko offer any longer, perhaps a cardiology placement would be offered somewhere? The seconds were ticking by fast and I needed to make a decision. I didn't have to accept the offer, but then I would have had to fill a gap somewhere else. So I said, 'That's great, I accept.'

I didn't finish my three-year placement. Halfway through, I was already in London, applying for psychiatry training posts. It felt natural; I didn't think of applying for any other specialty. I had become a psychiatrist.

ECT

My involvement with ECT also had an element of chance. I didn't always believe in ECT. In fact, I wanted to do research on better treatments that caused fewer side effects. I first started with transcranial magnetic stimulation (TMS), whereby a coil held over the patient's head produces low-frequency repetitive magnetic pulses that stimulate a small part of the brain and improve the symptoms of depression.

This research led me naturally to the next step, magnetic seizure therapy (MST) which uses the same technology, but with a crucial difference. The repetitive magnetic pulses are stronger and produced at a higher frequency, so they elicit an epileptic seizure, similar to ECT. The magnetic pulses are generated via a large coil (ours had a diameter of 11.5 cm) and create small electric currents inside the brain, just underneath the coil, to elicit a magnetically induced seizure. Instead of electricity passing through the whole brain, as during ECT, MST stimulates only a very small area of the brain. This was expected to cause much less confusion and fewer memory problems. My interest in this new treatment was provoked by a purely geographical coincidence: a small Welsh company, '*Magstim*', that was making this equipment, happened to be based not too far from Cardiff. It designed the first ever MST machine capable of producing

100 magnetic pulses per second, i.e. a 100Hz frequency. The treatment had been pioneered by Dr Sarah (Holly) Lisanby in New York. She came to Cardiff, together with her colleague who was also working on this treatment, Dr Mustafa Husain from Dallas, Texas, to help us perform the first treatment. They had used earlier versions of the machine that could only produce lower frequencies (40-50Hz) and the expectation was that the 100Hz stimulation would be more efficient. We treated the first patient on a very rainy morning in June 2006 in Whitchurch Hospital, our old, 100-year-old Victorian-style building with its extensive grounds, that I suspect created incredulity and doubt in our American colleagues, especially when they had to negotiate the puddles of water in front of the entrance and walk down the long and gloomy corridor.

But we had prepared well. The director of '*Magstim*' was on site together with the engineer who had constructed the machine. The sequence of events was rehearsed many times, the coils were cooled down to prevent overheating. The machine required a very strong electric current, so we had installed three-phase electric wiring to power it. The fluorescent lights in the unit still flickered from the strain on the electric grid in the hospital during the stimulations, and the noise created by the vibrations of the coil when the electricity passed through it was so loud that patients and staff had to wear earplugs. I personally thought that it wasn't that loud - any disco hall is much louder - but Americans are highly obsessed with safety, or rather with potential litigation, so they had introduced the earplugs into the protocols. There was excitement and anxiety in the air. I wasn't worried, I couldn't see any theoretical reason why this could be dangerous, at least no more dangerous than ECT. The patient was a 35-year-old lady suffering from depression, who was already going through a standard ECT course. The treatment went really well, with the patient having a seizure when stimulated for five seconds (half the machine output) and becoming fully awake and orientated four and a half minutes later, a very quick recovery time. Holly Lisanby put together a lecture for our colleagues in the hospital at the planned teaching session one hour later, together with the video taken during the new treatment.

A pilot trial went ahead. Patients were indeed less confused after treatment; they were orientated faster after their seizures, in fact much faster, at seven minutes on average, compared to 23 minutes required by ECT patients. They felt less confused, as if nothing had happened to them. They liked the new treatment. We were on a high, but the euphoria didn't last long. We couldn't elicit seizures in a couple of patients. In other patients, the seizures were so short, and the EEG traces were so poor, it was clear that they were not going to be therapeutic. And as we were treating everybody with the maximum setting of the machine - 10 seconds at 100Hz - there was no option of increasing the dose. I had to stop the trial. With hindsight, perhaps I had been unfair on MST: some patients in the trial had high seizure thresholds due to the medications they were taking (two of them were on anticonvulsants), or due to their previous ECT courses, which had increased their thresholds (most patients had on-going ECT courses). With improved equipment and perhaps better patient selection, there is now a prospect of this treatment finally becoming established.

I was trying to develop a treatment that was better than ECT, but during the trial I found that I was actually going through a gradual conversion to ECT. The treatments took place in the ECT unit and the regular ECT patients served as controls. Everybody was completing extensive rating scales. I expected to see cognitive problems among the ECT patients - this is why we wanted to compare ECT and MST. But with time it became clear, to my surprise, that the cognitive tests, those same Complex Figures, MMSE, Trail Making Tests and others, did not deteriorate after ECT courses. Yes, patients had memory problems, but their speed of reaction, concentration, executive functioning, working memory and other faculties, all remained intact once the acute post-treatment confusion had lifted. And, over a period of several years, I would observe desperately ill patients reaching remission with ECT at rates and consistency that I had not seen before in my psychiatric practice. I found myself working in a unit that was transforming the lives of the most severely ill patients, and I decided to stay after the TMS and MST trials had finished. I hope this book explains why I want to continue this work.

23

PANDEMIC

The events were taking place so far away and seemed almost irrelevant to us. A few cases of pneumonia in China that for some reason the press and the World Health Organisation deemed worthy of attention: one of those epidemics that spreads every now and then in foreign countries, in Asia or in Africa, and is contained there. Perhaps there would be a spillover into Europe for a while, just as swine flu had done 10 years earlier. Or more likely, it would stay away, like Ebola. It was going to be reported by the press for a while and then fizzle out and be forgotten.

China had fewer than 100 deaths when the whole 11-million-strong town of Wuhan was locked down. The West was impressed but also worried by this apparent violation of human rights. Were the Chinese over-reacting? They had only 414 deaths when they finished building the first new hospital for infected patients. Or perhaps they were not quite over-reacting: the death count was mounting and started reaching the thousands. This looked serious but surely was not going to affect us in Europe.

Then came Italy. Clearly, this country had got something terribly wrong. The numbers of infected people were rising alarmingly. Then the numbers of the dead followed in the same path. Why Italy? Was the death toll higher because they had many old people, as the virus was especially devastating among the elderly? Had the virus mutated into a more virulent 'local' form? Was it perhaps their lifestyle, with extended families gathering for meals and people kissing each other and spreading the virus, instead of just shaking hands? Our numbers in the UK were so much lower, the rest of Europe's numbers were so much lower, the death rate was so much lower. Poor Italians, they had either messed up something or were just so unlucky.

Then came the graphs. I was watching the process unfold on Twitter. Several people tracked the numbers of infected people in Italy, in the UK and in other countries and superimposed them on graphs. The numbers increased in every country, and the rate of increase was looking very similar, in fact stunningly identical. The size of the country didn't matter, on average each person kept infecting a similar number of people. If there were 100 cases somewhere, they would double after three days or so. The frightening fact was impossible to miss now: Italy wasn't performing worse than anyone else, it just had started its journey earlier, exactly two weeks earlier than the UK. And the number of deaths there was following the number of the infected by two weeks as well. What happened in the UK today had already happened in Italy two weeks earlier. It was becoming obvious that what happened in Italy today was what was going to hit the UK two weeks later. The graphs, when plotted, were so stunning; the correlations between the major European countries were nearly perfect. I had not seen such strong correlations in real-life medical data during my academic life. We were able to see into the future. The events were as predictable as the time of the sunrise in two weeks' time. A tsunami of very poorly patients was coming our way and it was going to hit our hospitals and our society, unless we acted quickly. Washing hands was not slowing this down. Italy was locked down on 9th March. We should have locked down on 9th March too, to avoid their fate.

But a crazy idea was being floated: that herd immunity would be developed, if we allowed people to fall ill gradually. The survivors would develop immunity and eventually this would stop the epidemic. The plan could work of course - 80% of the population would get ill, most of them mildly, and then the population would be immune. Without a vaccine, this was going to happen eventually. But if we didn't slow down the rate of the pandemic, 1% of infected people were going to die in the space of two to three months. And when the hospitals were full, the death rate would exceed the expected 1%, as patients would be turned away at the hospitals' doors. We had to slow down the speed of this plague, to allow the medics to treat the sick.

A study conducted at Imperial College London predicted the calamity too. Every day the Financial Times started publishing the most informative graphs of the epidemic spread. They painted a frightening scenario. All European countries were following the same trajectory. The movement of the graphs was slow, one notch every 24 hours, but the numbers for the next day and for the next week, were utterly predictable. You didn't need any mathematical skills - you could just use a ruler to extend the lines on the logarithmic scales and figure out the numbers. Politicians started to believe the graphs at last. Everybody was getting the message, unfortunately a bit late. The country was eventually locked down, but after at least a two-week delay. We were now following in the footsteps of Italy, but at least the hospitals were going to cope, just.

With the graphs torturing my mind, I could see our ECT service being put on hold, as non-essential. ECTAS collected data from all over the country that conveyed the feelings of resignation in many units: ECT was being wound down, like all other branches of medicine, to make space for the fight against the virus. Some clinics closed down, the majority reduced the number of sessions. The situation was similar around the world. In one country the decision to stop the ECT service was only reversed after one of the depressed patients jumped to her death from a high-storey building, after missing her sessions. A single personal case was more powerful than the statistics produced by the doctors and persuaded the authorities that ECT is also an essential service.

Anaesthetists were busy looking after infected people and connecting them to ventilators. Our own unit, equipped with cardiac monitors and intensive care beds positioned next to oxygen outlets at the walls, could be used for COVID-19 patients. For the first time I felt relief that we had an unusually low number of ECT patients. Nobody was refusing food or drink; nobody had frozen in catatonic stupor. We were able to wind down the treatments to one session per week and hoped that our patients were not going to relapse over the next two or three months. One maintenance patient didn't want to come. She was self-isolating, a wise move for somebody who had turned 80. She might stay well for a month or two. One patient who believes that she can't breathe, saw the irony of the situation when asked, as part of our orientation checklist, to name some interesting event that had been in the news recently. I hoped that she would avoid any real breathing problems in the coming weeks. For some, depression and loneliness were worse than the fear of dying: one lady preferred to be admitted to a psychiatric ward instead of being depressed and isolated at her own home. Yes, depression can feel worse than anything else, I keep telling my students.

I discussed starting a ketamine clinic, as a substitute for ECT. Ketamine is an old anaesthetic but, given at lower doses, has been shown to have a rapid effect on depression and suicidal ideation. It looked like a great short-term measure to put in place. But I was informed that there was a shortage of this drug. This was due to such an extraordinary coincidence, that I had to ask several people to confirm the facts. Ketamine is used during intubation of COVID-19 patients, so they can be attached to respirators. Ketamine was therefore reserved for these procedures and was already in short supply. I still can't get my head around this: the same drug is the best choice when intubating victims of the pandemic and for treating severe depression during the same pandemic!?

We would try to use ECT only on people who needed it urgently. I feared the epidemic could spill into the old-age psychiatric wards, therefore, by enabling elderly depressed patients to leave hospital, we would literally be saving their lives. Perhaps we could get them well with four or five sessions and send them home? Did we have this much time before the infection caught up with them? Probably not. For a few patients this looked like the right time to try to stop ECT, so we asked them to wait for a couple of months. They should pull through. Our patient with hypoxia must stay at home – it was just as well he had already stopped ECT. The patients with neurological diseases were also high risk: they were better off isolating themselves at home and waiting for a couple of months.

A depressed man had developed a classic delusion of guilt, that I had expected to come across: he believed that he had caused the pandemic. Not only that, he had stopped eating in order to prevent the food shortages in the country - he must have seen the empty shelves on the television screen. To my surprise, he wasn't crying or pulling his hair in despair, despite being unable to find any alternative explanation for the pandemic. But with both of us wearing masks, I probably missed some of the nuances in the facial expressions. We added him to our clinic list: I could justify that he was an urgent case.

There is a surreal feel to the clinic. Every patient is greeted at the entrance with a temperature check and questions about medical symptoms and contacts with infected people. Surgical masks are put over their faces. The relative or nurse who brings them is asked to stay out and come back later to collect the patient. We would not treat any infected patients – they don't need a further drop in oxygen during the treatment – but anybody could be an asymptomatic carrier and there is no way of knowing that without testing. We already have several nurses in the hospital who are infected: we can't trust anybody. The numbers of staff are trimmed down to the bare minimum – we are operating a skeleton staff, the joke goes. Doctors and nurses in the treatment room are dressed in full personal protection equipment (PPE), miraculously organised by Jess despite the shortages. They are at risk, especially the anaesthetists: they touch patients' faces and mouths, suction the saliva, breathe in any tiny droplets that could be forcefully expelled from the patients' mouths during the seizures.

The anxiety in the clinic is palpable, amongst both patients and staff. The introductions are more relevant than ever, as we are unrecognisable to the patients and look as if teleported from a sci-fi movie. Our voices are dull and hard to understand under the FFP3 masks. The plastic visors make the vision worse too. I mistake a male for a female member of staff and wonder how to apologise. We are still trying our best to pretend some semblance of calm and normality and avoid frightening the patients.

Somehow, nobody runs away, although one maintenance patient with frontotemporal dementia is getting agitated by the sight of masked staff. The person who felt responsible for the pandemic develops post-seizure agitation and stares with fear at the masked silhouettes around him, still unaware of his surroundings. I note with relief that he is not very muscular but I still pray that he doesn't develop full-blown delirium and doesn't start fighting for his life. The Midazolam enters his vein quickly and calms him down. We can carry on. A few days later I find out that this single strong ECT has sent him into a manic episode. He has spent the whole day in the locked-down city centre, celebrating his excellent mood with an enthusiasm that only manic people are capable of. A police car gives him a lift back to the hospital late in the evening. Is his transformation a good omen for an end of the pandemic?

We would keep this weekly clinic going until the end of the crisis, as long as we can get an anaesthetist and the hospital doesn't take over our unit. We have to wait and change plans one week at a time, even one day at a time. Who will survive the virus? And who will survive their depression? When will we be able to resume normal service? Life will not be the same for any of us. My book was ready for publication when the crisis started; I only need to add this last chapter. Surely ECT will continue to be used, so somebody might find this text useful when this is over. But the stories don't look as dramatic as they did only a few weeks ago. Everybody is caught up in a drama never seen before.

April, 2020

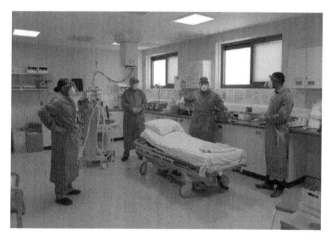

The ECT clinic during the pandemic. Magdi and Jess are in the middle, presumably.

Shocked

ACKNOWLEDGEMENTS

Several colleagues kindly offered to read chapters and discuss ways to improve them: Professor Nicol Ferrier, Dr Jonathan Waite, Dr Kathryn Peall, Dr Richard Braithwaite, Professor James Walters, Professor Rupert McShane. I owe special thanks to my boss Professor Sir Mike Owen, who has kept me in this department for most of my academic life and allowed me to do research in areas that I found exciting. In fact, he encouraged me to follow my intuition. This resulted in us working on some very promising findings in psychiatric genetics and in me pursuing my interest in ECT in my clinical work. My editor Fiona Marshall was not only meticulous in improving my writing and checking the scientific narrative, but also kept me on track when my jokes strayed a touch too far.

Above all, I want to thank my patients who so graciously agreed for me to use their stories for this book, driven by the desire that sharing their experiences could help others improve their understanding of this treatment, lift the mystery and preconceptions around it and ultimately help others to get better. They may not remember some details of the time they were very unwell with depression or were asleep during the procedures. I hope they will not be too distressed by the details, and they should not assume those exact things happened to them, as I have changed details to protect their anonymity and have even swapped some individual experiences. I wrote most of the stories when they happened, without much of a plan for publication, so I didn't ask patients for permission to publish at the time. I was surprised and humbled when the signed consent forms started arriving in the post, some from patients who had treatment many years earlier. I hope I have shown the respect that each participant truly deserved for bravely going through their ordeals.

Printed in Great Britain
by Amazon

43495301R00156

By the same author

FICTION
Five Rivers Met on a Wooded Plain
Turning for Home
The Vanishing Hours

THEATRE
Visitors
Eventide
Echo's End
While We're Here
Nightfall
We Started to Sing

The Remains of the Day *(after Ishiguro)*
Blood Wedding *(after Lorca)*
The Wellspring *(with David Owen Norris)*

Undercurrent

www.**penguin**.co.uk

Undercurrent

Barney Norris

doubleday

TRANSWORLD PUBLISHERS
Penguin Random House, One Embassy Gardens,
8 Viaduct Gardens, London SW11 7BW
www.penguin.co.uk

Transworld is part of the Penguin Random House group of companies
whose addresses can be found at global.penguinrandomhouse.com

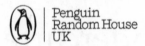

First published in Great Britain in 2022 by Doubleday
an imprint of Transworld Publishers

A CIP catalogue record for this book
is available from the British Library.

ISBN 9780857525734

Typeset in 11/15pt ITC Giovanni by Jouve (UK), Milton Keynes.
Printed and bound in Great Britain by Clays Ltd, Elcograf S.p.A.

The authorized representative in the EEA is Penguin Random House Ireland,
Morrison Chambers, 32 Nassau Street, Dublin D02 YH68.

Penguin Random House is committed to a sustainable
future for our business, our readers and our planet. This book
is made from Forest Stewardship Council® certified paper.

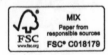

i.m. Sophie Christopher

Show me again the day
When from the sandy bay
We looked together upon the pestered sea! –
Yea, to such surging, swaying, sighing, swelling,
  shrinking,
Love lures life on.

Thomas Hardy, 'Lines to a Movement
in Mozart's E-Flat Symphony'

2019

A WEDDING IN APRIL. Most people wouldn't risk it, but there are discounts to be had, and Leah and Richard have been lucky: the weather's held off and the tents covering the tables and bar and the place where the band will play are unruffled by this still day. On the gravel drive outside the big house that's been rented for the reception, Juliet and I mill around among a hundred other guests, a mixture of friends and strangers, all bored and wanting to get through the photos so we can sit down to eat. We're at an age when weddings seem to happen every other weekend in summer, so even if an April wedding might be a change, the day still feels familiar in its rhythms: the ceremony, the drive to the reception, the photos, the speeches, the drinking, the food – pizzas or hog roast or cheese and biscuits, and cutting the cake – the band, the Airbnb at the end of the evening, drunk sex, a hangover the next morning, driving home to a takeaway in front of the TV.

On the regular occasions when Juliet and I arrive at these days, attending the weddings of friends and relations, enjoying some things, raising eyebrows at others, I often wonder how much she thinks about the day we'll get married, whenever that may be, if that day is going to come. The thought

1

always preoccupies me at these times, but we never seem to talk about it, not in any depth. We'll critique the wedding favours on a table, perhaps, or note the cheap wine, maybe say we'd never serve anything like that ourselves, but the conversation never goes any further. I suppose we've both known ever since we moved in together that marriage would be the next logical step. So perhaps we are poised on the rim of that next chapter in our lives, and trying to work out when to jump.

It's been on my mind for a while that I should make the next move, buy a ring. I only ever want to do it once, though, so I'm taking this thought slowly, letting it creep up on me, letting it grow. I might as well marry beautifully. So I've been saving money, a little here and a little there, and trying to work out how to do it right. It's not the easiest thing to do if you're a copywriter, saving for a wedding. Not if you're paying rent in the city, and your girlfriend likes date night, and date night is always a hundred quid of dinner and wine and a taxi back home, and I suppose I've let thoughts of money slow me down, an excuse to put off getting on with life. Because we never talk about the idea of getting married, I have no clear hints to work on as to what kind of ring I ought to be buying, either, or where I ought to kneel down and propose. So I've let that slow me down too. More reasons to let time drift by, just letting it happen to me, rather than me doing very much with it. We just go from one wedding to another, as if we're glimpsing our own future, hidden in shards among other people's days.

'She keeps looking at you,' Juliet says. I turn to her.

'Who?'

'The photographer. Look, she's looking right at you – see?'

I turn and follow Juliet's gaze in time to see the young woman, standing on a stepladder preparing to take a photograph of everyone, suddenly look away from me and up to the sky as if she's worried about the weather or the light. I almost missed the moment, but as I watch the photographer stare fixedly into the blue, I can tell that Juliet is right. I turned, and the girl was looking right at me. She's attractive, about the same age as us, dark-haired, slender. She looks like a yoga instructor, and hasn't dressed up in wedding clothes. Instead of making her seem shabby, this somehow has the effect of making everyone around her in formal dresses or suits and ties look slightly ludicrous, as if they're wearing their parents' things. It always amazes me just how far into life the feeling persists that everyone you know is only really playing at being grown up. Here we are in our thirties, inheriting the earth maybe, and I still feel as if everyone I know is putting it on.

The girl on the stepladder doesn't look like that, though. She seems at ease, set apart from the crowd, and not just because she's standing above them. As I watch her, she looks back my way again, and smiles, then turns away to talk to one of the best men, who's trying to organise us.

'See?' Juliet asks me.

'I saw, yeah.'

'Who is she?'

'I have no idea.'

'Looks like you've pulled, then.'

I glance quickly at Juliet. Her neck is flushed, and I can see that she's unhappy. The idea that, of all the young men at this wedding, I might be the one the beautiful photographer fancies is patently ludicrous to me, but things like this make Juliet uncomfortable. I put my arm around her and kiss her on the cheek.

'I think it's more likely I've got something in my teeth,' I say.

The joke's not very good, but she smiles nonetheless and pushes me away from her. 'Either that or your flies are undone.'

Then the best man is shouting for our attention, so we turn back to face forwards, ready to be captured for ever as part of this group who were here on this day. Whatever becomes of us all, this happened, we had this much in common, all of us here. My eyes are drawn again to the beautiful young woman on the stepladder, and once again she is looking at me. Some men might be used to this kind of attention. Some might be comfortable with the idea they're attractive to other people. I'm not one of those people, and can't help wondering as we smile and throw hats and plastic cups into the air what the explanation for that look might be. I'm surrounded by beautiful people. It's not going to be that. How could it be?

When the big group photo has been taken, the bride and groom and their families and whoever else wander off with the photographer to be captured in smaller groups down by the river, and Juliet and I drift away from the drive and the front of the house to scrutinise the seating plan and find our way over to our table.

'Was it just that she caught *you* looking at *her*?' Juliet asks.

'Sorry?'

'She's very attractive. Perhaps you were looking at her, and she noticed.'

'Seriously?' Juliet looks at me, and there's an atmosphere

4

between us now, as unfair as that seems. 'I'm here with you at our friends' wedding. I'm not eyeing up the barmaids, I'm not eyeing up the photographer. Don't worry. It's all right.'

Juliet shrugs and looks away. 'I'd understand, is all I was going to say,' she says. 'Looking isn't buying.'

We find our table and sit down together, saying very little till some of our friends find us and sit down on either side. The thought of the photographer has fixed in my mind. I can only half concentrate on the conversations going on around me, because I'm wondering whether I could have seen her before somewhere, wondering why she was looking at me, and whether there'll be a moment this evening when we have an opportunity to meet and speak. It doesn't seem to me that this would be disloyal. Isn't it natural to be interested in someone who shows an interest in you? Isn't it natural to wonder what they're thinking? Under the table I reach out and take Juliet's hand, and she lets me hold it for a moment, then takes it away, and smiles at me, briefly resting the same hand on my arm just below my shoulder.

'Too hot,' she says. And I smile, but I know she's unhappy, because it isn't hot under the tents at all. It's neither my fault nor Juliet's, not really, but something strange has happened and I know we're not going to feel close to each other today. Whenever she encounters things that make her uncomfortable, Juliet's reaction is always to withdraw. I don't know whether I'm the same; perhaps I am. It means our unhappiness always makes us feel alone when it comes, because we're careful to hide it, not to share it with each other.

We all eat together, and then there are some awful speeches, actually quite memorably awful speeches because the groom has appointed four best men, all of whom perform a forfeit in the course of the hour they spend talking to us, which involves downing shots and the singing of songs. Then music starts up, and the guests dance while the tables are cleared and the cake is brought out to be cut. That being done, we all eat the cut cake, then start to get bored till the drink kicks in and a band begins playing and the evening flows more quickly after that.

After half an hour of dancing, once we've worked up a sweat, Juliet and I walk away from the party, down to the bottom of the grounds, past the swimming pool and the tennis court and the little walled garden, till we come to the lake that marks the edge of the park; beyond it, there are cattle cropping the grass in the next field. There's a pontoon jutting out from the side of the lake into the water, and tied to the end of the pontoon is a rowing boat no one's thought to store away while the wedding's going on. It seems to me that the presence of this boat might become dangerous as the night goes on, if anyone finds it once they've had a few drinks. Then I feel disappointed at myself for responding to the boat in that way; why think of the dangers when I could dream instead of launching out on this water?

It occurs to me that the situation Juliet and I find ourselves in gives us the opportunity to be one of three kinds of people. We could worry about the boat, and fret, go and find the people who live in the house, and tell them they ought to store it away; that would make us responsible, rational, grown-up, absolutely divorced from the kids we used to be. Or we could do nothing, which I suspect is what most people would do, just take in the pontoon and the boat at the end of it, perhaps even walk out to get a closer look down into the water for a moment, but then step back and walk away, leaving the boat lying silent in the water. Or, there is a third thing. Perhaps the most irresponsible thing. Perhaps the least sensible or adult or logical. Which would be to get into the boat and cast off and row round the little lake for a short while. Thinking these options through, it seems to me that this is the choice you'd make if you still wanted to be young; if you still wanted as much of life as you could get, all it could offer you; if you still thought the reason you were here was to seek adventure. I turn to Juliet, her face only half visible in the dark now we've walked away from the lights of the party. It's early still, the moon is not yet up.

'Shall we go out on the water?' I ask.

She laughs. 'Why?'

'Might be fun. They've left the boat out.'

'Not because they want people to use it.'

'No one could possibly see us out here, though; we'd be fine.'

'That's not the point, though, is it?'

'Come on. It'll be like Bridget Jones.'

'No it won't, it's dangerous. Let's go back, come on.'

'Just quickly, come on.'

'Ed, I don't want to. Let's go back,' she says. I shrug, admit defeat. But I don't want to go back with her just yet. This thought snags in me slightly. I wonder what it means. It's not the first time this idea has come to me in the last few months.

It occurs to me as we stand there by the lake in the dark, a moment that ought to mean something, that ought to be happy, a secret we ought to feel like we're sharing, that some

kind of link seems to have unthreaded between us. I look at
the woman I've been living with for six years and realise that
sometime in the past year I stopped feeling like we were really
together. And I realise I've known this for a while now. I just
haven't quite acknowledged the feeling. I think of the way
we've been falling asleep the last few months; both of us have
started turning our backs to each other. I'd noticed it, been
aware of it. I hadn't drawn any inference from it till this
moment. But I've been waking up at the edge of the bed for
some time now, and I realise suddenly that it has to mean
something. We used to hold each other in different shapes.
Now, unless there's sex, we sleep alone on different sides of
our shared mattress. And what does that mean? Can you find
your way back from that? I don't know exactly what we've
stopped sharing. Unless it's love. Whatever love might be. I
wonder whether it's something to do with weddings; we're
not so young, after all, and things aren't so new between us.
Was there a tide we missed a while back, when we should
have done more than just live together? Should it have been
the two of us in front of everyone, or is that a stupid thought?
I look at Juliet and can't tell what's missing. But I think
she knows it's not there, too. At least that's something we're
sharing.

'I'll follow you in a minute,' I tell her.

'Why?'

'Don't worry. I'll catch you up.'

'What's your problem?'

'Nothing. I'll just catch you up in a minute, all right? I just
want to stay out here in the quiet for a while.' She shrugs, and
I can see that I've annoyed her. We're not in the same key

today, somehow. I can see now that I made a mistake ever thinking she'd want to get in the boat with me. Juliet's life runs on train tracks, and isn't easily diverted; surprises don't delight her, she doesn't like trying new things, she likes comfort and security, as I suppose most people do. As I suppose I do, mostly. But something about the lake has caught my attention, some deep silence.

'Suit yourself.' Juliet walks away from me and goes off to dance with our friends, and I'm alone in the dark. I turn back to the pontoon and walk along it to the end. The night sky reflects off the still surface of the water. I watch it rippling gently under me. I have stopped being happy somewhere along the way. When did that happen? And what am I going to do about it?

I get into the boat and the ripples of its movement spread to the edge of the water. The oars are stored in the bottom of the boat. I take them out and fix them in the rowlocks before untying the rope attaching the boat to the pontoon and taking an oar in each hand. Leaning forwards to reach for the first stroke, I launch myself through a new element out into the night. The idea comes to me that it might be as easy as this to leave my old life and go looking for a new one. Letting go of one's unhappiness might be as simple as pushing away from a lakeside pontoon. Cutting through new water till you reach another world.

When I've done a circuit of the lake and tied the boat up again, I head back to the party, and skirt round the edge of the festivities, a little downcast, because somehow I feel as if I've done something wrong, though I don't know quite what. In the back of my mind the thought is keening faintly that when

I got back on to the pontoon after rowing, I stepped into a different world. Something intangible about this place is different – or rather, it could be if I chose it to be so. A band playing at a wedding always sounds to me like the saddest thing in the world. The noise of our lives passing. Or perhaps it's just that I never learned the trick of having fun, and moments like this remind me there are aspects of life I miss entirely.

I collapse on a sofa someone has put out in one of the dining tents furthest from the marquee where the band is playing and the guests are dancing. It must have been put there for the elderly to get away from all the noise, but for now everyone more advanced in years is dancing with their kids. That's where she comes and finds me, the photographer, the girl who kept looking at me earlier.

Through the open side of the tent I watch her approaching across the lawn, cutting through the guests, her eyes fixed on me all the time as she approaches. I watch her figure in the clothes she is wearing, wide linen trousers, silk shirt, her dark hair flowing down over her shoulders. She is wearing sandals and her feet are wet. She sits down on the sofa, then turns away from me, looking instead across the lawn at the band and the dancers visible through the marquee's open sides. I turn as well, following her gaze, looking out across the night.

'Hi.'

'Hello.'

'My name's Ed.'

She smiles at me. 'I'm Amy.'

'I thought I caught your eye earlier.'

'You did.'

'Do you know them?' I point to Richard and Leah, the bride and groom, who are dancing together to the band's cover of 'Teenage Dirtbag'.

'No, I'm just a wedding photographer. They found me online. I've got to know them since, but I don't *know* them.'

We watch the dancing for a moment before she speaks again. 'Do you like Laurie Lee?'

'Sorry?' Her question is so unexpected that for a moment I don't know who she means.

'Laurie Lee. Have you read him? *Cider with Rosie.*'

'Oh. Yes, I have. Yes, I do.'

'I want to tell you a story about him.'

I can't quite work out what's going on. It's impossibly surreal to me, that this girl wants to talk to me, but only about poets.

'Go on.'

She smiles, and leans towards me, so that she's looking past, lips close to my ear as she speaks. The words become secrets only for me, and I feel the heat of her breath on my cheek as she tells her story while Chinese lanterns are lit on the lawn before us and released into the clear night air.

'Not all of the stories about Laurie Lee are beautiful,' she says, 'because he liked women a *lot*, so a lot of stories about him have a very similar narrative. Benny Hill stories, if you know what I mean. But as well as chasing girls, Laurie Lee also liked to take his violin into pubs and play to people. And one night, in the crowd where he was playing, he noticed a very beautiful young woman. A girl really, no more than about eighteen. She was standing at the back of the audience gathered round him, and didn't seem to know anyone else there, and she looked at him very intently all the time he played. Of course, he wanted to play it cool, like he hadn't noticed. I quite like that about Laurie Lee; he still played the game that women might want to go to bed with him well into his seventies. So he kept going with the tunes, and then when the barman called time, he saw the girl who'd been watching him turn and walk out of the pub. And suddenly he was seized by this fierce feeling that he had to speak to her, and she was leaving before he'd had the chance. So he called after her. "Have we met before somewhere?" he asked. And she smiled. "We have," she said. "I'm your daughter."'

Amy shifts and crosses her legs, angling her body away from me as she leans back against the arm of the sofa, and I want to ask her why she's telling me this story, but I don't speak because I'm afraid that if I interrupt her she'll stop talking and the spell will be broken. She looks at me and carries on. 'Laurie Lee, you see, had had a daughter with the wife of another man years earlier. He'd known her while she was small, but then when she was five or six, he stopped talking to her mother and they lost touch. This was her. Her mother had never mentioned who her father really was, but she'd seen Laurie Lee on the TV one day and thought, "That man's my father." Apparently, people sometimes just know. I don't know why. Maybe she'd already heard stories, and knew her mum had known Laurie Lee, and something about him made sense to her. So she went to see him play the violin one evening. And they knew each other for the rest of his life. Can you imagine that? Wouldn't that be the strangest life? I don't think I'd ever get used to it. I thought of that story when I saw you today.'

I try to work out what she means.

'Why? Do I remind you of your father, or Laurie Lee?'

She smiles and says nothing to that, simply leaning further back into the sofa, comfortable now, relaxed.

'I'm talking too much,' she says.

'You're not.'

She smiles at this, as if she doesn't believe me. 'There was a point,' she says. 'But I've started on the wrong foot.'

'No, you haven't,' I say. 'What were you meaning to tell me?'

'You sure you want to hear?'

'Absolutely. Go on.'

She takes a breath, searches the night sky above her for the thread of the thought she's been unspooling. Then seems to find it again, and continues, this time looking up and not at me, as if the whole experience is suddenly painful, as if she's trying not to cry.

'Reunions don't always go as well as that, though,' she says. 'When I met my birth father, it was very different. I assumed it would be a good thing to do. But not many people will give up a child for adoption if they're in a good place. I went and saw him when I was eighteen, as soon as I was allowed to, basically. I thought it would help me understand who I was. My adoptive parents had told me all along that I had once been another couple's child, and that always nagged at me while I was growing up. I always thought it must mean there were things about myself I wouldn't be able to understand until I knew the whole story. I think that really affected me, growing up. I did all kinds of things I regret. It was an excuse, really. I told myself that justified pretty much whatever I wanted to do. It was stupid. I fucked up my A levels and it meant I didn't go to university. So when I turned eighteen, I thought it would be good to snap out of that. It would be good for this not to be a mystery any more, so that I could make whatever decision I needed to make about who I really was, and get on with whatever my life was going to be. So I got access to my birth certificate. I already knew my birth mother had died while she was having me, and that was basically why I'd been given away. But my birth father was still around, so I wrote to him, and he wrote back. My adoptive parents, my real parents, knew all about it; they were supportive. Cautious, of course, but they understood it was something I needed to do. So I went. He lived in a horrible little town by the sea, in this empty little flat in a council building, and he had no possessions, really, a couple of kitchen chairs and an old armchair and a fridge. He let me in and I wanted to recognise him like Laurie Lee's daughter recognised her father, but it wasn't like that. He was just a man I felt sorry for when I saw him. I didn't feel much connection at all. He was quite a tall man, and furtive, very distant; he didn't like making eye contact with me. When he saw me, he just cried. He just burst into tears.'

As I watch her, I see the memory of the day take over, see the tears start in her eyes. ' "My God," he said. "My God, you look just like her." And I guessed he meant my mum. I didn't know what to say. I almost felt like I should apologise, because the way I looked had upset him.'

She pauses for a moment, breathing deeply.

I guess this must feel like someone walking on her grave.

14

The shiver of glimpsing the life she didn't have, the different person she might have been if she had been brought up by her birth parents. And how would that have changed them? What different lives would they have lived then? The possibilities become too many to take in at once. And the ghost lives that pass before your eyes in these moments are like very beautiful, very sad music. I find myself thinking of my own father, the last times we spent together before he died, and how keenly I wished things had been different then. I guess this young woman must be feeling something similar. Keenly aware of the lives she hadn't lived. She steels herself, goes on.

'I'd never thought of that before, you see. Because of course no one ever said I looked like my adoptive parents. So I'd never thought before about the way I walked round all the time actually looking like someone else. I still can't get my head round that, not really. My father invited me in and I sat down on one of the chairs. He put the kettle on, and apologised for the bareness of the house; he'd just been let out of prison and he was getting his life back together again, he said. He made me tea, and sat down in the other chair, and apologised for crying when he saw me, but he didn't even have a photo of my mum any more so it had come as a shock to see her again. That was the way he said it, "see her again". I was wondering all of a sudden whether he'd actually bought the chairs so that he could have me over, something about the way he sat down in them, something about the way they were positioned in the middle of the room with nothing to lean on, no table, not so much as a windowsill or anything, made me feel like they'd been specially set there, and he wasn't used to them. I felt so sorry for him then. This man was trying his best, he'd done what he could to be hospitable, and it was just crap, it wasn't nice at all, even though he'd tried. And I hadn't been gracious about it, I hadn't said anything about his flat being nice and clean or tried to make it OK between us. When it was very clean, actually; he must have hoovered and scrubbed all morning getting it ready for me to come round. And then I realised that this had been a terrible idea. I'm normally very careful about letting people into my life. Because once something's happened between two people, and it doesn't have to be a big thing – it could just be a coffee or a talk on a sofa in the middle of the night, or it could just be that you take the photos at their wedding – but once that's happened you have a kind of secret together. You've shared something no two other people have ever shared in exactly the same way. And that can last a whole life, it can bind you. But it was too late to back out of it by then. So I talked to him. I asked him about his life. And it was clear he'd been destroyed by the death of my mother. He gave me up for adoption. He had a job but he lost it, and then he assaulted a police officer one Saturday night – I got the impression he'd become quite a violent drunk – and was put away for a couple of years because of that. Then he'd come out of prison and got on with his life for a while, and actually things had been a bit better, he'd cut down the drink and the drugs and stayed in the one job, doing shelves at a branch of Tesco's, and he had an OK flat, better than the one we were sitting in now, he said. But then it went wrong again somehow. He beat someone up and went back to prison for another few years. I listened to him talking and it was just awful. I couldn't believe this was my dad.'

'I'm so sorry,' I say.

She shrugs and smiles. 'Yeah. It was hard. I envy Laurie Lee and his daughter.'

'Do you still keep in touch?'

'I do, yeah. I don't go and see him so much. But he's doing all right. Actually, he's doing better.'

'That's good.'

'I think it helped him to meet me, somehow. He'd never regretted giving me up for adoption, he said. Because it meant I'd had a better life, whereas he was sure he couldn't have offered me anything. But when he met me, I think that connected him with a part of his own life he'd lost when I left.'

'Did the same happen for you?'

'That's the sad thing. Absolutely not. I didn't learn anything about myself. Except that he said everyone had loved my mum, and she'd been very striking. That was nice, I suppose. And I realised what a complete idiot I'd been for the last few years, telling myself I could do anything I liked or as little as I liked, because I didn't really know who I was, so nothing really counted. That was always bollocks, it was always an excuse. Meeting him didn't make anything clearer. It actually made things stranger, I think.'

'Why stranger?'

'Just thinking of the other person I might have been. And having to confront how fortunate I'd been. And wondering where that other me was, and not being quite able to shake the thought that she existed in another ghost life somewhere else.'

'And can I ask you a question?'

'Go on.'

'Why are you telling me all this? I don't mean to sound rude. It's interesting. I'm interested. But I get the feeling there's a connection I haven't worked out yet.'

'Oh yeah,' she laughs, and her smile strikes me like an electric charge. 'Yeah, I should tell you about that.'

'I think you're about to say we've met before somewhere.'

'That's right. Can you remember where?'

'Not at all. I think I'd remember you if we'd met. I'm worried you might have the wrong person.'

She laughs then.

'I haven't,' she says. 'It just so happens that I looked you up not all that long ago. Just going down memory lane, you know? And I was looking at the photo list for this wedding yesterday and your name caught my eye and I thought it would be the weirdest coincidence if it was actually you. So I looked you up again last night, actually, then I saw you today and I knew it was you.'

'How do you know me, then?'

'Well, unless I've got this really wrong, I think you saved me from drowning when I was six years old.'

Memory rushes in. I look in amazement at her. I haven't thought of that day in a very long time. It comes back to me now like a dream after waking.

'That was you?'

'It was. I was thinking about it a couple of years ago. And I knew your name, because there was a little article about it in the local paper – do you remember?'

'I do. I've got the cutting somewhere.'

'So have I. I found it in a folder one day and I thought, "I wonder what became of him?" And I looked you up. So when I saw you in the crowd today, I knew it was you.'

A childhood holiday, ten years old. We'd gone to a town with a stretch of beach and a kind of swimming pool carved into the rock just below the high-tide line, I suppose because sometimes it got too choppy to swim in the sea. We'd been swimming in the pool quite a lot. The weather had been beautiful that whole week, and we'd spent a lot of time jumping into the pool then climbing out to dry off, lying on the rocks and looking out to sea. Then as the day waned and it got too cold, we'd walk back towards our holiday house along the beach or up over the rocks and the cliffs above it, and get chips from the little café by the car park, and eat them on the sand or in the car or once we got home. It might have been the most perfect holiday we ever had; my sister Rachel was only three years old, and I remember I loved those early years, following her progress as she learned to walk and talk, and seemed to turn into a proper person before my very eyes as if her life was some kind of magic trick. It was a lovely thing to be ten and have a sister whose wonder at everything could entertain you all day, but who would also go to bed early and leave you with time to play on your own, or go exploring round the garden or the now quiet rooms of the holiday home.

The day I saved Amy, though, Rachel had been playing up. This was probably the only reason the whole thing happened. We'd gone to the sea, and set up camp down on the sand because it was low tide and the beach stretched out for ever, but it was a hot day, and after an hour or so Rachel had begun to grizzle. We held out till lunch, eating the sandwiches we'd brought down with us in a picnic basket, followed by ice creams and cold drinks from the café by the beach, but by that time my sister was screaming, and Mum was losing patience and must have felt that all the other families on the beach were looking at us. So she decided to go back to the holiday house with my sister, in the hope that Rachel would be quieter if she could get out of the heat. Chris, my step-dad, offered to take my sister back instead, but I think Mum had had enough of the whole thing by then, the baking-hot sand and the time passing slowly as we all took turns to have a dip into the sea to cool ourselves off, so she said she'd go, and Chris could stay behind with me.

We helped her pack up and walked back with her as far as the café, then once we'd seen them off Chris suggested we move our camp, as the sun was beating down on the beach and we needed to look for some shade. He suggested we try the swimming pool in the rock. I wanted to go to the loos in the café first, so Chris said I should meet him by the pool when I was done.

As I came to the swimming pool, a movement in the water caught my eye. At the shaded end of the pool, out of the light and a little distance from any other swimmer, a child was swimming on her own. The end of the pool she was swimming in, being in shadow, was nearly empty; anyone who had got into the pool was trying to swim in the sun. No one seemed to be swimming with the child, who I could see now was a young girl, and who was splashing around a couple of feet from the edge of the pool without any armbands on. As I watched her, hardly concentrating on her because I was making my way round the pool and watching my step so I didn't fall in, it suddenly struck me that there was something uncoordinated and urgent about the way the girl was swimming. Even as I watched, I saw her head dip under the water. As I started to wonder whether she was really swimming at all, and might in fact be in some difficulty, my foot slipped on a slick patch of rock by the side of the pool, and I fell headfirst into the water, straight towards the girl I had been watching.

I realised before I hit the water what must have happened. The little girl had been walking round the pool like me, not looking properly at where she was going, just as I hadn't, and she had stepped on the same slick rock and fallen in. She wasn't swimming at all, and somehow no one had noticed she was missing, no one had seen her slip. As I plunged into the pool and salt water rushed into my nose and my eyes, I thrashed my arms and legs till I was the right way up in the water, and looked about, thinking I should call to someone who could help the girl, only to breathe in a lungful of sea-water and find I couldn't speak. It was as I coughed this up that it occurred to me perhaps the person best placed to rescue the drowning child might actually be me. She was only a couple of strokes away, struggling underwater still – she must have been under for a few seconds now, and I worried she'd be breathing in water just as I had. So I swam over to the girl and grabbed her as best I could, manipulating her flailing limbs till her head came back up to the surface again, where she took a deep, desperate breath and started to scream. Now several adults looked over towards us, and I cried for help as best I could, finding that I was being pushed below the

21

surface by the girl as she tried to scrabble away from danger. The next thing I knew, strong hands took hold of us both, and we were dragged forcibly through the resisting water and out on to the ledge around the pool. Chris had arrived by then, and rushed over to me where I sat and coughed up the last of the seawater I'd breathed in. The little girl's parents held their child, clearly in shock, a desperate panic setting in just as the emergency had passed because they'd only just discovered she'd been in danger.

I was accorded hero status for saving the child, who hadn't been able to swim, and shouldn't have taken off her armbands, and shouldn't have been walking on her own round the dark side of the pool without her parents, of course. One of the people who'd helped us both out of the water called the local paper to report the daring rescue, and I was both proud and embarrassed to see my name appear in print a couple of days later. The paper came out the day we were leaving to travel home, and Mum and Chris were triumphant, holding it up like a kind of trophy. This was too much for me, and I started to cry. They asked me why I wasn't pleased that I'd been recognised for my bravery in saving the little girl, and I said that I was, I was very pleased, but I thought I hadn't been honest as well, because I hadn't really saved her, I'd just fallen in and tried to save her but then discovered that I couldn't, and I didn't want to get in trouble for not telling the whole truth. This made Mum and Chris laugh, which confused me; but they told me there was no way that I could get in trouble, and when we got home, Mum gave me a rosette like the ones you get for horse-riding competitions, and said it was for bravery, and that I should keep it as a memento.

As for the girl I saved, I never spoke a word to her. She was quickly taken away by her parents, who were both terrified to discover how close she'd been to death, and mortified not to have noticed she was missing. Her name wasn't included in the article that mentioned me, as I suppose thinking back that the parents hadn't wanted social services reading what had happened, and I had forgotten all about her by the end of that summer, really. Years later, when I moved away from home, I had found the rosette Mum gave me, and remembered the day, and felt a little proud, I admit, because I realised that the situation might have been more dangerous than I realised. I kept the rosette because of that. But it was stored away in a box in the attic at Mum and Chris's farm, a buried memory; it wasn't like I took it out to look at all the time.

'That's extraordinary,' I say.

'I don't know,' Amy replies.

'Why?'

'Well, it just seems natural to me, somehow. It seems almost inevitable that we should meet again.'

Amy tells me she only dimly remembers the whole thing: a sense of panic, a sense she was going to die. She built up a picture of what happened through what other people had told her about it, her adoptive parents above all, who used the story to justify keeping her on a short lead for a while, and then, as time went by, made the story into something they could all laugh about. In their version, I was the hero who jumped in to save her. When I tell her I slipped just like she did, and my rescue attempt was more or less an accident, she's delighted. It seems wonderful to her to hear an old piece of family history reinterpreted so differently after so many years. These stories are how we understand ourselves, after all, she says – the scraps from which we build our ideas of who we are, of family and home. There's something magical to her about discovering this story might be made up, and that by implication every story she has used to work out who she is might also be a form of fiction as well.

We continue talking together on the sofa in the tent on the edge of the lawn for half an hour, till Juliet comes and finds me, clearly alarmed to see me sitting with Amy away from the rest of the guests, the photographer she suspected I was eyeing up a few hours ago. Amy is quick to explain the connection between us before Juliet even has the opportunity to ask; then she stands up, tells us both it was nice to meet us, and slips away.

Juliet watches me. 'You saved her life?'

'Sort of. Not really.'

She looks away. I try to speak as nonchalantly as I can, throw away the significance of that conversation, because as Amy walks back to the party, looking back once to smile at me, I feel suddenly certain it is very significant indeed, and I need to hide that, set that aside, wait till I have time to work out what it means and what might be happening.

'Small world,' Juliet says. The skin around her mouth is tight, and her eyes seem hard and dark as she looks away from me and over at the marquee where the guests are still dancing. And suddenly I wonder whether the reason I've held back from proposing to her these last few years might not really be that I'm saving up money; suddenly I wonder whether that's a lie, and the reason I've held back is something else, some absence I've known was there and never been able to name before tonight. I look at Juliet, and the possibility creeps up on me that I've had it wrong for years.

Strange, how these moments of clarity arrive, how they always comes so suddenly, how it's never when you'd think. Have I been a coward all this time for having known deep down there was something missing between us, perhaps even love, and not raising the issue, not saying anything? Have I spoiled this with my own detachment, which Juliet's had to live with, which she's slowly withdrawn from, until the two of us are walled off from one another now, miles apart with acres of silence between us? I feel almost sure I can hear in the silence between us that Juliet's feeling the same thing too.

How long have we both been feeling this way? How long since she last knew for certain that she loved me, and I knew that I loved her? When was the last time sex between us was a real connection? And how long have we spent pretending? I can't work out why these questions are coming to me now. What's so important about this night? Surely it can't just be one conversation with a stranger, one memory of a child-hood holiday long ago? Surely it takes more than that to turn a simple story into a fundamental questioning of the course of one's life? Or does it always seem this quick and easy when it happens, one chapter giving way to another with no more fanfare than the turn of a page?

My relationship with Juliet never recovers after that night. The day after the wedding I put Amy out of my mind, and Juliet and I go home to our flat and on Monday we both go back to work. I don't look Amy up online, don't scroll through her photography website, looking at the photographs she's taken of other people's happiness. I think of her a little, it would be a lie to say I don't. And I mention having met her on the phone to my mum, who remembers the time when I saved the little girl from drowning, and seems curiously relaxed about the fact we've met again, as if this is logical and natural, as if she always expected me to call one day and let her know we'd met. Other than that, Juliet and I get on with our lives, and nothing is outwardly different. There is only the single, crucial change that both of us know, I think we both know, that we no longer want to be with each other. When we're together in the evenings and I ask her how her day has been, she fobs me off with the briefest of answers. I do the same.

A day comes when she gets home from work and tells me she's booked a holiday that summer with her girlfriends, planning a summer without me, and I know we can't go on.

'When are you going away?' I ask her.

'Why? Do you have plans?'

'I'm only interested. I suppose I'm just wondering when we'll go on holiday.'

'Oh.' She shrugs, walking out of the room to go and shower and wash off the day. 'I don't know. I didn't know you wanted to. I suppose we can fit it around things if we want to go away.' She is planning her life after me, I realise.

'You don't want to, then,' I say. It's childish of me to feel hurt by this, because I realise that in a way I must have caused it, but I'm hurt all the same, so I think, fuck it – I'll be childish.

'Why do you say that?'

'I think you've made it very fucking clear you don't want anything to do with me at the moment.'

'I honestly don't know what you're talking about, Ed.'

'Fuck off, Jules.' Listening to myself, I think I must seem pathetic right now, resorting, so early in the argument, to swearing at her. The surest sign of a losing hand. It must be me who's in the wrong here. But it's she who's booking holidays like we'll have broken up by summer, so what have I done wrong?

'You fuck off, I've booked a holiday – why does that mean you're angry at me?'

'We both know.'

'Do we? What do we know?'

'Fuck off, Jules, we both know.'

'I know you've been withdrawn for fucking ages and don't want to touch me any more.' This is true, but seems unfair to me: since we came home from the wedding, she's been turning her back on me the minute she gets into bed.

'Why didn't you get in the boat?' I ask her. The question surprises me as I ask it; I hadn't known that was what I was going to say.

'What?'

'At the wedding. By the lake. Why did you go back? Why didn't you get in the boat with me?'

'That's what you took from that wedding?'

'I just want to know.'

She sighs, exasperated. 'It wasn't ours. It wasn't safe. It was antisocial to be away from everyone like that.'

'We wouldn't have stayed there all night.'

'I didn't want to, Ed. Is that OK? I didn't want to get in the fucking boat.'

And maybe in the end it's as simple as that. We had the chance to be one of three kinds of people. We made different choices. Now a fissure between us is opening up. Probably these choices present themselves to us thousands of times every day, and turn into our lives. I suppose we'd spot them time and again if we looked close enough. But most of the time we're not looking. Most of the time we don't notice the way our roads diverge. It was just something about that night, the lake, the reeds, that made things different, enabling me to see clearly for the first time what was going on, to see we were different people moving down different paths.

'You sure that's all you didn't want?'

She laughs at me, bitterly.

'Trust me, it's you that's leaving, Ed, not the other way round.'

We break up a month or so later, one argument having piled up on another till staying together just doesn't seem possible any more.

She suggests we meet in public for a drink after work, and I guess what's coming. I toy all afternoon with the idea of leaving her before she can leave me, starting the scene myself, or just not turning up, but it seems petty. She's the one who's suggested the drink, she should get to do the talking. We meet in a bar in east London near the office where I'm working, and she looks beautiful, all dressed up, as if she's going out somewhere afterwards. I don't know when we last dressed up for each other – not since the wedding, and even that wasn't really for each other, even that was just what the occasion demanded.

'I wanted to talk to you away from the flat because I think we have problems,' Juliet says. 'I want to ask you a very straight question and I hope you'll be honest with me when you reply. Are you seeing someone else?'

I've never been asked this before, and for a moment it throws me. It feels so like being in a film that responding in the moment is quite difficult. Too many half-remembered lines from the movies come into my head.

'No. Are you?'

'Of course not. I want to ask you as well whether you've been in touch with that girl who took the photos at Leah and Richard's wedding.'

'The girl that I saved from the swimming pool? No. I haven't.'

Juliet nods, taking this in. She's probably disappointed; it would be easier to leave me if I'd actually done something wrong. 'I'm sorry to ask, then,' she says. 'There was something about the way you were talking with her.'

'Nothing happened between us at all, Jules. It was just an extraordinary coincidence; I don't think you can blame me for talking to her about it. We've talked about this already, more than once.'

Juliet picks up her wine glass and half drains it. 'I know,' she says. 'I don't know what happened. I haven't quite come back from that night.'

'I know.'

She looks at me sharply.

'You do?'

'I live with you, remember?'

'It's not anything that happened. I just haven't felt OK ever since.'

I feel as if I would be able to spell it out for her if she really wanted me to. Something about that night at the wedding showed us both that we were treading water, that we'd been treading water for some time, that somehow we'd stopped being happy together, and very soon we weren't going to be living the same lives, our lives were going to travel in completely different directions. I don't know what it was, what forces were pulling at us, but we felt them all the same, and realised they'd been doing that for some time before that evening. It was one of those discoveries that couples sometimes make when they become conscious that things are going to end between them.

'I'm sorry you haven't felt OK,' I say. It crosses my mind that I should reach out and take her hand, but then the thought occurs to me that we might end up staying together if I try too hard, she might lose heart and decide not to leave me. I don't know when that was last what I wanted. 'I don't know why it means you've shut yourself off from me.'

Juliet looks hurt, and my stomach drops a little when I see the cloud pass over her face, because I don't want to hurt her or make her unhappy. But sitting here, drinking with the woman I've shared the last six years with, I know very clearly that I want to end this evening alone.

'Is that what you think I'm doing?' she asks.

'Yeah, pretty much. I feel like we didn't really come home from that wedding. Not as we were. I feel like parts of us must still be there.'

'I feel the same, if I'm honest.'

'I thought you might. I'm glad you've brought it up. I didn't really know how to.'

'So what's happened?'

'I don't know. I think something's gone.'

'Something's gone?'

'Don't you agree?' I can see she's really thinking about this. I watch her working through the implications of the thought. I might still be able to call this back, if I change tack now, if I beg her to love me. A part of me wants to. But it seems that there's a current that's carrying me away, and it keeps me silent when I could speak up; it keeps me from speaking while Juliet realises for the first time that she's not in love with me either.

'I think you might be right.'

'What do you want to do about it?' I ask her. 'Do you think we should have some time apart?' This all feels so civilised, so bloodless, so unreal. I'd almost rather we were screaming at each other.

'Is that what you want?'

'I don't know. You've asked to talk about this; I want to know what you're thinking.'

'I suppose maybe it would be good if we gave each other some time to work out what's happened, and what it is we want.'

I hold out my hands in a kind of shrug, as if I'm pushing all responsibility away on to her.

'If that's what you want,' I say.

She looks at me suspiciously. 'You're taking all this very easily.'

'Am I?'

'Is this what you wanted to happen tonight?'

'Is it what I wanted to happen?'

'I just wondered. You haven't answered, by the way.'

I shake my head at her. 'We don't have to argue, do we? We've both said what we want and we want the same thing.'

Juliet looks away, gets out her phone and checks the time. Perhaps she is going out. Perhaps she'll go on from here for drinks with her girlfriends. Perhaps she's even going to meet another man, someone from work, who knows? I wouldn't blame her. We must both have felt lonely these past few weeks. It occurs to me that I don't feel possessive of her at all tonight. As if that phase of our relationship is already long past. I wonder when it ended. What were we doing the last time I would have bridled at the thought of her with someone else?

'I can move out,' I say.

'That would probably be the best arrangement, seeing as it's my flat,' she replies.

I smile; she meant it as a put-down, but it strikes me as funny all the same. 'Fair point.'

'Where will you go?' she asks.

'I don't know yet. I haven't thought about it.' She doesn't respond. 'I'll be all right,' I tell her.

'Will you go back and live with your parents?'

'At the farm? God, no.'

'She'd want to help you if she knew, you know,' Juliet says.

'Knew what?'

'That you're homeless.'

'I'm not homeless. I'm just moving out.'

32

She shrugs.

'OK,' she says. 'I just think your mum would want to help if she knew what was happening. And maybe you should let her.' She puts her phone away from where it's been lying on the table, and empties her glass, and puts it down. I think of the Streets, the way this moment has been entirely colonised, at least for my generation, by a song, so that presumably no one lives through a break-up in a bar any more without hearing 'Dry Your Eyes' playing in the back of the brain, no one sees the scene for what it is, they see it through the filter of that music.

'This is all a bit civilised and grown-up, isn't it?' she says.

'I know,' I say. 'But thank you for saying it.'

'Life is too short. This is the only time we'll be alive,' she replies as she stands up from the table. 'I don't mean to hurt your feelings, but I don't think it's worthwhile pretending something's good enough, in the end.'

1911

I N THE BEGINNING there was noise, such noise. Chai sellers in the square and the chatter of hawkers, children laughing, drum of their feet against the stones where they ran and played, the spit and stutter of cooking always at the margins of each scene and the pleasant patina of human life around her house, all drowned, all dwarfed by the coming of the railways, din of their construction through the years of her childhood and the clatter and thrum of the trains passing through and the trains going into their sidings. All those years it was the trains that sang in her ears, changing everything, bringing goods from impossibly far away, carrying the produce of Hyderabad into the unknowable distance, out of the heart of India to who knew where else on earth, far away to the sea and the wide world beyond it, the sea she had never seen and could not even have imagined in those years long lost, so long ago. It always seemed to her like a miracle that the steam and oil and din of the trains brought forth the mangoes and spices and cloth that dazzled her so when her mother brought them into the house after shopping in the bazaar, that the living produce and bright dyes people made with such skill in Hyderabad could be packed away into crates that all looked the same, though they contained whole worlds within them, and loaded on to trains, and turned, as if by magic, into the same steam, oil and din.

Hyderabad was a place in between things, on the banks of the Musi, a city ringed by lakes. It used to smell alive, incredibly alive whatever hour of the day you breathed it in, the richness of its aromas a hymn to the miracle and the dream of civilisation, gathering together all human industry and endeavour into one complex, overwhelming bouquet: garlic and cooking, spices and tobacco, dung in the heat, sandalwood, smoke. All the city's colours were another celebration – the saris and dhotis rippling the surface of each street, flowers in women's hair like stars. The city's wealth rested on its status as a place for diamond trading, and for trading in pearls; though it was far from the sea, it was a great centre for the buying and selling of pearls.

Her father was never involved in those more ancient under-takings, the trading of pearls, the trading of perfumes – he lived among steel and packing crates, he was not a man of the bazaar. He came to the city after the arrival of the railways, when the factories were first being built, to seek his fortune in business while Hyderabad grew around him and new oppor-tunities presented themselves in industry, transportation, infrastructure, telecommunications. He tried his hand at every-thing, and enough of it proved successful that he came in time to be judged a success. He was a busy man, always chasing opportunities, chasing debts. She never saw very much of him. That was the way it was between fathers and daughters at that time. It never seemed strange to her; besides, her world was built around someone else.

In the beginning was her mother, a woman of extraordinary

beauty. Everyone who knew her said so – a woman people stared at, a woman who was listened to with a different quality of attention from that which was accorded to any of her friends. To Phoebe it had always seemed absurd, really, that the beautiful get more attention. But that was the world she was born into, that had always been the way of things wherever she'd gone in her life. It meant that her mother was used to finishing her sentences in a way few women of her class and background were in Hyderabad at that time, and that she had great influence among her friends. She used to hold parties, welcoming some of the most prominent people of the city into the home she had made with her husband. How she loved those sparkling, champagne evenings. That was how the family came to mingle with the British who lived in the city. Few of them ever came to the parties, but Phoebe's parents were recognised as significant people among the local population because they created that role for themselves, and were invited to the Secunderabad Club and the officers' mess, and in that way they mixed with the white men who ran things in Hyderabad. That was how Phoebe first met Arthur.

She knew from an early age that what her mother wished most of all for her was that she might meet a man from the British army, or failing that a businessman, marry him, and better the lot of the family in that way. As far back as Phoebe could remember, her mother always used to call her beautiful. She believed her own beauty had been reborn in her daughter, just as Shakespeare promised in the sonnets, and she hoped her daughter would secure success for the family by taking advantage of those charms, and meeting and marrying a British officer. She used to talk about that future with

Phoebe, over and over again on the long afternoons of her childhood, until it became Phoebe's own dream, until it became the only future she could imagine. So Phoebe used to go with her mother to the balls and gatherings at the officers' mess and the Railway Institute, which her father had recently been allowed to join, and her mother would teach her about the way to talk to a man so he thought you found him interesting, and by the time Phoebe was thirteen they were searching quite deliberately for a husband for her.

To Phoebe, her mother was the whole world. Of all the people who loved her mother and thought she was beautiful, no one believed it more fiercely than she did. She adored the wisdom her mother had, the elegance and refinement. She wanted to do whatever her mother wanted, to make her proud; she wanted nothing more than to make her happy. So she pursued this dream of her mother's with all her heart, made it her own, never really questioned where it would lead her if she saw it through to the end, because it was what her mother wanted and that was enough. She used to listen to the din of the trains, and watch the thin men in their billowing pantaloons loading all the wonders of Hyderabad into those endless, identical crates and taking them away from the city to distant, other worlds. She watched them and knew one day she would go the same way – packed, or so she imagined, into a crate of her own, her own vanishing act, whisked wherever her husband willed. And that thought used to fill her with happiness, because it was what her mother wanted, and making her mother happy was all she desired.

'Will I still live here with you?' she used to ask her mother when she was very young.

'Of course not. You will go wherever your husband decides.'

'But will I still be able to see you and Father and my brothers and sisters?'

Her mother shrugged. 'It will depend,' she said.

'On what?'

'On many things. On the man you marry, and what he is like, and what he makes of us, and where his work will take him. A family does not have rights over its daughters once it has married them off. I still see my mother, but that is because I am fortunate. I live close to her, and your father understands that it helps me to see my family, and he likes my family well enough. But there is one great difference between you and me.'

'What is that?'

'I married an Indian. You will marry an Englishman. So who knows what will become of you once that is done? No one in this family has done that before; you will be the first, you will be the one to discover it for us, and then we will know what it is like.'

From that single point of difference, their paths diverged so wildly that in the end Phoebe found herself a whole world away from the life her mother knew, and could not imagine the leap it would take for her to recover the young girl she had once been. She supposed that girl was gone.

Once she was thirteen years old she went along with her mother to every party her mother attended, as that was the strategy they had evolved for introducing her to the right English officer.

'You will have to be patient,' her mother would tell her. 'These people have an idea of themselves that is very high and mighty. They do not just go about marrying Indian girls as if it is nothing; most of these men think of going back to England and marrying girls from the villages they once called home. We will have to find a special one for you.'

Phoebe didn't mind that; that sounded much better to her than marrying just anyone. She thought her mother meant that they would need to find a prince.

She met her husband four or five times before it even occurred to her that he might be a man that she might marry. It took her so long to realise because he was so very much older than she was, well into his thirties when he first inclined his head towards her and offered her a smile.

'And what is your name, young lady?' he asked, the first words he spoke to her. At that time he was still a good-looking man, very tall and well built, and his moustaches seemed almost too big for his head, as if the weight of them might cause his neck to ache. Phoebe was most impressed by that moustache, but she could not say she was immediately attracted to him – it was at least another year before the thought occurred to her that it must tickle to kiss him, with so much hair on his lip, which she regarded as the first time she thought about him in any amorous way at all.

'My name is Phoebe, sir.' He did not take her hand and kiss it, or anything like that. He merely inclined his head with a smile, and Phoebe gave the smallest of curtsies, as her mother had taught her, knowing her mother was standing beside her and watching to make sure that Phoebe remembered. He turned from Phoebe to speak to her mother.

'The two of you could be sisters!' he said. Phoebe found this confusing; her mother was much older than her, after all, and they did not look very much like each other, as she had her father's paler skin. Her mother, however, seemed to think he had said something extremely funny.

'Yes, she is very grown up for her age!'

'I rather meant that you are very youthful for yours, madam.' And they both laughed, and Phoebe smiled with them, wondering what they were talking about and wishing that she was at home.

She met Mr French, as she was told to call him, three more times at various functions over the subsequent year before her mother started to talk to her seriously about him. She called Phoebe to her room one afternoon, and Phoebe stood in front of her where she lay on the divan bed, rubbing her feet surreptitiously against the carpet because her mother's room had the best carpet in the house and she liked the way it felt against her skin.

'What do you make of Mr French?' she asked.

'Mr French?'

'The man from the railways that we met last week. We have met him before.'

'Oh, yes. The man with the big moustache.'

'That's right.'

'He seems a nice man. Is he working with Father?'

Her mother thought about this for a moment. 'Not at present, no. He may do in future, though.' Phoebe said nothing to this, not knowing what she was supposed to say, so her mother continued. 'We think he might be interested in you.'

At first, she didn't understand what her mother meant – the thought of his interest being romantic did not occur to her, because there was such a great difference in their ages. 'What do you mean, Mother?'

'We think he might be interested in marrying you. He has said as much to your father. It would be a very advantageous match for all concerned.'

Phoebe, shocked beyond words by this news, began to cry.

'What are you doing?' her mother snapped, apparently irritated by her daughter's display of emotion.

'I'm sorry,' Phoebe said, hiding her face in her hands.

'Really,' her mother said, 'you have no idea how lucky you would be. What a great honour this would be for our whole family, if Mr French were indeed willing to marry you. You should go away and think about being more grateful.'

The next time they attended a social event, her mother let her know that Arthur – or Mr French, as she always called him, even after the wedding was over – would be in attendance also, and that he was hoping to speak to her. Phoebe replied that of course she would talk to him, she would do whatever her mother wanted. So she dressed up in her most beautiful clothes, and went with her father and mother to the British officers' mess, and took a glass from a tray as she walked into the party, feeling sophisticated and hoping she was at least passably beautiful that night, feeling very young and very frail and frightened. Arthur had already arrived, and was standing with a group of other men by an open window. Phoebe looked around for him at first, trying to see where he was, then spotted him at the far end of the room, and took him in, trying to see him differently, trying to look at him as she never had before, and see him as a lover, see him as someone who might become her future. But it was difficult; even as she saw where he was standing, her eyes seemed to slip past him to the evening beyond the window where he stood, the night sky over Hyderabad, the long lawn falling away to the street beyond, India, beautiful home, and the memory of childhood, and the parakeets in the trees, and the stones her brothers and sisters and she used to throw at the monkeys who came and perched on the garden wall, and the feeling that over that wall was a whole world waiting that could quite easily turn into anything. And was it going to turn into this? Was this, and nothing else, nothing more, what was to be given to her – was the rest of life in all its rich possibility about to be closed off? Would she ever see the real wild and teeming world, or was it all to narrow down to this man, those moustaches, the duties of a marriage?

Arthur saw her almost in the same moment as she noticed him, and smiled at her mother, and raised his glass to her father, but did not look directly at Phoebe, and did not come over immediately to speak to her. So she took up a position at the side of the room with her parents, and they all looked around to see who they could talk to. Her father was always keenly sensitive about these social relations, who he might be permitted to speak to of his own volition, who he would have to wait to be introduced to, who he should avoid at all costs. He lived in terror of giving offence, and of losing someone's business because of a misplaced remark, an inappropriate attempt at conversation, a smile or a nod to the wrong person. These kinds of things sometimes go over children's heads, but Phoebe was always acutely aware of the atmosphere of tension around her father whenever they were in company like this. His eyes were always bright with a panic he barely suppressed, and with a kind of desperation, as he tried to work out where he belonged in the pecking order of every room he passed through. It may possibly have marked him out as a small man, this obsession with rank, someone who placed no value in himself except that which was accorded to him by other people. But that never occurred to Phoebe until she came to England. In India, among the castes, rank was everything, as natural as breathing; in business, among the British, how an Indian man conducted himself was always a delicate game.

'Mr French has noticed you,' her mother hissed at her. 'When he has finished his conversation, I am sure he will come over. You remember what we talked about, Phoebe. You will smile and be pleasant to him.'

Arthur spent five more minutes laughing with his British friends by the window, then detached himself from the group he was in and made his way over to greet them.

'Good evening,' he said to Phoebe's father and mother. Phoebe watched him as he extended his right hand to shake her father's, and his eyes flickered for a moment to meet hers, then fixed again on her father's face. Did she feel anything? Any stirring of nervousness or excitement? Not really. Just the same slight sickness and creeping dread she had carried with her into the room. Was that normal in matters of the heart? Who knew? Who knew what love was really like? Not a girl of fourteen trying to negotiate its rocks and shallows for the first time.

'And good evening to you, Miss Phoebe,' Arthur said now, turning to her. She held out her hand and he took it, and kissed it, and a part of her wanted to laugh at them all being so formal together, putting on such a performance, but she kept a straight face and curtseyed to Arthur instead, because she knew it was what her mother wanted.

'How lovely to see you, Mr French,' she said. 'What a lively gathering.'

'Yes, it is, isn't it?' He looked around the room, the people talking, the light on the glasses and the dark falling slowly outside. 'It has been a lovely day, wouldn't you say?'

'Oh, I think they are all lovely days in Hyderabad.'

Arthur laughed at this, as if Phoebe had said something very witty. 'How very true,' he said. 'If you can stand the heat, that is.'

'Well yes, of course; it's no place for someone who doesn't like the sun.'

Her father said something then, and Arthur laughed again, and Phoebe was able to fade back to the edge of the conversation as her parents carried on talking to this strange man who had come looming over to them. She took the opportunity to have a closer look at him. He still looked relatively youthful; there was something quite boyish about him in those days. The trouble had not yet started with his knees, and she had noticed as he crossed the room that he had a strange walk, he seemed almost to bounce as he walked towards them. He seemed at ease with her parents, not too standoffish, and his clothes were nice enough. It was hard to see anything objectionable in him. Of course, he was as old as her father, and that was a little strange maybe, but perhaps that was only a detail. Lots of women married men who were older than they were. And lots of women weren't even that lucky, and never had the chance to marry at all. She watched Arthur as he

concluded his conversation with her parents, and tried to persuade herself that the situation she found herself in wasn't
really so terrible; there didn't really seem to be anything
wrong with him, after all. He was healthy and tall and he had
money, and some women never got a chance to marry anyone. Arthur turned back to her once more, smiling, and she
made herself smile back at him.

'I wonder whether you would care to dance, Miss Phoebe?'
he asked her. She felt suddenly tense and nervous. It was not
the done thing for a woman to dance with just any man at a
party; to dance with a man was to announce one's intentions.
She looked questioningly at her mother, who nodded sternly
at her. She realised, with some amazement, that already,
almost as soon as she had been acquainted with the idea of
Arthur, the moment had come for committing herself to him.
It seemed ludicrous; and yet her mother was nodding sternly
at her. What else was she to do?

'I would be delighted to, Mr French.'

'Very good. Shall we?' Arthur offered his arm, and they
walked together to the middle of the room, where a small
group of Europeans had begun dancing to the music of the
gramophone in the corner. She felt very afraid. She had not
had very much practice at dancing, and she had never danced
with a man before, and wondered whether she could do it
correctly, or whether she was going to make a fool of herself.
Arthur turned to face her, and held her to him, and looked
happily at her face, and they began to sway in time to the
music. She tried to smile for him. He did not seem to want to
try anything more complicated than swaying together, and
she was happy enough with that. She became aware, as he

pressed himself against her, that he was in a state of some tumescence, which did make her uncomfortable where he stuck into her side, but she did her very best not to notice or draw attention to the situation. She understood that men did sometimes find themselves in this predicament, particularly around young women, and did not want to embarrass her future husband. It was, after all, a compliment of sorts, she supposed. For his part, Arthur did not seem to be embarrassed at all; he smiled heartily, and pressed her close against him, until the song they were dancing to had finished, when they stepped apart, and he led her back to her parents at the edge of the room. Phoebe was surprised to find that she felt quite excited. She knew the whole room had seen them dance, and that was as good as telling them aloud that there was to be an engagement. She realised all of a sudden that she had been announced in public as having been chosen by a European man. It was a conspicuous honour, perhaps a great change in status for her, and, as it seemed to her then, the first thing that had ever really happened in her life. Arthur bowed to her slightly as they reached her parents, and he prepared to take his leave.

'It was very good to speak to you, Miss Phoebe,' he said. 'I hope we will be able to speak again before too long.'

'Thank you, Mr French. I would like that very much.'

He bowed his head to her once more, and then took his leave and went back to the drinks and the men on the far side of the room, who seemed to slap him on the back and whisper to him with bright, snarling grins, and Phoebe and her father and mother blended in with the other Indian guests at the party.

When she retired to her bed that evening, she thought a great deal about the excitement that had rushed through her when she returned to the edge of the room from her dance with Arthur. It had been a strange sensation, one that was not familiar to her. She suspected it had something to do with a change taking place within her from being a girl to becoming a woman; new emotions were revealing themselves as she encountered new experiences, emotions she had never suspected were waiting within her.

Her mother and father broke the news to her the following week that Arthur had proposed marriage, and following a discussion between them, both he and Phoebe's father had found the terms agreeable. Phoebe was told that she should be very proud, that this was a momentous day in the life of her family. The fortunes of everyone in the family would be changed by this match, and it would all be thanks to her, thanks to her beauty and her kindness and refinement, which had so enchanted Mr French. She listened to it all feeling like someone in a dream. They were married three months later.

The ceremony was undoubtedly very beautiful. Her father spared no expense, and for her mother, it really might have been the best day of her life, a day when the dream she had had for her daughter came true. She passed the day in an ecstasy, emotional and smiling, clutching her children to her as Phoebe went to the altar and exchanged the vows that made her and Arthur man and wife. Arthur did look very smart in his suit; really, Phoebe could find no fault with the day, it would be ungracious of her to do so. There was champagne that had actually been ordered from France, foie gras from the Army & Navy stores, and Phoebe's dress came all the way from a tailor in Bombay. It really was marvellous, all she was able to remember of it afterwards; but unfortunately that was not so very much, for she went through it all in a kind of stupor, a daze, and could not come fully to her senses until the end of the evening when Arthur arranged for them to be driven back to his house, and she stepped out of the carriage and into the home that was now to be hers, and found herself all of a sudden alone with a man she did not know, had barely even spoken to, and yet was supposed to stay by the side of for the rest of her life. She experienced, in that moment in the innocent year of 1911, a sense of crippling vertigo that she struggled to believe had ever really left her.

They were supposed to build a life there in Hyderabad, where Phoebe could have lived with her husband but still seen her family and her mother regularly, and still have felt part of the world she came from. However, things didn't turn out that way. Not very long after Phoebe married Arthur, a man named Gavrilo Princip shot and killed the heir to the Austro-Hungarian empire, Archduke Franz Ferdinand, and very soon afterwards the world changed for ever. The changes in Phoebe's life mattered very little, really, in the context of everything else that proceeded from that gunshot, but her life changed unimaginably all the same.

Upon learning that Britain had declared war, Arthur announced his intention to leave India and enlist in the navy in order to serve his country; Phoebe, naturally, had no choice but to follow him. So there was a rushed, traumatic journey out of India, west to Bombay on the trains Arthur had supervised, then by sea past coastlines that thronged with Bible stories.

Phoebe endured the journey in profound shock, hardly able to speak at this wrenching away that was happening to her, hardly able to take in the change that was occurring. She comforted herself as they sailed past the Holy Land with trying to identify places that were mentioned in the Bible, and avoided her husband, because she was speechlessly angry with him, and knew she had no right to be, and perhaps would not even be able to explain herself were he to ask what the matter was.

Her mother had upbraided her the last time they saw each other, and told her it had always been likely that Mr French would want to go home one day, and Phoebe should always have been expecting that. It was almost the last conversation the two women ever had; after that, they never met again, but only exchanged letters till her mother died five years later.

Phoebe recognised with hindsight that she should have realised she would one day go to England. But the suddenness of it, the mindlessness of it, and no one ever asking her what she might want or how she was coping, all of this shook and diminished her in ways from which she never recovered. Years later, she would remember that journey as the breaking of so much that had once been possible for her. Not because she had been taken away from her country, but because of the fractures that change had left in her. After she set foot for the first time on English soil there was less of her, and consequently there was less of life available to her, less to be done. It was not true, she realised bitterly, that experience made you stronger. It seemed to her more like an ebbing away of things, of what might have been possible.

2019

AFTER I'VE MOVED all my things out of the flat Juliet's parents bought her, I know what I'm going to do, though I don't feel very proud of it. I wait a fortnight, then call up Leah and Richard and get Amy's number. I call her, and we speak, and we meet, and go for dinner.

I get to the restaurant before she does, crossing Putney Bridge to the far side, wondering why I've suggested we meet somewhere so far from where both of us are living, wondering whether I was seeking neutral territory, somewhere neither of us were likely to have been recently with anyone else, unbroken ground for unbroken feeling. I walk past the church where the Putney Debates took place after the first civil war. 'I think the poorest he that is in England hath a life to live, as the greatest he'. That's all I remember from the Putney Debates. But it's a thing worth remembering all the same. The heart and source of every story, that every life is the centre of the world and weighs the same in the scales of – well, whatever we call God now that we mostly deny him, whatever scales we use instead. All that is etched into history at the Putney Debates.

I get to the restaurant, and give my name, and sit and wait at an outside table, thinking about all the better places I could have picked to meet, and how stupid I'm going to look when she turns up, and how I won't know what to say or what to do because I can never understand or believe this moment, I can never believe someone's interested in me, until Amy walks round the corner of the church and sees me. Then she smiles, and I smile too, and stand up from my seat, then feel ridiculous for having done so, but can't sit down again, so I wait, knowing I'm blushing, knowing I've overthought this terribly. Amy smiles as she approaches me.

'Did they make you stand up at school whenever a teacher walked into the room?' she asks.

'Yeah, I looked weird, didn't I?'

'A bit. Now it's going to be really weird if you don't kiss me, but I'm not going to let you, so we're just going to have to sit with the tension for a bit and see if it dissipates, aren't we?' Her eyes seem to flash with the mischief in her as she sits down at the table while I sit back down opposite her.

'How's it feeling so far?' she asks me, and our eyes meet, and neither of us looks away.

'I'm just sitting with the tension,' I tell her, and we smile, and we're feeling the same thing, and it feels like being alive to be here with her. I can feel my heart beating in my chest: not faster, just harder. The boom of a bass drum I can't always hear. What causes that, I wonder? What chemical is now coursing through me?

'How was your day?' she asks me.

'Fine, I think. It wasn't that exciting. I'm afraid I'm not an exciting person.'

'You should stop talking yourself up so much, I'll think you've got something to hide.'

'How was yours?'

'I stopped a mugging in the street.'

'Really?'

'No, of course not – look at me. But I thought I'd sound more interesting than you. You can tell stories, can't you?' She leans forwards suddenly, looking at me.

'I think so,' I tell her. 'When I've got a story to tell.'

'That ought to be always, if you're any good at it.'

'OK. What do you like to hear stories about?'

She shrugs at this. 'Anything. I'm not picky. People's families, people's lives.'

'Ask me a question, then.'

'No, not like that.' She leans back just as suddenly, as if I'd disappointed her. 'I'm not interviewing you. I just want to know whether you can tell a story.'

I think of the things I might be able to tell her. The family stories I've collected. The little pieces of my own life that might be worth saying out loud. There are fewer of those, it seems to me, though I don't know why. Every day ought to be worth retelling in some form or another, but I can't seem to find the trick of it. So many of my days feel just like time passing by.

'You tell me a story,' I say to her, 'and I'll see if I can pick up the trick.'

She tells me over pasta that she has a tutoring job that's going to take her away to Kuala Lumpur for most of the summer, some rich architect's kids she'll have to spend a couple of months bullying about their grammar and their algebra and the periodic table while they jump off their dad's yacht into the sea. Those endless not-quite-jobs my generation do and call our lives, because the money doesn't add up any more, because the jobs we were taught to dream for don't quite pay and all need to be subsidised by other work. Amy and I have done a lot of stop-gaps: bar work, call-centre work, café work, tearing tickets in theatres, cleaning offices, delivering free papers, clearing houses – all this has come up in the course of our lives. I ask her why her summer isn't filled up with photographing weddings, and she replies that she thought she'd like a change.

'I've done that for the last few years, and the money's great. It's robbery, really, what I get away with charging. But I do these tutoring gigs as well, and every now and then, they're rewarding. You know, if you help some kid understand something they didn't. Or just help some kid feel better about themselves. That feels good sometimes. So I was asked about this job, and I guess I was tired of the weddings on the day the call came in, or maybe I'd had a good session tutoring or something. Or maybe I just wanted to go abroad on someone else's credit card. I half regret it now, I think. But I'm back by the middle of August, and I've booked myself up doing weddings from then.'

What she's saying to me when she tells me about Kuala Lumpur, the story below the surface of her speaking, is helpful to hear. I won't be here every weekend, she's telling me; I'm not going to be free to meet up every time you call – if that's what's going to happen, that won't be what this is. That's all right with me. It seems like it might be what I need. It will be different from the life I've walked away from, and that must be what I'm looking for, isn't it? Otherwise I'd have stayed where I was. Otherwise I would have been happy.

'Do you have any plans for the summer?' she asks me.

'I hadn't made any yet, if I'm honest.'

'Maybe we'll go somewhere,' she says. Her eyes dance, and it seems like the bravest thing anyone's ever said to me.

'That'd be nice. Where do you want to go?'

'Well, I have my summer full of other people's weddings once I'm not in KL, like I said. So maybe we'll end up going to those.'

'Sure.'

'Do you ever want to get married?' she asks me. 'Is marriage something you believe in?'

'I don't think that kind of thing can exist in the abstract. I think it's going to be about a person you meet.'

'A lot of people know what their wedding will be like a long time before they meet anyone worth marrying.'

'No, they don't. Not really.'

She raises her eyebrows at this. 'Why not?'

'A lot of people think they know a lot of things. But it's not them, is it? It's everything around them. People are brought up around so much noise. Shutting it out till you can hear your own self is so fucking difficult. Lots of people never do it. They think they want a white wedding and a beach honeymoon, but it's not them. It's just what the world's told them they should be wanting.'

'The world might be right.'

'The world might well be right. But it's not the person wanting the thing. It's something different. Something else.'

'You talk about it like it's social conditioning. Like it's white noise drowning real things out. You might have it the wrong way round. What you're talking about might really be the evolutionary imperative. A desire to marry that's deeper than conscious thinking. An instinct that precedes our individuality.'

And I don't say anything to this. Because it suddenly strikes me as true, and it makes me wonder what I know about anything.

The evening is a kind of dance I haven't danced in years. I remember what I hated about dating, the uncertainty, the sense of performance all the time. But I remember what I liked about it too. The uncertainty. The unspoken thoughts that bloom between two people while they work each other out. Does that have to disappear once two people get to know each other? Or is it just that things between me and Juliet went wrong? Did we mistake falling into our relationship for the end of the adventure? Did we just sit in front of the TV and lose sight of what we'd thought was about to begin?

After I leave Juliet, I move into the converted garage of a friend. I never bring Amy there; when we meet, we meet in restaurants or bars, and when we go home together we go home to hers. The garage, after all, is never going to turn into my home, and the place is damp, and I've made great piles of everything I own because I'm too cheap to pay for storage. There are always clothes drying on top of boxes of books. I keep this secret, and tell myself I mustn't let this become who I am. When I was a kid I used to get like this about tidying my room. For weeks I'd say to myself that I didn't need to do it, and the mess around me was only superficial, a bit of untidiness, and one quick pass would have things back on their shelves and the room looking how it should. Until the day came when I'd be forced to confront the fact that the mess I lived in was actually several layers deep, that my shelves had been emptied, all my life was on the floor. I want to avoid that in the garage. But I don't do anything about finding a flat just yet.

I don't know whether it's dating Amy or feeling strangely comfortable in the little damp garage, but I don't really want to take another step in any particular direction straight away. I have this feeling that I don't know who I'm going to be in a few months' time, so it would be wrong to commit to anything. When Amy talks about the job in Kuala Lumpur, I wonder whether it will be the end of us, whether we'll drift apart before we've really started. Sometimes when I think of how likely it is that, by the end of summer, I won't know her any more, I wonder whether I've been mad to break up with Juliet for what might turn out to be a two-month fling. Perhaps I've been blinded by the romance of the past that suffused my first encounter with Amy, having suddenly been given access that night at the wedding to the deep dive of time lost and time recalled. When you meet someone who met you or knew you as a child, which to my mind is like them having seen you as you really are, the air between you changes a little. They knew you when you could have been anyone, when your life could have turned into anything, not just this. They remind you of things you've lost, and when you speak to them, the conversation sometimes has a different centre of gravity. Because the kid you used to be is buried under so many years and contradictory feelings. Until the very idea of a coherent identity becomes a bit ludicrous. But there was a time when it wasn't. And it's beautiful to meet someone who gives you access to the memory of that time, so that you almost believe in it again. All of that I feel very deeply, but it doesn't really mean Amy and I are going to be well suited to each other. It doesn't mean that I should have let Juliet go, and retreated from the future I'd been building for myself with her.

That particular door is closed on me before too long, though, and I'm forced to abandon any fantasy about going back. Online, as visibly and joyfully and aggressively as possible, it seems to me, Juliet charts the course of a new relationship that begins almost as quickly as I start seeing Amy. While Amy and I are still on drinks and dinners and theatre one or two nights a week, Juliet moves someone else into the flat we used to share. Her flat, of course, in her name, bought for her by her parents, but I can't help but think of it a little bit as mine, because I lived there; it became my outer layer, it was the shell that sheltered me for a while. I want to feel hurt, but I find that I don't. In fact, I'm glad she has someone with her.

Because what's happening between Amy and me is new, and is moving fast, so that before very long we're spending almost all of our evenings together, sometimes there are bumps in the road. Evenings where one of us is tired or stressed, and the other doesn't know how to navigate around it. If the person I'm with seems to be unhappy, I have a tendency to assume it's because of me. Amy always notices, and calls me out on this, and that tends to turn quite quickly into arguing.

'You're making it about you again, when it's not, when you shouldn't; it's not all about you.'

'Then why aren't you talking to me?'

'I just want to sit on my own for a minute. I just didn't sleep last night, and I was shit all day, and everyone's pissed off at me. I just wanted to sit quietly.'

'But I'm not pissed off at you, so why take it out on me?'

'I'm not, I'm just sitting perfectly still, Ed. Calm down. Can you make us both a cup of tea?'

I meet all of Amy's parents, the people who adopted and raised her, who she calls Mum and Dad, and also, just once, her birth father, the strangest meeting Amy arranges. I never quite work out her intention.

She drives me down there one weekend, tense and quiet in the car, the sound of Sunday morning Radio 2 filling the space between us while she cocoons herself and tries, I suppose, to order her mind, maybe to work out why she is taking her new boyfriend to meet this man, what she's going to say about us both when we arrive. She parks the car on a quiet road in the middle of a nondescript housing estate, and leads me to a low block of flats. Her dad has a place on the ground floor, accessed from a hallway round the back of the building.

She smiles at me nervously. 'I don't know whether I should have brought you now,' she says.

'I know. It's OK.'

'Just don't expect too much.'

'I promise you, it's OK.' I wonder at that phrase, 'don't expect too much'. As if she feels that she's on trial with me somehow. As if she needs to show me this man, this part of her life, before I will really believe in her. What have I done to make her feel that way? What could I do to let her know that's not how I'm feeling?

The council must have been round that morning or the

previous day, because the grass is freshly cut, and I can still catch a trace of its scent in the air. Amy knocks on an anonymous door, and her father shows us in and makes us instant coffee. I look around the room we've been led into. It is a little more lived-in now than the place Amy described that night we met at the wedding: a table, a pile of newspapers, a radio, a TV. But everywhere the air of the charity-shop bargain.

'You're Edward, are you?' he says to me, holding out his hand. I shake it and smile.

'That's right. Everyone just calls me Ed, though. It's Alan, isn't it?'

'That's it. It's good to meet you.' There's a watchfulness about him, as you see in people who've learned the world can fuck you over, who never quite trust that it's not about to do the same again. He lives his life as if he's ashamed of what he's done with it. He reminds me of my own father, who had his own problems in his turn. I'm always interested when I discover I share things like this with girls I'm involved with. Damaged fathers, or summers in haystacks, or whatever it might be. It always feels like an explanation of what we recognised in each other, and makes me wonder how we communicate these secret currents which align our lives.

'Take a seat, all right, and I'll get coffee. Do you take sugar? Do you take milk?'

'Just milk, thanks.'

I feel sorry for him and for Amy as well, because for as long as we visit, the two of them sit in an agony of uncertainty and tension, not knowing what they should be saying to each other, not knowing what they're supposed to do.

'You been all right then, Amy, have you? How was the drive, all right?' All these empty questions. Talk of the football scores, talk of the weather. Anything but the honesty of not saying anything at all, till conversations like this have no meaning, we've had them so many times before. How often do we break through this empty talking into real speech?

'The drive was fine, thanks. Have you been OK?'

It isn't an easy visit, but Alan does the best he can to make us welcome, and when we're leaving he seems to be almost on the verge of tears, grateful we've come. After that first time, whenever Amy visits him, she prefers to go alone. After that day, I avoid bringing Alan up. I get the impression she's said all she wanted to say about that part of her life.

Juliet finds out that Amy and I are seeing each other about a month after we first go for dinner. She doesn't confront Amy, or anything like that; she just calls me. I see her name on the screen of my phone, and it makes me happy at first, because I don't guess why she's calling, which I suppose is naive. So I pick up and say hello, not expecting the coldness I hear in her voice.

'Are you sleeping with her?'

'Sorry? With who?'

'You know who.'

'Oh.'

'I fucking knew it.'

'Jules.'

'I gave you the opportunity to tell me. Why couldn't you be a man and own up to what you were doing?'

'That's not what happened. I didn't lie to you.'

'Of course you fucking lied to me; I gave you a chance to tell me and you didn't.'

'We met up again after you left me.'

'I didn't leave you, Ed – don't change the story.'

'What do you mean? You left me. I remember it very clearly.'

'I just put us down. We did the dying together.'

'Jules, that's a really weird way of putting it.'

'I'm trying to say you made it impossible for us. I just saw it through because you wouldn't. Now I find out you were seeing someone else. You're a fucking snake.'

'I wasn't, though.'

'People who can do that aren't whole people, Ed, you know that? People who can do this to someone else. I'm going to hang up now. You don't deserve any more of my time.'

She hangs up the phone then, and I try to call her back, then text her later a couple of times, but I don't get through and she doesn't reply, and I guess she's probably blocked my number. I try to feel indignant, but realise I can't. The truth is that my conscience isn't clear, not really. This year has caught hold of me and carried me away with it, and I can't say for sure whether I've done the right thing. Perhaps it will be years before I know what happened, whether there are things I should apologise for. All I know is that I can't get back to the place where I started.

Most of the time when Amy and I are together we go to her flat and the area round it, but every week we make sure we do something like a date night – go out and walk after dark by the river, or watch the sun rise over a park, go to dinner or into the city to see a film or a play, go for drinks, just the two of us, and talk to each other.

'Do you want kids eventually?' she asks me one evening.

'Yes,' I say without thinking, and the thought surprises me, and I suppose that surprise must pass over my face.

'What was that look for?' she asks me.

'I just never realised I did till this exact moment,' I say.

'Did you never talk about it with Juliet?'

'No, never. It never came up.' I look at Amy and realise for the first time that one day I want a family. As if I've suppressed this thought for some time, and now it's rushing up in me with great force for having been hidden away. 'I'd like to foster too, wouldn't you?' I ask her.

'What interests you about that?'

'I don't know. A chance to help someone. Like my friend Joe is helping me. He's let me keep my things in the garage. When I move them out again, I'll thank him, and we'll go on with our lives. I'd like to do that for people one day. I'd like someone to know they could always come to me.'

'That's a nice thought.'

'Would you ever foster?'

'I've looked into it actually.'

'Really? How come?'

'I just think it's something you can do that makes a difference.'

'I think it's been on my mind this last year because I haven't had very much for myself. Do you know what I mean? When you're feeling itinerant. You pack up your things and you realise there aren't many of them. You don't have walls around you, you don't have much permanence. And that makes you think about how valuable all that is. And it makes you think it would be a good thing to offer shelter to someone.' It occurs to me as I speak that I'm sounding pathetic, and I start to feel anxious, start to worry that I sound like I'm asking to move in. But Amy smiles, and reaches out, and takes my hand, as if she can see everything I'm thinking.

'I'd say it's strange that we both want to do that,' she says, 'but it probably isn't, really.'

'Why not?'

'Well, I don't believe in soulmates. Soulmates in the abstract. But I do think people are suited to certain other people. And at nineteen or twenty you date whoever you can get your hands on. But as you get older, here we are, we're thirty, basically, we've been in the world a while. Well, it stands to reason that we'd have started to know ourselves a little better. And spend our time in places and around people who are closer to who we'd like to be. So it would make sense if the closest thing we might ever have to a soulmate would be someone who moved in a similar circle. It would make sense if the closest thing we'd ever have to a soulmate were sitting with us, in this room.'

The day I tell Mum that I've started seeing Amy, she hangs up the phone on me. As simple as that. I call one evening to break the news, instinct telling me already that it would go badly.

'Hello?'

'Hi, Mum.'

'Hello, Ed – is that you?'

'Yeah, you OK?'

'We're all right, love. I'm just making dinner. Is there anything you need?'

'Oh. Actually, I just needed to tell you something.'

'Oh right?'

'You know that Juliet and I were on a break.'

She hesitates a moment before speaking again. 'Yes?'

'Well, it's not a break any more.'

'I see. You don't mean you've got back together?'

'No. I'm sorry.'

'I see.'

'And I have some other news that I wanted to tell you.'

'Right?'

'You remember I told you I met that girl, the girl I saved from the pool when we were young?'

'I remember.'

'Well, we've been seeing more of each other. And we've kind of got together, I think.' Mum's silent for a second; then the line goes dead.

I think Mum's first instinct is to reject the idea that Juliet and I might have needed to break up at all. We'd thought we were happy just a few months before; surely we could have gone on being happy together? But life has changed, and she will have to let that go. The life she imagined me having with Juliet was simply one of many alternative futures that are never going to come into being.

For some time afterwards, Mum makes it very clear she's not at peace with what's happened. When I call, it's always Chris who answers, and Mum can never speak, she's always busy. I don't know why she doesn't just want to talk. Perhaps because she knows deep down that she's being unreasonable, and there would be no way to argue out what she's feeling.

This new silence is also complicated because it feels like the continuation and evolution of a different fight we've been having for the last year or so. Although saying we've been fighting for only a year seems disingenuous; it was a year ago I said to her that I wasn't sure I could ever see myself moving home to take over the farm where I grew up and on which she and my stepdad still lived and worked, but that wasn't the beginning of things by any stretch.

I'd felt unsure since I was quite a young child whether I wanted the life I'd been born to, the hardship and money worries and the labour of shepherding. I'd put off thinking about it over the years. Easier to let time drift on without making decisions, knowing there'd be years still before I needed to make my mind up. But a year ago, Mum had tried to talk to me about wills and about inheritance, and that had become a moment of fracture between us.

'I'm just calling because I'm updating my will,' she said when I'd answered the phone and we'd done with the pleasantries. 'And Chris and I have been talking about how to write it.'

'All right.'

'The thing is that it's simpler just to leave the farm to one person, rather than leave it to both of you kids.'

I think in the moment she spoke I was shocked by the assumption that either Rachel or I would want to do what Mum and Chris had done. Phone calls can surprise like that; they come out of nowhere, into ordinary days, changing the weather without warning. I didn't know why Mum talked about us taking on the farm one day as if it was a given. Both Rachel and I lived in the city; we had both drifted away from the world of our childhood, and had never said anything about wanting to drift back.

'I don't know whether either of us is sure about taking it on,' I said. I heard the quality of silence change at the other end of the phone. I could feel Mum's focus intensifying as she sat, presumably at the big window in the cottage, with the wire of the home telephone trailing across the room from where the phone sat on its little table by the door. I imagined her looking out the window at the fields beyond, a cloud passing over her face as she listened to me.

'What do you mean?' Mum asked.

'Mum, we've talked about this before. Rachel and I don't know whether we want to do that.'

'Why not?'

'We're not sure whether that's our life.'

'It's your home, it's the world you come from.'

'No, Mum. You shouldn't think you're there to hand it on. You should be there because it's where you want to be. Don't think about what will happen to it after your lifetime; we'd both rather you thought about what you want to do, about your own lives.'

'But this place is our life.'

'Good. That's good. It's not necessarily going to be ours, though.'

'It's the history of our family.'

'But one day our family won't live there any more.'

The conversation went downhill from there. I suppose Mum had just never listened to me or Rachel when we'd told her before that it wasn't what we wanted. She had shut out a future she didn't want to contemplate, and assumed she might be able to force her wish through if she held to her course, fixed her eyes on what she wanted. But what becomes of your one and only life isn't something you can easily give way on, so I didn't, so Mum was talking about betrayal by the end of the call. Despairing at the thought that she had raised two citizens of nowhere. She then called up Rachel and tried the same trick. Rachel, I think, handled it better than I did, but she stuck to her course as well.

I felt guilty for not particularly wanting the life Mum had laid out for me. I knew it was what she wanted for me, I knew it was something she'd planned all her life. And I knew as well that my reasons for not wanting to go home were not because I had something lined up that was demonstrably better. I hadn't built much of a life at all. But that didn't mean I'd want to move back to Wales and farm sheep for a living. The work had always been hard and draining, the money had never added up; the idea that the land had meant a lot to my family over many years had never counted for ever so much when set against the way I felt about the way it made you live. That lean, hillside farming, losing money on the lambs each year, relying on the single farm payment, out before dawn and back after dark, always lugging dead bodies to fires because so many of the sheep died, and the dogs died, and the farmers died from time to time as well, the dogs in their kennels barking in the night, the cold and the foot rot and the mud caking the whole of you – all of it was a backbreaking life that belonged, it seemed to me, to the past. It wasn't who I wanted to be, it was just the life I had been born into, and I didn't know exactly what I did want to do with my time, but it wasn't that – that hardship, that solitude.

Above all it was the solitude I shied away from. To live around no one but the other old farmers, who all hated each other and all hated you. Nursing ancient hatreds while their lives passed by. In our valley lived a farmer who had run over his neighbour's dog some forty years ago. The neighbour, another sheep farmer, had fired off a shotgun into his chest in revenge. Grapeshot, probably, only meant to wound, but it had happened, and forty years on they still farmed side by side, not speaking to each other, never having gone to the police. There was something extraordinary about living in a place like that. Like living in a myth. But it was essentially mad as well, and I didn't want to go back to it.

Of course, all this wasn't the real fight either. The real fight with Mum was buried so much deeper than that; it was as old as life, fundamental enough that I could probably have sat and thought for a year and never quite got to the heart of it. Something about the scrabble for survival. The way kids end up effacing their parents. The way parents try to ensure their kids will be faithful palimpsests of them, and not rewrite the story too much, not dispel the meaning of the family when it's their turn to decide what that meaning might be. The fight that comes with all our surviving, and the fight of trying to be yourself, not just one bead in the necklace of a family, not just who your mother wants you to be, fulfilling her wishes rather than your own, a thought she had once that lives on after she does rather than a person in your own right. The fight we were really having encompassed everything, and the farm was a face and a name we'd put on it, and now Amy seemed to be about to become a face and a name we'd put on the fight as well.

Just as Amy shared the story of her family with me, I try to tell her the story of mine. Whole evenings pass telling stories to each other; it's something I've never quite done before with any other girlfriend. There's an intimacy to it, a quality of listening that seems to heighten the atmosphere between us. I suppose each person's family and the world they come from is a kind of secret, and the way to let someone into your life is always to share your secrets with them. We lie on the grass in the park near her flat, drinking Rekorderlig and swapping stories, and I try my best to unfold the history of who I am.

'So in the beginning was the farm, kind of thing,' I say to her, lying with my head on her lap while she lies back on the grass as well, both of us staring up at the clouds that are scudding across the light, across our vision. 'That's been ours for a very long time.'

'How long is very long?'

'I don't know completely. Two hundred years? I think the house is about two hundred years old. I don't know whether it was us who built it.'

'How can you not know that?'

'I don't know. Two hundred years is a long time. Not everything survives that long, does it?'

'But knowing whether it was your family who built the place.'

'Maybe my Mum knows. I'll ask her some time. If there's ever a good time.'

'Ask her now.'

I laugh at this. 'Not a good time.'

'Why not?'

'She's decided now that I have no interest in it. If I text her now, I'll just be starting a fight.'

'Or putting a stop to one.'

I think about this. 'Do you reckon?'

'I don't know. Only one way to find out.'

I try to imagine the way it would go. Pulling my phone out, and getting the text right, sending it off to Mum to get the story. I ought to get all the stories from her one day; there'll come a time when I've left it too late. Those sorts of jobs get set aside in families, and they shouldn't. Families really ought to write the stories down. I try to imagine Mum writing this story in a text, and sending it back to me, filling in a gap in the family history. But other scenarios crowd into my mind. The snide response; the questioning as to why I care right now; the silence that gets a bit harder to break every time she stretches it out across new moments. There are too many ways it could go wrong. Better not to write to her, better to say nothing. If you say nothing you can't get hurt.

'Maybe another time.'

Amy doesn't say anything for a moment. 'Fair enough,' she says in the end. 'So tell me what you do know.'

I try to bring my mind back to the story I'd started to tell, having lost the thread for a second. What was I going on about? That was it. In the beginning was the farm.

'So I think my family had already been there for a couple of generations when my great-grandfather, whose name was Arthur, made a break with things and went away to work in India for a while.'

'Why India?'

'I don't know, really. I suppose there was work. This was at the start of the twentieth century. He went over to be involved with building the railways in Hyderabad. It was just that his father hadn't died, I think. And Arthur, my great-grandfather, was quite a bright man, and he didn't fancy just working for his dad till his dad died, so he went and did something else for a bit. And when he was out in India, he met an Indian woman called Phoebe, and married her, and they lived over there for a while.'

'Phoebe isn't an Indian name.'

'I think she was Goan. Christian Indian. She was christened with a Western name. I don't know the whole story, really; I don't know all that much about her family.'

'What was a woman from Goa doing in Hyderabad?'

'Her father moved them there because of the trade. He was some kind of trader. Buying and selling. So she grew up there. She was quite young when she married Arthur. In India then, women married quite young. So she lived with him in India for a few years, and then when the war broke out they came back to England.'

I am watching a cloud cross the face of the sky, a cloud that seems to be taking on the shape of a rhino. I watch its shadow pass over our bodies.

'What does that cloud look like to you?' I ask. Amy is silent for a moment.

'A ship,' she says. I look, but I can't see it. 'They'll have come to England by ship, I suppose; is that why you mentioned the cloud?'

'I didn't see a ship,' I say.

'What do you see?'

'I don't know, really,' I tell her, even though I do. But I don't know why I've changed the subject, and I think perhaps I should go on with the story I'd started to tell. 'They did come back by ship, though.'

'Port out, starboard home.'

'That's it, yes. And then Arthur enlisted in the navy, and left Phoebe living on her own in east London for four years, looking after their son, my grandfather, who was born just after Arthur went away.'

'Really?'

'Mad, isn't it?'

'Can you imagine how alone she must have been? There by the docks in a place she didn't know with a child to look after, and no one to talk to.'

'If I'm completely honest, I can't really. But I agree with you. I know what you mean.'

'And he was at sea for the whole of the war?'

'Yes. Then after the war he came home. And they didn't go back to India again. Arthur took over the farm after his father died, and went there to live with Phoebe and their child, my grandfather.'

'What was your grandfather's name?'

'Leo. Poor man.'

'Why poor man?'

'I don't think he got to have much fun, really. He had a long enough life, but didn't get much out of it.'

As I've been talking, the feeling has been growing that, for some reason I can't quite put my finger on, talking about all the family history is making me unhappy. It's strange, how anxious it's making me feel. I suppose because Mum used to tell me all these stories. But there's also the feeling of time running out on me while I'm talking: all these lives that seemed as long as mine to the people who lived them, which are all gone now, which can all be summarised in half a dozen sentences. I suppose it makes the idea of breaking free of this history seem futile. How could I ever make time to live my own life, and set my own parameters, and choose the person I want to be rather than just inherit where I came from, when lives pass so quickly, when there's so little to them? How can I ever resist subsiding into this long-running story, and being just one more brief anecdote about to be forgotten? Telling my history makes me feel I'm running out of time, and the things I have built up are ending, they are going to go away.

I have found in my relatively short experience that life has a way of giving me springs and autumns, one thing always following another and all seeming to vanish as quickly as they come. Ephemerality is what everything feels like in the end. I think I got the idea from Mum when she told me the stories of our family, the stories that had shaped us and brought us here. What the relatives she spoke about all seemed to share was a life that ebbed and flowed around them, one tide always giving way to another, so they were caught and pulled in different directions, every move they tried to make for themselves beset and foiled by some counter-movement, so no matter what they tried to do to change their worlds, they always seemed to end up back where they started. Back on the farm. What became of their lives seemed to be out of their hands. They were just drawn through time by deep, irresistible currents.

Mum, like Amy, loved to tell stories. In the evenings or on long afternoons when I was very young, she'd sit and yarn with me, remembering, imagining. I'll never quite know how true her stories were; they became the cloak of memories around me as I grew up, so they had that much truth to them, but they might have all been plucked from the clouds. I remember nights when Rachel and I would sit by the fire, while Chris and Mum nursed drinks and Mum imagined the world for us, making it seem so vivid and real, so much more charged than the everyday around us.

'The saddest thing about wanting to find out who you are is that, by the time you start asking questions, it's already getting to be too late,' I remember her saying to me. 'I think the reason any of us get round to asking is a kind of sixth sense that the answers to our questions have begun to disappear. It's when you realise the people who knew them are dying and you've never sat down and asked for their secrets that you wish you'd started sooner in collecting the tale of who you are. Then you set off searching. Or that's how it was for me, anyway. When I was a girl I never thought about who it was that walked round in this body of mine, looking out through these eyes at the world.'

I remember her sitting in front of the fire at home, the old iron stove that heated most of the house through an intricate, arcane system of pipes and pumps, a few drinks deep in her evening, talking poetry the way she sometimes did on winter nights.

'I think the reason my father died the way he did is due to what happened to my grandmother when the first war came. When she was made to move to England from India, and washed up here without her husband, having to live by herself in a place quite unlike anything she'd ever known. That was what drove her mad. I'm sure that's why there weren't more children. After my father, she just couldn't manage it. She didn't have the strength to be a mother any more.'

'Did your dad talk to you about your grandparents?' Chris asked her, careful not to look at her, fixing his gaze on the fire. Thinking back to conversations like these, it seems to me that sometimes eye contact would make Mum think more carefully about what she was saying, and she would discover that it upset her, and then withdraw into herself.

'Not very often. Not ever so much. But I know that when he was a young child it was more or less his grandmother who raised him. Isn't that a strange thing? He must have felt so close to the long ago. His grandmother was born in the 1840s, I think that's right. She'd have brought him up with the values of that time. And he'd have been so out of step with his world, without even knowing it, just because of the start he was given. No wonder it was difficult for him to fit in. The child of an Indian woman, living out here, brought up with the manners of seventy years before. He'd have seemed like an alien to everyone. He didn't say all that much about his parents. I have two photos, though – hang on, let me find them.' She stood up and crossed the room to take a photo album from the shelves. She leafed through it for a moment, then walked back across the room to us. 'Here we go – look at this.'

She put the album down in front of me and Rachel, and I saw two photographs side by side on opposite pages. In the first photograph, two people, a man and a woman, were looking at the camera. He was seated, and she stood beside him: a much younger woman, very beautiful. The man was well dressed, and had a big moustache about the width of his face. In the second photograph, the same man was seated in the middle of a group of about a hundred Indian workmen. He had the same moustache, but seemed much older, his pale suit making him stand out among the thin men sitting round him.

'That's my grandfather with everyone who worked for him,' Mum said. I looked again at the photograph of the couple. The woman standing beside her husband was dark in complexion, but dressed in Western clothes. I had hardly thought of her as Indian when I looked at the picture the first time. More than her race, the photograph expressed the moment it was taken in. She looked more Edwardian than anything else – strapped into the period, bound indelibly to the moment she had lived through. 'They were married just a few years before the war.'

I remember my mum's unease, the tension in her body as she showed us those photos that first time. I try to imagine what she must have been feeling. She was trying to show Rachel and me who we were, of course. And weave that tapestry of inflections and secrets that would shape how the world looked through our eyes, becoming the way we saw, creating the unconscious, instinctive reflexes that underpinned all our actions, that made us who we were. But when I remember how tense Mum seemed as she leaned over us, showing us the photos, I think she must have also been feeling the same way I felt when I told Amy my family's story. A kind of grief would have been roused in her, a panic that soon her time would run out, it would all go, just as it had for the couple in the photo. I think she took the album out in part because she didn't want to die.

'Did your dad never want to go somewhere else?' I remember asking. When I think back to this night, this conversation, I feel sure this was the first time I formed the thought that I didn't want to always live on the farm. So I think it was very important, this question, though I didn't know it at the time.

'He didn't have the chance,' Mum said. 'By the time he was thirteen and leaving school, his grandparents had both died, and his mother was more or less an invalid who never left her room. His father wouldn't look after her. He didn't know how, I don't think. Who can blame him? I think his wife lost her mind. What does a farmer who once worked on the railways know about that? No, my grandfather didn't stand a chance, so my dad looked after her. He stayed at home and kept house, while his father was out on the hills with the sheep, summer and winter, and that was their strange life till my grandfather died.'

'There has to be more to it than that,' I said. 'He can't have just never done anything. Never gone anywhere.'

'The world wasn't like it is now, Ed,' Mum answered. 'He worked keeping the place together till the year his father died. Then he took over the farm, and married my mother, and then his mother died, and then he had me.'

It was strange, how our family spanned the century. My grandfather Leo had been well into his forties by the time Mum was born, so it was only necessary to go back a couple of generations to be speaking of a hundred years ago. He had been introduced to my grandmother by a man he knew at the livestock market in Hereford, so the story went. Grandma was younger than him, a farmer's daughter, without much of a plan in life, and she was happy to move to another farm and continue to live the life she knew. She brought up my mother very well, and in every story Mum ever told about her, the two appeared to be very close, they had shared a lot together. I didn't remember her all that well, because she had died when I was young. A woman who used to give me sweets; a woman with a laugh that shook her whole body, as if it came from deep inside her.

'You try your best to get on with it. But I think life happens too quickly for much recovering; there isn't time. That's what I felt myself when I found out I was having you,' I remember Mum saying as she smiled at me. 'How strange, I thought to myself when I learned I was pregnant. Because I'm still just a girl. And none of the things I wanted to solve have moved on even an inch for any of my thinking about them in the time I've had. But life's going on anyway – now I will be a mother, and I'll just have to go along with it, I suppose. Because it all keeps happening, one day at a time. Sometimes I find myself feeling very small and frightened, and I think of the day my father died, and I don't know how I can ever be all right. But it's happened before. It will happen again. So it stands to reason that there must be a way to keep going on, because others have managed it, billions must be managing it even now.'

Because Amy and I found each other at a wedding, it makes me strangely nervous, just a few months later, to be travelling to another wedding with her, although this time it's different, and Amy's just a guest, and won't be taking photographs of anyone. But this is how it started, I suppose, so it's hard not to wonder whether this could somehow be how it ends. But two of Amy's friends are getting married and she says I should come, so we travel to the coast for a weekend to stay with a group of her school friends in an Airbnb. The place we've rented all together for the weekend is a seventeenth-century farmhouse with a nineteenth-century front built on, surrounded by a couple of acres of grounds and set back from a narrow country road. There's a half moon of lawn at the front, fenced off with elegant ironwork and a scrubby hedge. It was planted as an orchard many years ago but hasn't been maintained. Half the apple trees are no longer producing and the only new tree growing is a young oak. The idea this place exists and yet has been left to fall into neglect is unimaginable to me. When the day comes that I have a home of my own, one of the things I'm most looking forward to is planting apple trees in the back yard. I dream of this moment. I imagine it will feel like coming fully alive.

After breakfast the first day, Amy goes to take a shower before getting ready for the wedding. An hour and a half till the taxi comes. Too soon for the men in the house to start dressing. I take my coffee and a book outside, go into the forgotten orchard, lie down under a russet apple tree.

We arrived the previous day before most of the others, and the couple who had got here before us had gone on already to the wedding rehearsal, so for a few hours we had the place to ourselves. We made dinner, then chose a bedroom, undressed and got into bed together, then dressed again to greet the next couple arriving. For half an hour we all tried to put up the sofa bed one of Amy's friends would be sleeping on that night, then accepted the thing was broken and did the best we could to cover it over with a sheet instead. Half an hour later, two more people arrived on the back of a motor-bike, then the last three returned from the wedding rehearsal. We poured out drinks for each other and sat talking together for a little while, then Amy and I took ourselves off to bed again, this time to sleep. I was tired after four hours travelling up the motorway, weekend traffic, warm Diet Coke from the services. The beginning of summer. In the morning we were woken by the alarm on my phone, and those who had to get to the venue early left us, and the rest of us made breakfast and ate together round the big dining table.

I've been lying on the grass for no more than five min-utes when I hear a voice calling my name from the front door, one of the girls asking whether I want a glass of some-thing. The first cork popping will be the sound of the start of the day.

I close my book and start getting up to go inside and help make drinks, then the same girl who called out to me comes back to the door and her voice has changed; there's a sense of real and sudden urgency in the air as she calls out to me. She tells me Amy's hurt herself and I'm needed upstairs right now.

I don't guess at first that it might be serious. I go inside and climb the stairs and walk through to the ancient back of the house where we slept last night, old boards, low doorways, not knowing what I'll find but guessing a stubbed toe, a nail pulled back; I have no intimation of what's waiting for me. Which is strange, because most of the time I tend to assume the worst, but in the summer sunshine where all life feels lazy and welcoming, the idea of real danger seems impossible.

Then I reach the doorway to our room and the day changes. There are four people kneeling round Amy where she is slumped on the floor, holding towels to her head, and all of their voices are panicked and their faces pale, so I walk round to see what's happened and Amy's face is grey, she's shaking and her breath comes in gasps and the towels are soaked in blood and there is blood pooling on the floor and a spatter pattern reaching all the way to the bed across the whitewashed floorboards.

I kneel and ask what's happened and if she can tell me when her birthday is, and she can hardly speak. Someone tells me she hit her head on the doorframe coming back from the shower and there was this crack like a gunshot.

I call an ambulance while her friends start to mop up the blood where it's staining the white-painted boards and the call handler asks to speak to Amy, then tells me to maintain pressure on the wound and that an ambulance will take two hours. I ask where the nearest A&E is and we find it on a map and then we set off, Amy insisting she takes her dress in the back of the car though I can't imagine she'll need it now, driving away from the ceremony we surely won't see, the vows exchanged, the life embarked on, driving through green meadowland past osier-lined brooks and little villages, driving with a police motorbike on our tail for a dozen miles of the journey, following us closely, as if he knows there's something wrong with us, as if he knows I'd be flooring the accelerator if he wasn't there, finally reaching the town with the hospital after forty minutes, funnelled through one roundabout after another on the ring road encircling the town, then parking up at A&E and passing through the sliding doors, and I think of the time I had my skull fractured, a fight I didn't ask for down a backstreet one Saturday night, and the stabbing pains that still come to me sometimes ten years later, like a knife in the skull, and feel a growing panic about Amy, a fear in the pit of my stomach that anything could be happening to her now. We get to the front desk and a doctor takes her away.

The day doesn't feel real. We've all watched too many films; sometimes when things that matter are at stake, we feel as if we've walked into one. Such a sense of detachment is dangerous. It makes people feel they're invincible, when we're not, we're all one crack like a gunshot away from life changing. It is so brief, this thing we're in, so fragile, and only one thing is certain – the end approaching each of us.

The beginning of summer. Perhaps it crosses my mind even now while I wait for news of Amy that something is coming towards us. Like sighting the first slow swell of a wave. And in this moment, I don't know what it's bringing. Because the image of the blood spattered over the floor is still in my eyes, and what if she dies now, what if she's keeled over even now? I press my hands together between my legs, because it feels like they're shaking, and I don't want her to be dead on the other side of those doors, I don't want her to be gone before we've even started, and we had no chance to be happy together; I had no chance to stop her hitting her head on the doorframe, so how could this be taken from us, when we have done nothing?

As I wait, I start to feel desperate, and I want to get up and go to her, walk through the doors, demand I'm allowed to be with her while she's seen, but I do nothing.

I sit and wait. I try to control this urge to make it about me.

She comes back out into the waiting area thirty minutes later, pale and slightly dazed, blood still caked in her hair. I stand up when I see her, walk towards her, and I can feel tears starting in my eyes, because I'd begun to wonder if I'd see her again.

'Are you OK?' I ask her. She looks at me, but not quite at me, as if her vision's blurred.

'Fine.' And her voice is quiet, she seems withdrawn, and I can see she's not fine, she's shaken.

'So what happened?'

'They glued me up. My head, I mean. I can't wash my hair for a week while the glue's in. I can't wash the blood out of my hair.' She raises a hand very gently to her hair, touches the blood that's matted and dried there, then winces, lets her hand fall back down by her side.

'And what are we supposed to do now?'

'We'll go to the wedding.'

This sounds very unlikely to me. Surely she shouldn't be out around people now? Surely they've told her she ought to go home?

'Are you sure?'

Amy looks at me and I can see she's suddenly close to getting angry. 'Do you think we're just going home? I'm not missing my friends' wedding, Ed. They've told me what's safe and it's fine.'

'And it's totally safe? But presumably you can't drink, can you?'

'They've told me what's safe. Come on.'

I suspect her of lying to me, of course. Deciding she's willing to take a risk because she wants to be with her friends. It's her choice, to a point; part of me thinks it's selfish too, but in the end I suppose it's her choice, and I wasn't in the consulting room, so I don't know what they've told her. So we go to the wedding in time for the meal. Amy changes on the driveway of the big house that's been rented for the wedding reception, standing in her underwear on the drive, defiantly alive and determined to be present at the wedding of her friends, the life in her shining, dazzling me, too beautiful to put into language.

In the evening she dances and it makes me smile to see her laugh, makes me feel almost dizzy, because the blood spatter all the way to the bed is still before my eyes while I watch, and suddenly I realise this is happiness, this has been happiness all along. I know this with a clarity I haven't felt in years, and it runs through me like drink, like a chemical high. But I can't join in with the dancing. It feels too ghostlike tonight, this luck we've had, this being here.

When the night ends and we lie down to sleep, I find that I'm holding my breath, as if listening for footsteps, as if something might be coming to claim us. Sleep takes me in the end, but I fight it. Something is waiting at the corner of my vision, and what is it that's coming towards me exactly? What can I almost see? The briefness of this place is suddenly too brittleclear to bear; what seemed this morning like the whole, real world now resembles little more than a dream, ice across a lake that could give way at any moment, plunging us into other worlds, unspoken underneath.

Every minute we live could change our lives. But even though each minute carries the same potential charge, there are nevertheless certain days that seem to shine brighter than others, days when our lives seem to be shaped and decided. Lying in bed next to Amy, looking at the matted blood clotting her hair into ropes on the pillow, I feel like I'm living through one of those days. Right now, right here, my life is changing and I can feel the current that's drawing me inexorably on. I look at Amy as she sleeps and see this is the person I want to be with. Her and no other. Perhaps I hadn't realised that till now. We'd fallen easily into one another's lives, and discovered a rhythm together. But things seem suddenly different tonight. This morning when I saw the blood spattered across this room, for just a moment I imagined she might die. And I discovered as that thought passed over me like cloud shadow that this, the life welling up between us, has come to mean a great deal to me, though it hardly seems we've been together long enough to speak of love, to speak of lasting. It's so new, and it's untested, and if someone had asked me yesterday, I might well have said our relationship was just the two of us going with the flow, but when we were in the car going to the hospital, I felt I simply couldn't lose this woman who was sitting beside me, cradling her head as the blood dried on her hands. We're playing for keeps, I see this now. We have made moorings of each other.

In the morning we wake and eat breakfast with the others, and then I drive us home because Amy is now feeling the effects of the previous night and of the accident before the wedding. The day is a brilliant blazing, bright sun beating down on the apple trees and the house, which makes everyone's hangovers worse. Magpies chatter and flit among the trees. A jay swoops through the shadows, hunting.

'Does your head hurt?'

'Not really.'

'What does that mean? If your head hurts, then we need to see someone.'

'It's a Sunday morning.'

'That doesn't matter.'

'I'm just hungover.'

'Are you sure?'

'No.'

'Then should we go back and ask to be seen again?'

'At the hospital?'

'Yes.'

'It's miles in the wrong direction.'

'That doesn't matter.'

'No, I'm almost certain I'm just hungover.'

'Are you sure that they said you could drink?'

'They told me I wasn't concussed.'

'That's not the same as saying you can drink.'

'They said that too.' I know then that she's lying and I wish I'd gone into the consulting room with her.

Amy stands impatiently, looking at me. 'Can we just go home? I just want to get in my own bed again.'

She sleeps in the passenger seat beside me as we travel back down the M1. At Watford Gap services we stop for coffee. I look up at the bridge over the motorway, and imagine my father standing there. He used to live in a village two miles away, and every evening during his teenage years when he was waiting to escape from this place and make his way into the wide world, Dad told me that he used to walk out to the bridge to smoke his pipe, and look to the north and then to the south, and wonder what was going to become of him, what life was going to offer. He thought by doing this he would avoid his parents, my grandparents, ever finding out that he smoked, but I imagine they knew very well what he was doing, and smelled it on him, and simply let him get on with it. There's no one on the bridge today. This road is so much busier now; I can't imagine anyone ever stops up there any more to look down over it. It's strange to think that if all time was suddenly made visible, and every day in the life of the world was allowed to rub shoulders together for just a moment, I'd be able to see my dad as a young man standing up there, smoking, looking around him, wondering what the future would bring. Like sighting the wave that came before you.

After that weekend it feels like something has to change. I don't quite know what to do about it, but the rhythm I've been in, going round to Amy's and then going back to the converted garage I've been living in, seems suddenly ludicrous to me. Moving into the garage had been natural enough, I suppose; the idea was always to retreat for a time before finding a way to go forwards in life again. But now the adolescence of the present situation feels embarrassing to me, and I'm anxious to do something about it. Amy's due to leave for Kuala Lumpur in a week's time, and I feel like we're running out of something, I suppose we're running out of time, and I don't know how to tell her before she goes that, if she didn't mind, if she didn't object to it, I'd like to still be there for her when she gets back.

How do you say that? Tell someone you love them? Isn't that just banal?

In the end I do the only other thing I can think of, the thing that Amy's already done with me; I take her to meet my parents. Pathetic, really, but it seems like a way of saying, here, look – this is my life. You can share it with me if you like.

Because Mum hasn't really talked to me since I told her Amy and I have got together, I feel more than a little apprehensive when we get in the car to drive to the farm to visit her and Chris. But I know I need to go over there and fix what I've broken, and I can't think of any other way to show Amy that I don't want her to forget me, so I call Chris and invite myself over to Wales for the weekend. I realise after we've finished speaking that it will be the first time I've gone there in almost a year.

Since I left home, I've always gone back in the spring to help with the lambing, but the argument Mum and I had about her will meant that didn't happen this year. It did feel like there was something missing from the year. I stayed in the city and worked instead, and work doesn't feel very much like my real life. All the work I've ever done has only really been a way to pay for living – answering the phone in an agency for a long time, working in the bar at a theatre and, for the last two years, writing advertorial for a website that sells watches and other things people don't need but spend a lot of money on. In the last half a year they've started letting me file my copy for them from home, and I've been able to make some money on the side writing listicles for other websites, but for a long time they made me go into an office every day to make sure I stayed productive. So when I didn't go home for the lambing this year, I sat in a cubicle in east London writing about watches instead.

By coincidence, I hadn't visited at Christmas either; Juliet and I used to have a system of alternating who we visited on the day, and last year it was her family's turn, so I called Mum and Chris and talked on the phone with them, and told myself that was enough, and that they felt it was enough, they wouldn't mind that I hadn't done more to see them. It must be similar with every family, I suppose. Once the children have grown old enough to move away, we all enter the endless dance of how to navigate that week between Christmas and New Year, never in the right place, never all together, all of us wondering how to get that week right. This is where the idea takes hold, I think, that somewhere there's a centre, there's a place called home that's the rootnote of your life. And the search for that starts to consume you, as you try to work out what that strange word means. Home, an idea which is constructed out of place, people, and stories above all. A synonym for love. It's the memory of Christmases when no one had to worry where to spend them, where to go. The memory of a childhood when nothing was complicated. If such a thing ever really existed at all.

Realising I haven't been home to see Mum and Chris for almost a year makes me a little more anxious about visiting, but it doesn't change my decision about travelling out there; in truth, feeling uncomfortable about going back home isn't anything new. Almost every visit I've made out there in the last ten years has been a little awkward, and Mum and I have long ago become used to biting our tongues when we're together. That's partly why Mum liked Juliet, I think; Juliet was nice to her, and wanted to involve her in our lives, so she became a bridge between Mum and me, a way for us to reconnect at a time when we seemed to have lost our connection.

Before it was arguing over wills and inheritance, the face the fight between me and my mother wore was over my father when, in the year after I left university, I let him come and live with me and then looked after him while he died. Dad slept in the spare room for that terrible last six months, and Mum kept her distance, causing a big silence to open up between us.

The way I'd seen it, I didn't have a choice. Dad had already lost his battle with drink by then; his life was already over, and he just needed a place where he could finish the process of dying. He never actually asked me to help him, but we had coffee one day, and I saw the state of him and guessed he'd lost his flat, so I asked if he needed a place to stay, and he moved in with me. I was living at that time in the flat of a friend who'd moved abroad for work and needed a house sitter, so it was easy enough for me to take him in – I had no flatmates to upset.

For the last half a year of his life, Dad sat on my sofa and drank. I'd remove the bottles and take him to the doctor, cook him meals and collect his medication, do whatever I could for him, but I was years too late really. I knew within a month of him arriving that his liver had more or less failed.

After a while he had to go into the hospital, and I would go and sit with him, and then it all came to an end. There was nothing much left for us to talk about by the time he was in hospital, so I read to him instead, a chapter of a book I'd then leave by his bedside with a bookmark in so I could pick up where I'd left off and carry on reading the next time I visited. I suppose I left the book because I hoped someone else might want to go and see him, and find the book there, and be grateful for it because it would mean they could read to him, and wouldn't have to think of anything to say. But no one else ever went, I don't think, and the bookmark was always in the same place when I returned. He liked children's stories. I suppose they took him back to his own childhood, and that comforted him. And I was his child reading to him as well, and I guess he found some kind of happiness in remembering the time when it was the other way round.

When he died, I was reading him *The Magician's Nephew*, about the portals in the attic that led into other worlds. When I got to the hospital that last time, and found that his bed was empty, I took the book home with me. I still have it somewhere on my shelves. He was a bastard, my dad. The things he put himself through traumatised me and Mum and everyone who knew him, and there was a lot we might have wanted from him which he was never able to give. But he was my dad all the same, so I keep the book and I keep the bookmark in the page where I left it. Many years from now, when I die, someone from a house clearance firm will pick up that old second-hand copy of a C. S. Lewis book, and see it was read by someone who never finished it, decide it has no resale value and throw it away. But for now it's a doorway into the memory of my father.

Mum kept her distance all the time he lived with me. I suppose she had to. The fact was that the trigger for Dad's drinking had been their divorce. I suppose it must have been hard for her not to feel some guilt, some responsibility. After the divorce she built a life that made her happy, and looked like permanence, and was filled with children and friendships and the open air, moving back to the farm to live with her mother for her last years, then taking the farm over, and meeting Chris, and marrying him, and moving on. Dad drank, meanwhile, and lost his work because his hands shook, and lived on benefits and odd jobs and moved from flat to dirty flat, and sometimes when I visited him I would take a bottle of gin with me, knowing that he'd kill himself one day, but knowing as well that, until he was two drinks deep, he could barely string a sentence together. I'd sit with him, have a drink myself to normalise the situation. I tried to make it seem like I was keeping him company, like nothing was wrong. After a couple of drinks, his hands would stop shaking and he'd talk in sentences again. It was natural for Mum to keep her distance from all that. But in the last months, that meant she also ended up keeping her distance from me, and after the funeral, which in the end she didn't come to, telling us she didn't think Dad would want her to remember him like that, I found it was difficult to restart things between us.

I don't think we really spoke again till I met Juliet. Then there was someone to introduce Mum to, a new person in the room to listen to the stories, and we were able to build an alternative narrative about our relationship through telling Juliet the story of who we were, rewriting our family history so it wasn't overshadowed by drink, by the marriage that had failed, and other things came into focus instead, parts of our shared history we might otherwise have forgotten. We left out the failures and hidden darknesses, and talked about the farm and childhood and holidays – the stuff of life.

There were things we couldn't get back, of course. There was the problem that even after Dad's funeral I still felt like his representative on earth somehow, responsible for his memory, trapped on his side when the wind had changed. I felt as if I brought him with me whenever I came to stay at the farm. These visits only strengthened the sense I had that one day the farm would stop being part of my life, because it was only half my life, the place where Mum and Chris had lived, not Dad. Knowing that changed the way I saw the place when I went back. It started to seem like a crime scene to me – my childhood was marked out there in chalk outlines, but the body was gone.

My parents had met at college, and got together, and married about a year after they left and started work. Probably too quickly, as it would turn out. After the marriage, they didn't go back to the farm, but tried living away in the south of England. Dad worked in the building restoration trade, and Mum took in people's sewing and worked as a typist for an agency. It isn't so very long ago, but it was a different world; money stretched further, so jobs no one even does any more used to be enough to make ends meet. They made their home in West Sussex in a disused hunting lodge in the middle of a wood, two miles from the next living soul. The lodge belonged to an earl who lived in the big house in the middle of the estate we lived on the edge of, and who had taken a liking to my dad when he did some work on the house, and let him have the lodge for a peppercorn rent because no one was using it, and having someone in it would help to keep it from falling down. It was during this time that I was born and I think both my parents liked the idea of bringing up their child in a wood in the middle of nowhere: the peace, the seclusion, the freedom of no one watching.

For a while it was just the three of us alone there, and I think we were happy. Then Dad started to travel more for work, and then one winter a six-week job turned into the best part of half a year, and the marriage ended, in the way marriages do when a husband and wife are pulled apart like that. Dad moved out, and I stayed in the lodge with Mum for a while, but there was a feeling once Dad had gone that everything was temporary. Mum didn't want to stay any longer than she had to in the ruin of the life she'd tried to build, and money was a problem, and I guess the isolation must have been a lot to cope with once it was just her and me and the ghost of her marriage out there in the woods. So, in the end, she decided to go home.

I remember it seemed to me when we arrived at the farm as if we were walking into a dream my mum had had years earlier. When she was pregnant with me, she had made a blanket that looked just like those hills in Wales. She stitched together squares of wool and felt in different shades of green and russet for the fields, with little border hedges in dark green, and a blue woollen river running through it all, and a road with a bridge in grey-brown, and little sheep sticking up from the blanket made from tufts of white wool that looked a bit like clouds, and this was the blanket I used to lie on in the big room in the hunting lodge before I learned to walk. The farm looked just like the blanket. The same patchwork of fields, the same greens and browns and sheep and hedgerows. I remember taking in the valley we had moved to for the first time, ruined barns that dotted the hillsides and seemed to be caving into the grass like ships going under, like memories sinking back into the long withdrawing furl of time. Of course I didn't take in the meaning of those old ruined buildings at the time, my thoughts were simpler, I doubt I even put them into words, but I do remember knowing those places had sheltered people once, whole families, and now they were nothing. And now we were here, and we'd do the same thing. I remember feeling I could see back in time.

Once we settled there, I learned that time kept different rules in that valley. There were days when changes in the weather seemed to make time move faster; we would watch a weather front scour the valley in the space of an hour, swooping over like a buzzard so that all of a sudden there was snow harrowing the ground. Then it would be gone, and the sun would shine, and the snow would disappear as if it had never happened. The sun burning off the last clouds in the valley would pick out rainbows in the threads of cloud it scattered, so they looked like oil slicks smudging the light. It seemed sometimes as if the sky spent its days in drafting and discarding wild masks of light, riotous and diffuse, the most beautiful show you could ever imagine, searching for a true face, trying to find its real self, never deciding what that might be in time for nightfall, then having to give up for another day when the stars and the moon came out.

It was always the valley more than the cottage that I loved. The cottage itself was nineteenth-century, with an extension built by my great-grandfather, and another lean-to added by my grandfather later on. There were eight rooms, a living space you walked into through the front door where the stove had been joined up to a radiator system through the rest of the house, which was where my grandmother used to sit all day in the short time she was living there as well, before she died and it was just me and Mum again. Either side of that room was a kitchen where the walls were always wet with damp, and the sitting room my great-grandfather had added, which was the biggest room in the house, and heated by a separate stove. At the back, the lean-to served as a utility room, always filled with washing on lines and things that needed to be cleaned, and a small toilet that had been put in and boxed off from the rest of the room. Upstairs were three bedrooms and a bathroom, the older two bedrooms barely larger than the double beds in them, memories of a different time, of the modest spaces claimed by the people who first came here and made this hillside habitable. Stretching up the hill in the field nearest to the house were a few outbuildings for timber and machinery, straggled all the way to the top of the field where the water tank was housed, all of them thrown up over many years as and when they were needed. It was an isolated place, half a mile from the next farm and a mile from the nearest village. In summer it was very beautiful, but in the winter the place became lonely. The cold months always seemed to be trying to drive us out, and something in them spoke to the stone of the farmhouse, enlisted the slate flagstones. Because of this I never quite trusted the farm in the summer. In its heart, I believed that it wanted us gone.

An old school friend introduced Mum to Chris at a dinner party. He was living in the area and had worked on the farm for a time when it was just my grandmother living there, when my grandmother had hired a manager to run the farm, and the manager had occasionally brought in hired labour at lambing time. Mum and Chris liked each other straight away, they've both told me, and Chris says it was the boldest thing he'd ever done when he asked Mum for her number. After they first met, he didn't call for a couple of days, because he said the whole thing just felt too unlikely to him. But an evening arrived when he gave in and called her, and Mum picked up, and everything started.

There followed a strange period in both their lives. The beginning of love, when what you want is in the air but no one's said it. Every evening they'd sit on the phone and talk to each other. Mum said she started to feel as if all day she was waiting for their phone calls, as if that was the real centre of her life. The conversations everyone has when they're trying not to say I love you.

Eventually it happened. It was the phone bills that made them cross the invisible sword that lay between them and find a way to put their dreams into words. Chris said to Mum one night as he stared at the fire in the grate that, seeing as all his money was going on calling her, maybe he'd be better off if they tried living in the same place for a little while. Maybe that would at least help the phone bills, if nothing else.

I was very young when we moved to the farm, but perversely I think of that as the time when childhood ends in my story. I felt like I'd lost some part of me back in the woods after we drove out of them for the last time, the quiet woods that sheltered us for those first few island years, when I have no memory of any other face except my mum's, not even Dad's, as if the world was only two souls wide. The world was never so perfect again, though of course we found happiness out on the hills at the farm; but ever since we left the hunting lodge, I've known there was another life, a ghost life, happening just under the surface of my own – a boy I'd left behind in the wood who never grew up, who no one ever went back to rescue, who couldn't even be reached if someone tried to find him now. Like a record playing in another room. That's what became of my childhood. I've never done anything about it. I've never gone back, or sought out a therapist to talk things through. The only concession I've ever made to the memory of that boy is that every time I move out of a flat or a house and into a new one, I always make sure that I leave a day early. I'll spend the day moving boxes into the new place, and then after dinner on the day I move, I'll go back to the place I've left, and let myself in with the key I've kept, and check the rooms and cupboards one last time. I've rescued some useful things that way. A jacket I left on the back of a bedroom door. A scarf on a coat hanger. A crystal glass that belonged to my grandmother. What I've always hoped I'll find, though, is the real original self I left behind. But that boy is never there waiting for me. I always leave the old places for the last time on my own.

On the day we travel to visit Mum and Chris at the farm, I find myself hoping to put off the moment of our arrival, praying we hit traffic, praying we might get lost down some side road. I think Mum had got the idea fixed in her mind of Juliet as her future daughter-in-law, and I think that particular casting became important to her. Living out in the wilds, the farm being so far from other people, Mum's world can sometimes come to feel quite small, I think, so the people in it take on great significance. I think Mum had imagined the talks she'd have with Juliet in the lead-up to our wedding day, the first visit she'd make to our home when we settled down somewhere, all that. And she thought Juliet brought out the best in me, moderated the behaviour of her son, who she'd been half estranged from, made it easier for us to have a relationship again.

Amy and I both feel the tension on the drive, and snap at each other, but I can't find the words to tell her how I'm feeling. I end up telling her the story of how my grandfather died instead. The story makes me feel ashamed as I tell it to her, and I suppose that's why I tell it. A way of expressing my shame at being irritable towards her as we drive, even if I can't actually explain the emotion.

'Part of why I don't really ever want to live there again is that my grandfather killed himself on the roof,' I tell her.

She turns to look at me. 'Jesus. I'm sorry.'

'It was before I was born. He climbed up there with a shotgun one morning and killed himself. Took half the roof tiles with him when he fell, and he landed in the back yard and my grandmother found him.'

'Why did he do it?'

'Why does anyone do it? He just struggled, I think. He had to look after his mum for a long time. And she wasn't well. She was an invalid, really, her mind had gone. I think that kind of thing builds up in a person.'

'But to kill yourself.'

'It's farming. A lot of farmers kill themselves.'

Amy looked at her hands, and didn't say anything. I could

hear that I was being aggressive, shrugging her off, telling the story so that it would sound shocking. I didn't know how to tell it any differently. 'None of us ever step on the spot where he fell. It just wasn't something you ever did when we were growing up. So the weird thing is that you can see where it happened, because the weeds grow up differently in between the flagstones. You can almost see the outline of the body in the middle of the yard.'

'Jesus. How did your family stay there after that?'

'I never really understood it. I asked Mum about it. She said you can't only see the bad.'

'But that's pretty terrible.'

'She said that leaving would have been like forgetting him.'

'It's pretty terrible all the same.'

'The coroner recorded it as an accident so he could be buried in consecrated ground. And so that Grandma could claim his life insurance. He said my grandfather accidentally climbed on to the roof, took off his shoe, put his shotgun in his mouth and fired it with his big toe. A lot of suicides used to be put down as accidents like that. If the coroner wanted to do the family a favour.'

I immediately regret telling the story, but it's too late to take it back, and I don't know what to say to make us feel better.

We pull into the front yard with sinking feelings, and see Chris open the door to the house and open his arms to welcome us in. Mum follows him outside, smile fixed on her face. Can Amy see the determined look she carries, the watchfulness in her eyes? How well do you have to know her before you can spot that she's acting?

'Ed, hello.' Chris shakes my hand as he always has since I moved away. Mum hugs me, and then turns to Amy and hugs her as well.

'And you must be Amy. I've heard so much about you. It's lovely to meet you. I'm Angela.'

Amy, who has heard too much about Mum, not enough of it complimentary, smiles and hugs her back.

'It's lovely to meet you too, Angela.'

We dump our bags, then all four of us take the dogs out for a walk. We talk about house prices and the weather, public transport and the dogs, then turn for home, and then we're shut in the house for the rest of the night, and just have to hope we can get through it happily. I deal with the tension in the worst way possible, drinking too much, and have to go to bed by ten.

Amy follows me up to bed, but once I'm undressed and horizontal, she says she'll go back downstairs to help wash up the dinner things. I hear her walk back down, the floorboards creaking with each step, and then I hear her in the room below with Mum. Chris has gone outside, I think, or gone to the bathroom, or gone to bed. The two women find themselves alone together, as I suppose both of them knew that at some point they might do, and Amy doesn't yet know how thin the floors are in this house, that I can hear every word they say to each other.

'He'll be asleep in a minute,' Amy says. I can hear the sound of the dishwasher being stacked, and wonder whether Mum has looked up when Amy came down, whether she's smiled at her or turned her back.

'He doesn't normally do that,' Mum says. 'Drink that much.'

'No, he doesn't. But he's home, I suppose.'

'Does that make a difference?'

'Perhaps it means he can relax.'

'I just find it unsettling, really. Because of his father.'

'Oh, yes. Of course. Is he like his father?'

'In some ways. Isn't everyone?'

'Can I do this bit of washing-up?'

'If you don't mind, that would be very kind, thank you.'

I listen as Amy turns the tap on and runs it till it starts to get hot. Then the sound of the water changes when she puts the plug in and the kitchen sink starts filling up.

'I enjoyed dinner.'

'I'm glad.'

'It must have been a strange evening for you.'

I hear Mum stop clattering the cutlery around, a hair's breadth of silence. 'Why strange?'

'Because I'm not her, am I? The person you'd thought he was going to be with.'

'Oh. I see.'

'Ed told me you were very fond of her. Juliet, I mean.'

'I was. She's a lovely girl. We've kept in touch, actually. Just the odd text.'

'I only met her once.'

'At that wedding.'

'Yes. That's right. She was very pretty.'

'I don't know how important that is. She's a very considerate person, that's what I liked about her.'

'Of course. You're right, it's not important. But there's nothing else I can really say about her. We've barely ever exchanged a word.'

'Could I ask you a question? I don't want to seem challenging.'

'Of course.'

'Did you know he was going to leave her for you?'

Amy doesn't answer for a moment. 'That's a difficult question.'

'Is it?'

'In some ways. I didn't know he was going to leave her. I couldn't have really, we only spoke for half an hour and we didn't exchange numbers; I didn't even know if we'd see each other again. But I suppose I did know, as well.'

'It was quite a charged half an hour, then?'

'I suppose so, yeah.'

'I might just dry those so you've got space.'

'Oh, thanks.'

'Thank you for rinsing. Ed never rinses.'

'I know, I criticise him relentlessly for it, but it just makes him more stubborn, I think.'

Mum laughs. 'That's him exactly.'

There's silence below me for a short time.

'I hope we'll be able to be friends,' Amy says, 'even if I'm not her.'

'Of course. Whoever Ed wants to be with is a friend to me, as long as they make him happy.'

'It's so difficult, isn't it? In-laws and girlfriends. I've seen so many people get together with terrible men and women who were awful to them, and all of their family would know and say nothing for fear of causing a rift. It happens all the time, I think. And how do you know the right time to step in and say something? So many relatives must put up with girlfriends and boyfriends they really hate, because they haven't crossed the red line that would allow open warfare.'

Mum laughs again. 'I've seen quite a lot of that, yeah.'

'It's strange to me, really, that people so often seem to get together with people who don't make them happy. It's probably very naive of me, but I'd sort of like to believe that any two people in the world could make each other happy if they tried. I'd like to believe that. Some would be better matched than others, but if everyone was kind, it should be possible for any two people to be happily married. But it isn't, is it?'

'No, it's not.'

'I think I'm sounding very naive.'

'I don't know. Idealistic, maybe. I think you could look at it the other way as well.'

'Yes?'

'I think really, when you think about how difficult people are, and how many fears we all have and insecurities, how much we hate ourselves, how unsure we are, and how jealous we get, and how hard all of us find it to talk or even really to know what we're feeling at any given time, I think really you could argue it's miraculous that any two people do manage to make each other happy. And winkle each other out of their shells.'

It occurs to me then as I listen that Chris still hasn't come back into the kitchen to clear things away. I wonder whether he's stayed away deliberately, to let Mum and Amy have this talk, and whether he's somewhere in the house now, listening like me to what they are saying, and whether Mum knows he's listening, or whether she thinks she and Amy are alone.

Mum's already up by the time I wake the next morning and

head downstairs to make coffee. She's sitting in the kitchen with a cup of tea, watching the steam rise up from the cup.

'Morning,' I say to her, keeping my voice low.

'Morning,' Mum says, and smiles at me.

'Couldn't sleep?'

'No, I never can, I'm not very good at it.'

'I'm sorry.'

She shrugs. 'I'm used to it. Getting up is hard when you're always tired, but once I'm up, I find I can keep going.'

'Mind if I make a pot of coffee?'

'Of course, help yourself.' I put the kettle on and reach into the fridge for the coffee and the milk. 'Amy seems nice,' she says.

'I'm glad you think so.'

'I'm sorry about the way I reacted when I first heard.'

'That's OK. It was a shock.'

'It was. But I understand. Things had reached a point with Juliet, hadn't they?'

'How do you mean?'

'Well, you'd been together for quite some time. So there comes a point where either that's for ever, or it's not, I think.'

'You mean marriage.'

'I suppose so. But more than that, really. You just have to ask yourself at a certain point, is this who I'm going to be? Am I ready to commit to this? And you're a young man. You probably shouldn't have reached that point yet. It's like with this place, with thinking about the farm. You probably shouldn't have reached a point yet where you know what you'll want to do with it when the time comes, because all that's still to come.'

I don't know what to say to this. It seems like a wilful, contorted misunderstanding of who I am and what I think and how I've been living since I left this place, and it feels strange to listen to Mum turn the whole life I shared with Juliet into some subordinate clause of the question of whether I'll ever want to live here again. As if that was the only thing that mattered. But perhaps it is to her. I hold my breath, say nothing. Mum notices that I'm not replying, and glances at me, checking the impact of her words.

'I just mean that I support what you're doing, that's all,' she says.

'So are we OK now?'

'I hope so.'

'I think we are.'

'Well, let's say we are, then.' And she smiles, and I smile back, and the kettle boils, and I make the coffee and take it with me as I go back upstairs, wanting to believe her.

1925

L EO WAS WHISKED away from his first world while he was
still just discovering it, and though he never did go back,
though the call of the past never got so loud he felt the need
to act on it, retrace his steps and revisit that lost world by the
dockside, a part of him missed it for the rest of his life. Indeed,
that might have been exactly why he never returned to Poplar
and wandered around. To go back would have been to have
seen the place had forgotten him, had changed and moved
on, and that it wasn't the place he missed so much as that
moment in his life. That state of innocence when the world
was just one place wide and he knew all of it. To go back
might have taken away the feeling that everything he had left
behind was still in the world somewhere, and that he might
one day find it again. And he liked his nostalgia, it made
things beautiful to him. He didn't want to let it go. Instead he
liked to remember the noise of the docks and the faces pressed
together, the great shout of the streets of London he had
thought of as his birthright. Later in life, when he visited London again, the city came to seem mad to him, too loud to
hear itself, and he despaired of the idea of ever trying to live
there, but it had been intoxicating to a small child to always

be among such energy, such life, as if you were really part of something and not just a person on your own in the world. That lost London, the London of the mind, remained always beautiful to him forever after.

Perhaps that memory of the city was why he felt loneliness so keenly later on; he was introduced to solitude late, so it could never seem natural and fade into the background of his life, as he suspected it did for many others, becoming something they accepted, like the weather. Leo always had a horror of the loneliness that followed him through his years, because he couldn't break out of thinking of it as an affliction.

'We have some news,' his mother said to him one day in 1925, calling him into her room where she sat at her dressing table. Leo stood to attention as best he could in the doorway, hands behind his back, trying to look like the boy she wished him to be. His mother didn't turn to look at him directly as she spoke, but fixed him with a look in the mirror on her dressing table instead. As if she was shy to really turn and face him. Or as if they spoke in some mirror world, not the real world of flesh and blood and bodies. 'I'm afraid to tell you that your grandfather has died. Your father has gone down to Wales to see to his funeral.' Leo felt the rush of shock in his belly, which felt something like embarrassment, and something like being punched quite hard in the stomach. He wondered what it meant for his grandfather to be dead. The thought had never crossed his mind before, but it occurred to him in that moment that he wasn't absolutely convinced that there was such a thing as heaven. Could his grandfather be in some other, better place? Leo couldn't work out why, but instinctively he doubted that somehow. It seemed more likely to him that his grandfather simply no longer existed. He wondered what he was to feel about that. It was difficult, to be sure. He hadn't really known his grandfather, had only met him once. But he supposed it must be important when people related to you disappeared. 'That is going to mean a change in our circumstances,' his mother went on. 'We are to leave London and move to the country.'

'Why are we doing that?' Leo asked, seeing no sense in it. What could the city lack that the country offered? For a small boy in love with the life of the river, it was impossible to comprehend.

'Your father is to inherit your grandfather's farm, and we are going to live there,' Phoebe said, picking up her powder brush to cover up her face, as if the matter was finished.

'Is it very far from here? Will we come back to visit?'

'I don't know why we would ever need to come back here, but it's not too far. It's in Wales, on the other side of England, but it's not so far really.'

'The other side of England sounds like quite a long way.'

Phoebe laughed, but still didn't look at Leo, focusing instead on applying the powder that would make her face seem pale. Leo wished sometimes that she wouldn't do that. There were boys at school who made him feel less than them because his face was darker, as if his skin meant he couldn't fit in. When his mother worked to whiten her face, it made him feel as if the boys were right, and the shame was real, not just his invention. He watched her in the mirror, creating a new self, covering her real self up. Through all the years of his growing up, it would remain his mother's habit to tell him difficult news without looking at him, often while sitting at the dressing-table mirror. He guessed it was simply a way of avoiding him, avoiding the confrontation that is always inherent in admonishing someone, or giving bad news. Years later, Leo would learn that painters sometimes liked to look at their work in the mirror as it developed, in order to see it in a new way, from a new angle, and simulate the moment of its being looked at by others after they had finished their work and gone. When he heard that, he thought of the way his mother and he used to look at each other in the dressing-table mirror, and wondered whether that had been part of what they were doing as well. Rehearsing a time when they wouldn't be together. Imagining the world the other would live in when they themselves had left it. Or if that was at least what his mother had been doing to him.

'Before you were born, your father and I crossed the whole of the world so that he could live in this place. I sat on the deck of the ship each day for weeks, and watched the countries going past. We sailed past all the places in the Bible, and he pointed them out to me one by one. As if we were sailing through the whole of that book and the whole ancient world. Once you've done that, you'll think nothing of moving across England for a better life. And it will be a better life, Leo, I can assure you. Inheriting the farm will make your father a wealthy man, and in time it will make you a wealthy man as well.'

So they moved, and Leo grew up a country boy and not the boy he wanted to be, watched his father struggle and fail to get used to the work he'd grown up around but, through India and the railways, lost all the instincts for. What his father couldn't understand was that, working with sheep, things sometimes just weren't fixable. Sometimes sheep would get maggots breeding in their bellies, and die. And that could not be remedied by an engineer. Failure was simply a part of life, the farming life especially, and it had to be borne and accepted. Leo was young enough to take this on board and see it for a fact, the way that some things just didn't work out. But his father had got too used to being able to find solutions to problems, and he never came to like the work he did, the better life he had supposedly inherited.

Leo hated his school. His face seemed much darker in Wales than it had done in London. He trained for a life on the farm when school was finished. He grew up thinking of life as a series of inheritances that were taken away from you, or otherwise thrust on you when you didn't want them. A place where you had to put up with what happened to you. It was a view he would later discover was shared by many of his generation. Strange, how ideas seemed to move through the air. As if they got into the water supply. On an average day, Leo felt quite independent in his mind, and then from time to time he'd come across something that would make him question whether such independence was even possible.

The little escapes he managed, when he could, were into the pages of books, where no one could get you. There it was possible to hop from world to world at great speed and with great variety – all you had to do was change the book you were reading to go to some new and previously unimagined place. And Leo liked the way that a book, once read, stayed in your head for ever, as if your head became bigger, and gave you more places to hide when you didn't like your life. No one could get to him inside his head. So he could go off into worlds no one knew he contained and kept hidden about his person, like secret stones sewn into his coat lining, and be safe there, and find relief from his loneliness. His favourite worlds, of course, were the island dreams, *Coral Island* and *Treasure Island*, and books like that, where people were given the chance to start their lives over again; he liked that more than anything else, and the heat, and the palm trees, and the light on the water, which were all so many miles away from Welsh rain. But any place could be freedom if no one else knew you were there, so he collected all the secret worlds he could, and went back to London in the pages of Dickens, or back into the past in the pages of Hardy, or over the top with Siegfried Sassoon. He would sit in the garden on dry afternoons, daydreaming his way through these different worlds, and no one ever suspected what he was up to. It was the closest thing in his life to freedom, and it grew all the more necessary as the years went by, because to his surprise the person who did worst out of the move from London into the country turned out not to be him, but his mother. The way she slowly collapsed in on herself as Leo grew up became unbearable to him as the years rolled by. Like a plant that had been pulled out by the roots and left lying on a path somewhere, because someone had forgotten to replant it.

Once they left the city it was like a light went out. Leo had known for as long as he could remember, of course, that England was not his mother's home, that she was having to learn the place just as he was, and finding that harder in many ways because she had to unlearn another country at the same time. When they moved to Wales, it seemed as if some thread connecting her back to the girl she had been was snapped and lost, so she couldn't find her way home, even in memory, even in imagination. Her head no longer seemed to contain any secret rooms that she could escape to, as Leo's did. She hardly ever went out into the local towns once they left London. For a while Leo wondered why she'd wanted to move at all. Only slowly did he realise that she hadn't. Only slowly did he realise that just because someone was a grown-up, that didn't mean they were in control. When it finally dawned on him that his mother was a long way from where she wanted to be, that she hated her life and where she lived and really recognised no part of it as the life she would have chosen, he came to wonder whether anyone was ever in control of anything at all. Who could be powerful, if not your own mother? Life was a series of inheritances taken away from you one by one, or given to you when you least wanted them, and there was no question of controlling any part of it, so it seemed to him.

Discovering how lost and sad his mother was, and watching as she withdrew from the world and spent her time in the house supervising the maid, ensuring that things were kept clean and meals served on time, and not doing much more with her life than that, brought out two strong and strongly opposed attitudes towards his mother that Leo struggled to reconcile. The first was that he came to love her very much. She was so vulnerable, and because she was always forgetting to eat, she turned into this frail and birdlike thing, so easily hurt, always cold, always wrapped in blankets and crying for the memory of her own home, that he wished he could be stronger, with an income of his own, and protect her, and take her back to India, leaving his father behind in this wet place that made his mother unhappy. Then, on the other hand, the more she retreated into herself the more he wondered if really he hated her, and that was the source of all his own unhappiness. Hated her inability to accept the life she had, and get on with it, make something of it somehow. Hated the fact that she needed his strength, when it ought to have been him who needed hers. Hated the weakness as if it might be catching, and pitied his father, who had to put up with her, had to get through all the work of the farm and come home each evening dreading what would have happened, what state he'd find his wife in, and whether she might have broken something in a rage, or whether she would have got out of bed at all that day.

2019

Amy leaves for Kuala Lumpur a few days later. The period that follows is a strange dreamtime. Waiting for her messages, working out the time difference, staying up late so we can message each other. It gets hard to keep things in perspective when you're worlds apart, and for us, only beginning to know each other, still uncertain, still constantly nervous of saying the wrong thing, the experience is like being caught in a boat in bad weather. I read too much into everything she says; half of our interactions are explanations of what we wish we'd said and what we meant by our last message.

Hey.
Hi, how are you?
OK thanks. Good day?
Only just started.
Course. Sorry. I get mixed up. What day is it there?
  Thursday?
Tuesday.
Told you I get mixed up! What are you doing today?
Theoretically trigonometry. Actually sunbathing. But I
  will try!

Try what?

Try to do some tutoring. But they won't listen.

Why not?

Don't worry, it's boring. Tell me a story.

Erm . . .

What did you do today?

*Oh, nothing too much. Went for a walk and saw the wild
  garlic still in blossom.*

Did it smell good?

It doesn't really smell that strongly.

Could you do me a favour?

Sure.

*Could you drop into my flat and check it's OK? Just been
  worrying.*

Anything specific?

No, just worrying! You can stay there if you like.

Thank you. I don't think I will but you're kind.

Why not?

Just might feel invasive.

Oh.

Sorry, is that the wrong thing to say?

*Well, I've said you can stay there if you want, so why would
  it feel invasive?*

Sorry. Didn't mean to say the wrong thing.

I watch day and night for the message that will persuade
me she's changed her mind, she's gone away for good, and
think I see it all the time, when a message gets left on read,
when I send her a joke and she doesn't find it funny.

I feel stupid asking for her permission to be at the airport

when she flies back, worried that she will want to see someone else, but she says yes like it's an easy thing.

She comes through the gates half an hour after I get there,
and I confess my stomach seems to turn over when I see her,
my body betraying the way I feel. I'm nervous as she walks up
to me, rolling her eyes at the sign with her name on it that I'm
holding as a joke, and kisses me there in the middle of the
airport in front of everyone.

The first weekend after Amy gets back to England, she goes
and stays with her parents, and picks up her dog, which they've
been looking after while she was away. It surprised me the
first time I discovered Amy had a dog – I don't know why; I
suppose because pets root you in places, and at our age the
idea of putting down roots seems hard, anti-instinctive, a luxury most of us can't yet afford. But having a dog seems to
work for her, a little Westie called Ivan, and when she comes
back to the city after a weekend at home, Ivan's with her
again, and he seems to remember me when I see him.

For the next few days, Amy complains of feeling tired all
the time, and it's clear the time away has taken it out of her. I
get the sense, as well, that she has mixed feelings about coming home. The flat where she lives is in one of the city's more
discarded far-flung corners, a place to sleep rather than a
home, and she's done well to find somewhere she can afford,
but I'm not sure how much she likes it. After a couple of days
of watching her stare a little fearfully at the surrounding walls,
the idea comes to me of taking her away. A holiday somewhere. A chance for us to reconnect. Perhaps a chance to have
the conversation about what might be happening between
us, and what we want to be doing together next.

So we trawl through Airbnb till we find somewhere we can afford, then make a few calls to clear the following week, and we leave the city, back in the car and devouring the long tongues of road that disappear endlessly beneath us. How many days of our lives are spent this way, doing nothing at all except watching the road? Are these the stillest hours of our lives now we live the way we do? Sometimes it seems more peaceful than sleep to me, to sit behind the wheel of a car and perform the Rumpelstiltskin trick of turning distance left to travel into time lost, time billowing behind you as it scatters and frays.

These escapes. These brief freedoms that come round like choruses in the song of our long, loving goodbye to the life that has been lent us. I never quite know what they mean. Are we really travelling outwards when we drive into the country-side, or are we trying, somehow, to return home? Is the journey really back and in, a reach for memory? John Berger wrote a trilogy of novels about the drift of the French peasantry from the near-feudal state in which they lived at the start of the last century into the cities, into the dirt jobs and shanty towns that turned into the suburbs as the century ended. If he were still here now, I wonder, would he make his fourth story about Airbnbs? The way those peasants' children pulled themselves up by their bootstraps, and spent their spare money on take-away coffee, then went out once or twice in a year to look at the places their ancestors worked in, sleep in converted barns where hay was stored once, and marvel at the quality of the ice cream, and feel moving powerfully within them like a current but never quite put into words the hardship and the toil remembered just below the surface of the scene? Is that the fourth act in the unfolding story of the rural working people – to drive out for long weekends, haunt the landscapes they called home?

On the way down to the Airbnb, Amy and I stop at Fleet for coffee. The pines all around us make the place feel unreal, like a film set somehow, like a dream. We are secluded from everything here, and the light strafes through the pine branches palely, as if it were only the memory of light and not the real thing we were seeing. I always feel as if I could spend for ever in this place. I could grow old walking round these shops hidden in the middle of the woods, then return to civilisation after what felt like decades there and find no time had passed at all.

'I feel like these places exist outside of time,' I say to Amy. It's not quite what I meant to say, but I can't find the right words for the feeling I have, so I say what I can instead.

'Like Brigadoon?' Amy asks me. I smile at her. Perhaps I've made myself understood after all. *Brigadoon* is a film I love, a fictional world I would love to walk into or discover in real life. In the story, a man goes away for a very literal-minded stag weekend, shooting deer in the Highlands with his best friend. They walk through the hills all day, and then can't find their way home and walk all night as well, until, at dawn, still lost in the wilds, they stumble on a village hidden deep in the middle of nowhere. What they don't know at first about this village is that, just yesterday, it was cursed by a witch who decreed that, for the rest of time, for every night that passes in the village of Brigadoon, a century will elapse in the world outside. So the man and his friend on the stag weekend walk in to discover a community of people wearing the clothes and living the lives of a hundred years ago, people who are just starting to get to grips with the implications of this new curse. The men spend the day there; the groom, who is on the brink of a high-society New York wedding, accustomed to a life lived in bars atop skyscrapers, falls for the simple, unadorned charms of a local girl, and then night comes, and he has to make a decision. He's been given a glimpse of a different life – a life with a woman he is completely at ease with, and a possible love unlike anything he's experienced before. His own life in New York seems suddenly shallow, hollow, to him – it's that life, not the village, which has come to seem like a dream. So he is faced with a choice. He could stay here with the girl he met just this morning and live in what now feels like the real world, having broken through the surface of his life into a true depth of feeling; but if he did, if he fell asleep just once in this village, a hundred years would pass in the world outside, and everyone he ever knew, everything he ever lived and worked and hoped for, would be gone.

The man makes his decision. He returns to New York. Which of us wouldn't, in the end? He goes for a drink in a bar atop a skyscraper. But the whole place has changed, and he can't believe it's real any more. All of it seems to him like no more than the surface of something, like a dream. So he flies back to Scotland, and walks out into the wilds, even though he knows that because of the witch's curse the village of Brigadoon won't appear again for the rest of his lifetime, and because this is true love we're talking about here, and also a schmaltzy Hollywood musical of a certain era, the mists part for just one last moment, and he sees the woman he met that day welcoming him home. The man – who, incidentally, has been Gene Kelly all along – walks into the mist and vanishes. I hope that once a century has elapsed since the original film was released, someone will make a sequel where not only the Scottish village of the mid-nineteenth century but also Gene Kelly from the mid-twentieth century will emerge into the cold light of the twenty-first century and try to comprehend what we've all done with the place in the time since they left it. The technology will presumably exist to allow Gene Kelly to still play the role by then.

We drive on. Hours pass, and Ivan's sick after a while, so we stop the car to clean the back seat. The roads grow narrower. We know the journey's coming to an end. The sun is ahead of us now, beckoning us into the west. We arrive at the barn we've rented to hide in while Amy recovers her sense of herself, and unpack the car, and let Ivan out into the yard by the farm next to the barn, and he plays with the dog in the farmyard, and we watch them, and we're happy.

On the first day of the holiday, armed with an Ordnance Survey map, we take Ivan to walk on the moor to the south of the place where we're staying. There's a smell of dry earth in the air from the mud we kick up as we walk. Cornwall for me is Radiohead country, I suppose because I know the singer has a house nearby. Something about the emptiness of this coastal landscape seems to leave spaces and silences that long for filling in. What I hear rushing into those vacuums is that spare and spectral music of longing, displacement and desire. Within half an hour of setting off, we take a wrong turn and find ourselves walking through a farmyard. A girl of about six runs out to look at us, as if we might be the circus passing through. A woman who looks like she might be the little girl's grandmother comes out of the farmhouse.

'You two all right?' she asks. She seems friendly but her voice is raised almost to a shout, as if she's mainly used to talking to people who are half a mile away.

'We were following the bridlepath, but I think we've gone the wrong way,' I say.

'People do that. You wanna go back along the path and turn left down the lane you passed.'

We thank the woman and turn to leave. The girl watches us go. I wave goodbye to her. I know what it's like to start your life so remote, what this solitude and silence does to a mind, to an imagination. She is like a glimpse of someone I used to be. I want to take a moment to tell the girl: all your life there's going to be a secret room in your head no one else will ever know exists or know how to get into, a room filled with the silence and freedom of your childhood. Sometimes it will seem like a miracle to you, and sometimes it will seem like the purest loneliness. There's nothing you can do about it; the secret room will always be part of you, it will always be there, and sometimes you'll need to go into it and sit quietly for a little while. It will be the only way you ever find to feel like you've come home. The rest of the wide world with its sound and fury is never quite going to feel like home, it will always resemble a dream, and you'll never truly convince yourself that all of that noise could be real.

We turn away from her and retrace our steps, then open the gate for the left turn, and the lane beyond is shadowed by trees overhanging us. We walk on for half a mile until we come to a tree that's fallen and been left across the path, blocking the route. I try for a moment to find a way through, but the branches are thick and we can't fit under. So we clamber out of the lane into the field on our left, walking round the tree. In the field a few dozen young bullocks are grazing. They watch Ivan, uneasy. Amy slips back into the lane, and I follow her out of the bright light of the field back into the shadow of the trees. The bullocks come right up to the hedge as we walk away from them, but they don't come through.

We come to a fork in the path. There are no signs, so I look at the map, and we take the right branch that should lead us up on to the moor. We walk into dense deciduous woodland, the light on our faces dappled by oak leaves, the ground soft and loamy under our feet, and the path begins to peter out as bracken and moss encroach and claim the space, until all we can see are a few scuff marks from other feet that walked here before us. The ground grows steeper, and after a while we find we have to start climbing, grabbing on to branches and roots growing out of the hillside and making our way ever more slowly towards the light we hope will mark the edge of the moor, which ought to lie just past this wood's liminal margin. We stop for breath, and I get out the map, because it seems clear now that we've taken the wrong path; I've misread our location. I look at the map, and don't understand why the ground here is so steep; the lines on the page give no indication of this climb. It seems as if we must have been on the wrong path all this time, and travelling in a different direction; but I can't see where we've gone wrong. I realise the map's no use to us any more, until we get out of the wood and see where we are. Drowned in this woodland, there are no landmarks to orient us. So we keep on climbing. After another ten minutes we pass out of the wood into a clearing of long grass, parched by the summer heat, and fall down on our backs, and stare at the way the grass falls away from us till it reaches the next hedgerow, where trees rise up again beyond it. I look at the map once more, and now I can see where we must be: another path, almost parallel to the one we should have taken, has brought us out half a mile to the west of where we thought we were walking, to the same stretch of Radiohead country, the same place that's been awaiting our arrival all this time.

'Isn't it strange?' I look at Amy, and follow her gaze to see what she's staring at. She only seems to be looking at the space ahead of us, the grass and the trees and the sky. 'All this was water once. All of this was underwater. Not even that, it didn't exist. There was water here instead where this view would appear one day.'

'And one day this won't exist again, and this will turn back into water.'

'Will there be anyone here, d'you think?' she asks, turning now to look at me. 'To see it when it goes?'

Neither of us speak for a little while. Neither of us need to say anything, as we lie back on the grass together with Ivan lying behind us, as walkers have rested on their way for thousands of years, and imagine the end of the world.

After a while, when we've got our breath back, we stand up again, heave our packs back on to our shoulders, and go on.

I try and imagine a future with Amy, and it plays out compulsively in my imagination, like a movie rising up unbidden. The film of our life would be made up entirely of these holidays, these adventures, our lungfuls of freedom away from the rest of the world. That's how they'd tell it in the movies, the romantics' version, and up to a point they'd be right – that's how we try to live. Always the next adventure to be planned and looked forward to, always the memory of the last one just gone for us both to retreat into when work gets hard, more secret worlds that are ours alone, where no one else can reach us, just like the pool where our lives first collided. In the film of our lives, we'd take that idea even further. You'd never even see our home, our families, the offices we worked in. We'd be played by two very beautiful actors who would walk together through one European city after another, through forests of vast redwood in backwater Maine, talking all the time about how hard it is to feel you belong anywhere on this earth, talking about the way we met, and the sacrifices we made in getting together. It would be pure Richard Linklater. Beers and weed on Prinsengracht in Amsterdam, rye bread and tomatoes from the little supermarkets, padlocks on the bridges, Amy wanting to linger in the red light district and take it all in, me wanting to get away from the women in the windows and the tired, lonely figures queueing to go in and see them. Dinners on Kollwitzplatz in Berlin, days lost in the English-language bookshops and among the tattooists who ravelled their stories in blue ink over our skin. Then a train to Leipzig, the wide-open square in front of the beautiful station, and going from church to church to visit the graves and trace the lives of great composers round that city. And on again, further east to Prague and soup served in bread bowls and walking up steep hills to look down on the city, then to Dubrovnik, baking in the sun, diving off concrete platforms busy with Croatians selling beer to each other from cool boxes, diving and losing ourselves in the sea, the sea. Then back west to Ireland, walking out from Knocknarea to Sligo. Stopping the car to watch the Glencar waterfall fly into the air. Sitting in the bar of the Grand Hotel while the Irish dancers come in and out with their parents, young girls dressed like nothing you've ever seen, their hair done up like wedding cakes. Orkney in the pouring rain. Then south again and the view from the slopes of the Atlas Mountains, lasting for ever, lasting till the end of space and time. One image of freedom after another, and the two beautiful actors walking through all of it like Adam and Eve, sharing all this life, talking beautifully and filling the screen with ideas, but none of them really mattering, because the real narrative would be the move from one location to another, the passing of time, the change from scene to scene. Perhaps when we're old that will be how we'll remember our lives. All of the dailiness melting away, only the red-letter days still shining.

When we've finished exploring the fields around the village where we're staying, we get back into the car to travel further afield, and make our way, inevitably, to the waiting sea.

English summer weather rifles through its moods and many faces over this stretch of coast like a spell. Over these rocks the weather of childhood still dances changeably and seems to be always drawing you back into memory, like a radio left playing in another room, music reminding you of something you'd forgotten when you hear it through the walls, down a hallway, through an open window as you walk in the garden.

Change down into third gear for the hill, foot always poised over the brake in anticipation of the vehicle coming in the other direction that will mean you have to stop and back up to the last passing place. These old lanes are maps of the history of a place as much as they're a way of getting any-where. The route from one village to another the cowherds once took, or farmers with their carts, or trudging labourers. Now they are made to take the mad, impossible strain of this century, too narrow for our needs and not getting anywhere quickly enough. Emerge from the tree cover and see, ahead, the ocean, the idea that can never be caged within words, the largest thought that's ever put to us until the day of our deaths. Amy spots the car park to the right while I'm still dis-tracted by the sat nav, and we slow down too quickly, turn off the road. There's no signal on our phones, as if the parapher-nalia of our world were losing its grip out here. I feel as if I'm in the middle of some enchantment. We scrape together enough cash between us to pay for parking, get Ivan out of the car, and head down the hill towards the old fishing village.

'Do you know which way?' Amy asks.

'I think just follow the steepest road down and we'll get there.'

'Everyone's going the same way, aren't they?'

'Yes. We'll follow them.'

'Is it how you remember it?'

'I don't remember this car park at all.'

I have been here before. A friend's birthday in a field by a house overlooking the sea that his parents had bought when they retired down here six or seven years ago. I thought of looking the family up while we are here, but in the end it seems too complicated, and I worry they won't remember who I am. While we've been in this part of the country, we've been revisiting places. Twice we've gone to a place whose name Amy remembered from a childhood holiday, and found she didn't recognise it, then driven on to the next town to find it was in fact the place she had in mind. These are memories dating from when she was eleven or twelve years old, and the mind doesn't keep complete tapes from those years, or any years, I suppose – it compresses and cuts out and sticks things together, so our memories are montages of things that have no more to do with each other than the fact that they happened about the same time. What we find Amy has remembered each time is the name of the town where she stayed; but her richer memories, the places she recognises and in which she feels she has been happy, seem to have been day trips she went on with her family on that holiday. They were the exciting days, the prettier places, out of the ordinary, vivid and new. Each time, in the memory, for some reason she's given them a different name. There is a pleasure for both of us to hunting the real site of what she remembers, seeking out the places that feel alive to her, trying to second guess where she might have been happy, in what feels to her like a different life.

On my previous visit to this town I never made it down into the harbour. Amy has seen this place in a film, though, so she knows what to expect: the shelter of the harbour cleft deep into the coast, streets of old cottages rising like wings on either side up the cliff-like flanks that shape the village like a potter's hands. Every second person walking down the hill has a dog on a lead, and ours is still practically a puppy, and desperate to play. He yips and strains at his harness, skittering his claws on the pavement. The road grows steeper and turns to the left, and then we see the harbour lying below us, the gift shops, ice-cream parlours, local crafts and pottery, tourists making their way up and down the narrow streets as if on pilgrimage. And this to me is everything beautiful I love in people, this little postcard spread out beneath us: all of us dutiful and patient, making our way through one place or another on our holidays, soaking up what's been laid on for us and finding in it the peace and freedom we need to go back to our real lives and face them next week or the week after that. An ice cream, a mug with the name of the village on the side, a walk on the beach; we take these small offerings and somehow find in them the restoration and the courage and grace we need to face the world's indifference. Here, in a place like this one, you can see the agreement we've all made with each other playing out: that we'll observe some kind of system to keep things moving; we'll be civilised, and lay these small rituals over the untamed surface of the world, and lend some pattern to our time here. Holiday towns always fill me with love. We all appear to have made a pact with each other: I won't stove your head in, and you won't stove in mine; instead we'll agree to set boundaries, say that this is a place where we come to get away from things, and that is a place for farmers, and that is a place for office work, and we'll accept these limits on our lives because they will make our lives possible.

The shops here sell the merchandise of three different franchises which have been filmed around this harbour, an electric shock provided to the local economy by storytelling. As we walk round the horseshoe of narrow streets, we hear people talking about each of the shows in question, pointing out one house or another to indicate that this is where a particular scene was filmed on one of those shows. People chasing the ghosts of stories over cobbles, in and out of the light and shade of the cottages. Halfway up the hill on the other side of the harbour from where we came in, the home of a doctor in one TV drama stands right beside the B&B where a record producer stayed while visiting the town in a different film. People gather to stare at both, as though celluloid characters might become flesh and walk out into the street to be among them. What are we hoping to see when we go on pilgrimage to former film sets? We all do it, when visiting those places that have been turned into stories and sold to us elsewhere. We stare at the spot where a shot we know was captured. Is it that we want to see some ghost of the magic? Do we want to be able to see as if through the eyes of the director, somehow acquire her fierce clarity by looking at the same things she did? Or do people just like collecting things, and collecting places is as good a hobby as any other?

We take Ivan down the harbour slipway and on to the sand while the tide's out, because he's burning to be let off the lead and allowed to run round. There are boats lying beached on the sand as if dropped there by children; by the water, a jellyfish is in the same state. Ivan takes no interest in the jellyfish; it's dead and can't be played with. Instead he hares over the warm rock pools and ridges of barnacled stone and the soft sand to be among the terriers already playing there, so there are three dogs suddenly together in the belly of the harbour, suddenly running, springing into action like a flock of pigeons leaving a square, breathless mad energy bursting around us. We stand and watch them, laughing, with no intimation that the day holds anything for us but happiness like this. Amy's eyes drift past the dogs, and now focus on the sea.

'There must be a moment somewhere out there in the water where the tide turns and an ebb becomes a flood again,' she says to me. 'When the tide meets itself coming back the other way, you know what I mean? How does that happen? What does it look like, do you think? I think it must look like the centre of the world, the place where the tides change.'

I stare out across the water with her. 'They're always both out there, aren't they? Just pulling in different directions all the time.'

She turns to me. 'How do you mean?'

'It's always high tide somewhere. And low tide somewhere else. Everything just gets pulled from one to the other.'

'But the water we can see must get turned around somewhere.'

Ten minutes pass with the dogs dancing in and out of the water, attracted by the water, yet also afraid of it, shaking themselves when they get wet, then one of the owners has to leave, so we catch hold of Ivan and put him back on the lead, and it's while I'm doing that, ruffling his head and giving him a treat, that my phone rings.

I take it out and see that it's Chris calling. I answer the phone, already uneasy, because he never calls me; whenever I speak to him it's because I've called the phone at the farm.

'Hello, Chris.'

'Hi, Ed. Sorry, I know you're on holiday.' I can tell from the sound of the call that he's out and about, not at home. He sounds as if he's walking.

'Is everything all right?'

'I think so. I just wanted to let you know that your mum's gone into hospital.'

'What's happened?'

'She was having breathing difficulties over the last few days. And she assumed she just had a cold – well, we both did – and she hoped it would pass. But she hasn't been able to sleep, because when she lies down it feels worse, so she went in to see the doctor about that, and they've said she's got pneumonia.'

'Right.' The call feels suddenly unreal to me. Dad got pneumonia too, before the end.

'She's in Abergavenny hospital, and she's totally fine, she's on oxygen and they're putting her on antibiotics.'

'Are you with her?'

'I'm in the hospital but I've just stepped out to get a cup of tea and make some calls.'

'Are you OK?'

'I'm fine. Bit scared, if I'm honest.' It occurs to me that this might in fact be something serious; I don't know whether I've ever heard Chris describe himself as scared before.

'What are the doctors saying?'

'Not much, really. I mean, it's too soon for them to say much, that's what they say. They've put her on antibiotics, but it'll take a couple of days before they know they're working. In the meantime, they've said that she could be in hospital for a few weeks.' I think of the work that Chris is going to have to do while Mum is in the hospital: the endless, backbreaking work of the hill farm where they live, and the visits to Abergavenny, forty minutes in the car each way. My sister and I both miles away in the city. Should we be dropping everything, I wonder? Should we be going back home?

'We'll come and see her.'

'She doesn't want you to cut short your holiday.'

'It's all right. We're due to travel back. We'll come to you instead.'

'I know she'd love that.'

'Of course.'

'I'd better go, I think, better call Rachel.'

'Do you want me to call her?'

'No, it's best I do it.'

'OK. Will you give Mum our love? And we'll get to her as soon as we can.'

'Absolutely. All right.'

'Love to you both.'

'All right.' He rings off then, and I look at Amy, who has guessed what's happened from hearing my side of the call.

We walk up off the beach. The day has turned against us now, the rain is lashing in from the sea as we drive back along the coast towards the place where we've been staying. The trees bowing low over the road loom larger in this weather, darker against the shifting sky, the progress of the afternoon bringing different things into focus. The day we knew two hours ago has vanished, scattered and drowned in wind and rain. The hedgerows seem closer on each side, windows of the car steaming up, all colour drained from the face of the sky.

'Do you want to go tonight?'

'No, there's no point. We won't get there till after visiting hours.'

'You're sure we shouldn't go anyway?' I know what she means. Am I sure we don't need to get to the bedside? Am I sure visiting hours still apply? In truth, I don't know. But if I pretend this isn't an emergency, then perhaps it won't become one.

'He hasn't said that. He just said it was too soon for them to know what's going to happen.'

'And you don't think we need to be with him?'

'He doesn't want us to be with him tonight. Turning up in the middle of the night.'

'If you're sure.'

I'm not. But I don't want to go, and I don't know what to say to explain that irrational feeling, so I say nothing, and the silences stretches out between us.

Along the cliff road with the sea roaring to the left of us, incoming waves volley and thunder, Atlantic breakers tearing at the strand below, a few lonely cars huddling down in a car park by the side of the road on a gorse-littered hilltop, people eating their sandwiches in front of the sea, or having sex, or making calls, or waiting for their shifts to start. Whatever people do in parked cars. All these lives like islands we'll never set foot upon. As we drive home, we see an arrow of Canada geese heading north-west, out over the sea and carving fearlessly into the weather. In the car park we left behind, there were seagulls stalking up and down as if they were guarding the bins. Is that what it will be like when all the humans are gone? On these islands, the bigger predators wiped out long ago, will it be only the birds still stalking the deserted landscape, pecking at the rubbish till even that has been consumed? Perhaps the birds as they eat the last remnants of who we were will become a kind of forgetting, a benediction. And will the ghosts still be there for the birds to see, the ghosts of our lives that seem to be always trailing after us – are they part of us or do they stay behind here, trapped and lonely, when we leave?

A ghost can appear to you anywhere. I am certain that ghosts are walking with us everywhere. But there are also places where ghosts are more easily seen. At the edges of things. The coast, the first fingertips of a forest closing round you, dawn and dusk, and time away from the familiar. In liminal places and times like these, where we are shaken out of the stupor of the everyday by the prospect of things changing, a great deal can appear to us more clearly, as we are forced to look more closely at what is around us and take life in.

We get back to where we're staying and I sit in the main room of the barn in silence, thinking of the gulls in the car park and the geese in the air, like lost souls crossing the earth, and the day wanes and disappears, and I know I won't sleep, so I tell Amy I'm going for a walk and head outside.

I pull on my jacket and set out into the dark with my head down, listening to the crunch of gravel beneath my feet. The absolute dark of a moonless night in the middle of nowhere. I leave Ivan inside to keep Amy company; even though it's stopped raining, he won't want to be out in the dark, and I don't want to have to entertain him, reassure him, rein him in. At first I can't see my hand in front of my face. But there's always a light source somewhere, even on the blackest night, so as I stagger forward my eyes adjust and my pace gradually increases as I start to make out the shifting gradients of the ground underfoot. I am listening to the different qualities of silence: the sudden rushes of sound like the sea that come from the hazels and oaks surrounding me when the wind picks up, the rustle of mice among the ground ivy audible in the lulls. Out the gate and left up the hill, and I suppose I might as well visit the church as it's only a short walk and unlocked all night, and that will allow me to sit somewhere silently. Above my head the clouds are moving quickly, and now they are starting to fray, and here and there I catch a glimpse of stars. Should I feel afraid of this dark I'm in now? Is there something in it that's waiting to meet me?

I come to the church and open the gate and walk into the graveyard. I listen to the wind in the trees sounding like the sea, and watch the skies clear till the stars are spangled all above, layer upon layer of faint yet brilliant ancient light lapping like waves across the darkness. When does it start? A day comes when you lie on your back in the grass and wonder whether this is the closest you'll ever come to happiness, whether the long slide away from this moment begins now. The rest of your life a falling away from this point. When do we first know that might be what's happening? Is that what's happening to me now?

It gets colder the longer I'm out here, but I don't want to go back to the barn just yet. I open the door to the porch of the church, and step inside, looking for shelter. The view of the sky through the open door is shadowed by holly trees blocking the night. The leaves of the holly trees' higher branches are smooth-sided, with none of the spikes on the lower leaves. As I watch the silhouettes of the trees moving gently against the night, a different movement catches my eye: a spider is moving over the porch doorway, trying to spin a web across it. The frail bright threads are visible and sharp against the darkness. I watch, still and silent in the church porch, for what feels like an hour but might only be ten minutes, as the web spools out and shuts me in, like a blanket, like a concealment. I am alone in here. No one can reach me. No one else has ever stood like this before and watched a spider stitch them into this place.

1933

ARTHUR NEVER DID quite work out what he had done wrong. Except that he disgusted her, except that he wasn't what she wanted, except that it turned out long after it was too late that he had taken her away from her life. And that was his fault. Somehow, though he hadn't known he was doing it, that would always be his fault; there was nothing to be done that could change that simple, sad fact. Eight years after he moved the family back to Wales, a day came when he accepted she would never get better. She would live upstairs in the cottage, and continue retreating into herself, until finally there was nothing left.

He remembered the way they met in Hyderabad. Of course, she had been much younger than him, of course he could see that was so, but no younger than the women many of his friends had been marrying at the time. And she had seemed to like him, she had seemed to want to marry him back then; she was kind to him and seemed to think he was an interesting man. It was only later he discovered that, in her eyes, he very much wasn't. In her eyes he was just a conqueror who stole her and took her away, like a looter, like a common thief. That hadn't been the way her mother and her father talked about it when the marriage was negotiated. They talked about her kind nature, the way she would grow to care for him as they shared their lives, just as she had always cared for every person she was close to, just as she was always kind to animals or the poor. And she would bear him children, which was the reason Arthur could not have married a woman of his own age; the women of his own age were past childbearing by that time, and it was his responsibility to his family to try and carry on the line. He remembered the way Phoebe's mother and father talked about the opportunity he was giving to her. And if he had made a mistake, if he could put his finger on one moment when it all went wrong, perhaps it was then, when he assumed their feelings would be hers as well.

Of course it had started slowly. The idea of intimacy between them had been as embarrassing to him, he guessed, as it had been to her; at least she was beautiful, after all. At least she had no reason to feel any shame. Whereas Arthur, trapped in the prison of his middle age, had a very great deal to be ashamed of. He knew going to bed with him couldn't possibly please her; he tried to ask as little of her as he could, and respect her instead, let her have her own bed and her own room, let her spend her days as she wished, and go back to visit her family, where happiness seemed to lie. He had believed in time that kind of respect, that kind of understanding, would lead to a deeper connection between them. But perhaps he had done all that wrong as well? Many years later, she would tell him he had never shown her love, and he would think back to those days, the way he tried to give her space. And he wondered whether he should have done it all differently, whether things might have ended up better for her in the end.

The trouble was that he did come to love her. He really did. His beautiful wife. Her life, her fragile life, that he had been tasked to watch over. It might have been easier if he had never fallen in love.

Had it been wrong to heed the call of the war, and come back to England? He supposed that it had. He supposed he should have stayed out in India and supervised the railways, and then Phoebe could have stayed in the place where she was happy, and even if he never became someone she loved, at least there would be love around her that kept her safe. But he had never intended to stay in India for ever. And he had said that to her parents, back when they were negotiating, and they had raised no objections to the idea of her going to England with him. They had said it would be a great opportunity, he seemed to recall. And yet, even as they got to Bombay, even as she took in the men working naked on the docks and the way the dogs scavenged round them for scraps, and were chased away, the savage starving animals, he saw a light start to go out in her. Some kind of connection to the soil of home. Some faith that the world was a good and decent place. Such faith struggled to remain strong in the face of the evidence of Bombay, and the subsequent stink and sickness on the ship, and the docks of Poplar where they made their home.

That, he admitted, had lacked imagination. They had rented a house more or less where they first alighted in England, and he accepted it must not have been the best place to have a child and start to raise him. He rented that house at the time because he was in a hurry, he was going to the navy and didn't have time, and a friend of his father's owned the house, and let him have it with a maid for a good rate. He thought Phoebe would be safe there, and to an extent he closed his heart at that time to the thought of her unhappiness. There was a war on, after all. Many people were unhappy at that time. It was a mistake to think of life as all spices and roses. But then when he came back, once the war was over, perhaps they shouldn't have stayed so long. She withdrew a lot from him then, and seemed to give up on the youth he'd always loved in her. Though she was a young woman, she acquired more than a touch of Miss Havisham in that time, always alone and flitting round the rooms, always staring like a ghost through the windows. He used to watch her reading and rereading *Wuthering Heights*. Is that what she saw reflected in the glass when she looked out over Poplar, he wondered? Did she imagine the glass shattering, rude hands reaching in and snatching her away from the silent world of their home?

By the time his father died, and he decided to move back to Wales and take up the birthright he had expected for so long, it was already too late, he came to realise. Her mind was going, her happiness was already gone; nothing he could have done would have helped her. It was those years in London when things went wrong, and the poison of that time simply seeped out once they had got away to the hills and the farming. He was too old for it by then, of course, and his father had half bankrupted the place without telling him, mortgaging and remortgaging it to get through the post-war depression, so Arthur couldn't afford the help he would have wanted to make a success of the place. He knew very early on that it would be the work of the farm that drove him before too long into the grave. But he didn't regret that. It became very hard to do so. At least he wouldn't be here to hurt her, was all that he thought. At least he wouldn't torture her any more if he was under the grass. It was enough to make a man think of taking his own life, but Arthur had no more interest in suicide than he did in divorce. A life was a series of responsibilities. You took them on and then you saw them through. These things were not to be backed away from. That was not how to be a man.

And anyway, he couldn't have left; Phoebe wouldn't have managed. This, always, hung heavy over his head, as she withdrew to the upstairs rooms, as she walked round the house at night and he was left with nothing but the memory of her brown eyes when she was young, and her hair, and the way she first looked at him those evenings in the club when they danced together, and the air was thick, and the scents of India came in through the windows. He couldn't give up on her now all that was gone. The light had gone out, and his leaving would not have reignited it. His leaving would have just left her alone. She was his responsibility, and he had to make sure she ate and washed and stayed alive. Who else was going to, after all? There was only Leo, and one thing he could still do was save his son from having to do this for as long as he could. He had nightmares about predeceasing Phoebe. He knew it was likely, but feared it all the same. It would pass all the weight of this care on to Leo. It would pass all this lovelessness down the generations. He dreamed of lasting long enough to get his beautiful wife to the end of her life, though she didn't love him, though she would never thank him for being here, just staying in her haunted attic, day after day. That was the only way he could see of making sure this sorrow lasted only one generation. And preventing a longer cycle setting in. And after all, why should he let her go? He loved her; he couldn't help that. He wanted her near him. So he stayed, and he worked, and felt it wear him thin, and said nothing of their poverty, and nothing of his misery. If he could take it all upon himself, then perhaps he could take it with him when he came to the end. That would be right, he liked to think. After all, it must have been something he'd done.

2019

I N THE EARLY morning, a light rain falls till it has exhausted itself in patterning the gravel, till the sky is drained and quietened, then clouds are scudding over the lonely farms. We pack without saying much to each other, and walk through the rooms doing idiot checks. The morning is gorgeous and pristine; we imprint nothing of our own on to it, no thought, no inanity, no disagreement. I start to imagine the air I'm moving through as something perfectly white, tablecloth white, wedding-dress white, which my thoughts spoken out loud could only muddy. Like dirty fingerprints on the sleeves of a shirt. How could any thought of mine add anything to this place, this quiet? My head's full of things that could never matter like the morning seems to matter as I live it and watch it vanish and prepare for the car and leaving this moment behind me, the sound of the birds outside, the heat rising up as the day develops its themes. I hope Amy is feeling the same things too: the preciousness of this hour spent packing, the day like pure clear water we are holding cupped in our hands for as long as this silent moment lasts, before saying good-bye to it. I hope she is alive to the magic of this farewell to our holiday, and loving the feeling, loving the intuitive choreography of our shared packing, our quiet dance through the rooms as we check them one last time. The peace of the morning is broken only when the farm dogs bark to each other across the fields, and Ivan joins in. At the end of the lane where we've been staying, two Basset Hounds make sounds like Judgement Day.

We walk Ivan one last time round the woods, under the apples ripening early in this strangely balmy climate, and pass the church on the way home, and I say nothing to Amy of having sat there in the porch last night, and a small scar of silence forms between us, a part of my life I'll never tell her. But love is not the act of consuming the whole of a person. These scars and silences are also part of love. Amy had wanted us to get straight in the car and leave, but I insisted we should walk the dog first, or he'd grizzle in the back seat. The reality is that I think I'm trying to put off leaving. Trying to persuade myself this isn't the emergency. People will do anything to locate the emergency later than it is.

Cutting through the woods is the filled-in ghost of an old railway line, closed off and shut up before we were born. On our first day here we followed it through the fields until it broke away from the slope of the ground it had been passing through, a bridge to nowhere, a raised escarpment built long ago by men who will all have vanished now, who broke their backs to throw this bridge up into the sky, and whose work came to nothing when the railway line closed. It must have taken months, chucking up enough earth from the surrounding fields to keep the train travelling level through this shallow valley. Now the overgrown spit they made jut into the air seems to grieve their memory, the time they lost and wasted, the time they could have been doing something else. Still, at least they were paid for it. And the work would have been hard, but they would have gone home at the end of the day knowing the bills were paid, and there are worse ways to make a living.

Strange, how the labour of a handful of men who were simply doing a job of work for the wage it earned them can become the landscape you walk through, shaping the hills and valleys. Every place we pass through is so much more than the scene as it appears to us. Every place is held up, patterned and formed by a latticework of choices, decisions, memories. Everywhere is made out of ghosts.

I think of the road running past the school that I went to. To walk down it today would offer the casual observer one or two points of interest – the restaurants, the B&Bs. But the life under the surface of that street is infinitely richer. I can pass its houses knowing a marriage ended in this room; a drunk threw a spice rack at a group of boys from that window; a boy was killed crossing the road just there; a priest was arrested in that house, for the reason priests are always arrested. All this only a heartbeat, a fraction of the life of that place. All these chance happenings become our history, more or less random, more or less unplanned, but growing all the same into the reason a place is like it is, and the world is like it is.

How far does that history reach into us, control us? Which of us ever really knows whether we're making our decisions for ourselves, or whether our days are finally shaped by these ghosts? If we knew the whole stories of every family in the world, I think we would discover the secret sources of everyone's actions. If most of the history of the world wasn't lost, allowed to vanish because no one wrote it down, we might be able to understand how it came to be what it is now. But the world is too big to ever catch all these stories. We can only observe the way these memories work like pain bodies for ourselves, the way we retreat back into the pain body of family memory whenever we confront something important, and act out of fear of what's hurt us before, and guess at the way that affects everyone else around us, all the time.

Life like a coastal shelf, built up, layer upon layer, like minute upon hour upon day, till it looms over you, till you come to fear its falling, because when the end comes and it finally falls, it will cut you back into the ribbons of minutes and hours and days that made you, and you will be dissipated, and ebb back into glimpses, fractured and diffuse, and you will be nothing at all, scattered memory, a ghost.

Days that feel like going home pattern the years like clouds, like occasional rain. The visits to parents, the visits to graves, the occasional return to childhood places, like finding tucked away at the back of a drawer something you thought you'd lost. Or simply coming together with the people you feel closest to in life – that becomes a kind of homecoming after a while as well. As I get older, I feel more and more as if these moments of togetherness, of happiness, provide the real and secret rhythm of each year. They take me under the surface of my days into the real story. In the company of friends who really know you, who know where you came from, what you used to dream of when you were young and how it measures up to this life you're living now, your world can take shape as you see it through their eyes, and you can make out more clearly where it is you might be heading.

Amy drives today, which is always the best option really, because she's a better driver than me, and a worse passenger – she becomes angry and irritable sitting shotgun when I'm driving. I sit holding on my lap the new teapot we bought in one of the ceramic shops clustered round this county, and the plates and bowls we bought a day earlier in between my feet, and we listen to the radio, and I try and chart the way my legs seize up, the stages of stillness, stiffness, discomfort. When we stop to refuel at a service station after about an hour and a half on the road, I limp like a pensioner.

There's a closed-down, slowly collapsing old diner by the petrol station, windows with signs still hanging in them that haven't been lit for what looks like a year or more. When I see the old adverts for chips and beans, I feel a rush of nostalgia for that disappearing old culture, the world of bad fry-ups, fat swilling on the plate, cheap bacon and the ketchup in the Heinz bottles replaced with own-brand stuff that tastes like vinegar but costs less money. One by one those roadside places will all shut down, replaced by franchised Jamie Oliver sausage rolls, and Costa Coffee machines. And people will forget the terrible filter coffee you used to pay a quid for in the Happy Eater, and the kids' slides shaped like an elephant that I used to play on in the deafening fenced-off spaces people called gardens that sprang up outside diners on the side of motorways. Shit Britain, old Britain, where the commercial travellers and football supporters would nod to each other, and hold the bathroom door while avoiding eye contact, because they knew what they'd just done. I miss that world. Even as it's disappearing, I already miss it. Not because there was anything good or wholesome or life-improving about it.

It just reminds me of when I was young, and nothing had gone wrong yet, and things were easy. It reminds me of my grandfather taking me out for the day and letting me get a buzzcut at the barber's, then buying me a milkshake in a roadside café and taking me home to Mum, who almost cried when she saw my hair.

And I think, as well as the memory of youth, there's a kind of innocence to all these shut-down cafés that we'll never have again. This is where we gulped down bacon rind, and never thought about calories, never thought about sustainable, ethical meat or where our eggs came from, or the ecological holocaust we were creating. We were idiots. But it was a very simple time, and I know that we'll never live it again. When chocolate bars were massive, and a two-thousand-calorie breakfast seemed OK. And then we'd get back in our cars and motor on down to the seaside, to leave litter on the beach. Imagine being so thoughtless, so carefree. Of course, we can't now. I can only see the damage it's all done. But it must have been wonderful while it lasted. Once, people used to worry about E numbers. That was the problem that needed solving. I'd give a lot to have a conversation about E numbers over a Big Mac in McDonald's again. In the windows of those old, shut-down diners, I see the equation between ignorance and bliss. There'll always be traces of it, of course. The cafés on industrial estates, the little roadside vans, and the places outside football grounds. There'll always be people who need real fuel for a day putting up scaffolding, or just don't care about the modern world's discoveries, the modern world's attempt to take back some of the things that were said and done in the wild, American moment of the eighties and nineties. But for most of us, for those of us who separate our rubbish for recycling and only get takeaway once a week or so as a treat we regret later, those days and that innocence are gone.

We look for something to eat in the petrol station, but none of it seems edible, so we head into one of the towns the road takes us close to and where we guess there'll be better cafés, and while Amy shops I walk Ivan round the multi-storey car park, trying to find a way out and into the town centre that doesn't take me through the shopping centre, where dogs are banned. It's difficult, and I have to turn back twice before I find a back staircase that gets me down to a service road, and follow that round till I get in among people again. Clearly, no one who planned the car park or the shopping centre gave much thought to what people would do if they were travelling with dogs. I have half a mind to stop searching for a way out and just let Ivan shit on the car park floor. Once we're out in the streets, I distract myself with being attentive to Ivan, and wait to catch Amy on her way back into the shopping centre. This is when dogs do the greatest good for their owners. It helps at times like this to lose yourself in another life, to be kind, and not need to speak, not have to put what you're feeling into language. It's immediate and present to be kind to Ivan, anchors you in the here and now, and keeps you away from the twin, grim precipices of the future and the past that are lurking always at the edge of your vision.

Another dog approaches, young like Ivan, straining on the leash to say hello. The woman holding the lead is missing some teeth.

'Don't mind him, he's friendly,' she tells me. 'He's only nine months. Ten. Sorry, I'm not sure. He was my partner's dog, but my partner died last week, so I'm taking him on. Keep him in the family.'

'I'm so sorry your partner died.'

'Thank you.' She watches our dogs as they playfight. 'Yeah, I took him to the morgue to say goodbye.' I don't know what to say to her. She doesn't seem to want me to say anything; she says it like it's merely a statement of fact. 'I better go now. Have a nice day, yeah?' She walks away then without looking back at me.

Amy finds us as she walks back to the car park from the shops and we get back in the car, and the rest of the journey passes in podcasts and toilet breaks, stopping to take out Ivan and walk him, the traffic disappearing once we cross the Severn Bridge into Wales, the empty bridge, no toll booths, no money changing hands, just the long grey tongue of the road leading us on into a new emptiness. Up through the country on the winding roads past ancient slate-grey pubs. Every town disfigured by the bad architecture of the late twentieth century. Every 'For Sale' sign has been up for months.

We clean our hands at the door to the ward and walk inside, and I see Chris sitting in a blue plastic chair before I see Mum lying in the bed beside him. Chris stands up when he spots us. Mum can't. She has a mask clamped over her face, plugged into the wall, getting her oxygen through a tube. As we approach I can see that her face is red and there's sweat running off her. Her breathing is quick and shallow, like a fish on the bank. She looks emotional when she sees we've arrived, and reaches out an arm towards me. Her hospital gown is hanging off her shoulder. She turns her head to look at us but doesn't raise it up off the pillow. I sit down with her, take the hand she's holding out towards me. Amy stands behind me and the thought crosses my mind for just a moment that this must be so strange for her, very new to this family, pitched into this bedside *pietà* in reverse.

'Hi.' She doesn't speak, but smiles instead, and I realise that perhaps with the mask and shortness of breath, speech is difficult. I turn to Chris while Amy leans in to smile at Mum and say hello.

'I'm sorry we didn't get here sooner,' I say to him.

'Don't worry. It's wonderful that you've come.'

'How are things?'

He searches for the right words for a moment. 'Pretty scary right now, actually. They've pumped the oxygen up as far as they can go without putting her in intensive care. She's running a temperature and she feels very hot. We don't really know what's going to happen.'

'What's she on? What are they giving her for it?'

'They've put her on antibiotics, but apparently it takes two or three days before they know if it's working. So for now we just have to wait.'

'But once the antibiotics kick in, she'll start to recover?'

'That's the hope. As long as they're the right antibiotics. Different forms of pneumonia need different treatment. They won't know whether they've got it right for another day or so.'

'So they might have to try her on something else?'

'That's possible, yes. We just have to wait and see.'

It's hard to know exactly what it is I'm feeling as I listen to him. So many of the most dramatic moments in our lives can feel very ordinary, because they happen too quickly for us to take in. And we've seen them all so many times in films that sometimes we can't help feeling like we're in a dream, watching ourselves from above as we act out our lines as best we can. I feel numb, almost calm, as if none of this is real. I turn back to look at Mum in the bed.

'Are you in pain?' I ask her. She shakes her head.

'Just my breathing.' Her voice, when I hear it, is shocking to me – all the strength stripped out of it, all the life. She is speaking with the voice of an elderly woman. Now I've heard her speak, she seems suddenly much more unwell than I thought she was a moment ago. As if I've just discovered that a part of her has vanished.

'They're looking after you, though. They're making sure you can breathe OK.' She nods. There's fear in her eyes. Her gaze wanders. It occurs to me that she might be a little delirious. 'Are you able to sleep?' I ask her.

She shakes her head, listless, exhausted, terrified. 'I can't. Not for days now. I'm so frazzled, I feel like I can't see straight. When you came in just now, I thought it was a dream.'

A nurse comes and talks to us, checks Mum's oxygen levels and her blood pressure and asks if she's feeling all right. Mum does what everyone always does, and says she's fine, though it's clear to all of us that she isn't. A porter brings a plate of food and I chop it up so it's easier for Mum to eat. Watching her try to eat is agony. She has to take the mask off her face to get the forkfuls of food to her mouth, but without the mask she struggles to breathe, so she can only take a couple of mouthfuls at a time before she has to pull the mask back down and get her breath back and recover. So the food cools as she eats it slowly, slowly. I remember the way she used to tell me off at mealtimes when I wouldn't eat what was in front of me. 'Don't you know there are children starving in Africa?' 'Well, why don't you send it to them, then?' The hospital food disgusts her. Before long she gives up, pushes the plate away. She still feels hot, so we hold a cup of water to her lips, and she sips at it. Chris finds an electric fan, and turns it to face her, and turns it on, and that seems to help a little. The water makes her calmer. She stares into space and shakes her head, and the look in her eyes is desolation. We are sitting around her in postures of supplication, leaning forward, hands resting on the bed. We turn our faces to her like moths to the light.

'I don't know what's going to happen,' she says to no one. 'I don't know what's happened.'

I find it hard to stay in this moment, not to think ahead, my mind is racing forwards now to the troubles I feel sure this illness is going to cause both Mum and Chris. Pneumonia is one of those illnesses that takes a long time to get over. When she gets through this, I wonder whether it will be possible for her to recover on the farm, or whether she'll need to stay somewhere else. Surely there'll be too much work waiting for her if she goes home, too much struggle? And surely it must have been the farm that made her ill in the first place? I think of the black mould on the kitchen wall, damp and cloying from lack of ventilation. Just stepping through the door of the place made Amy start coughing when we visited. Rachel's the same these days, though she grew up in that environment; years in the city have made her sensitive to it, and she coughs whenever she goes home. Surely that will be why Mum picked this illness up as well?

I know part of my reason for asking myself these questions is selfish. I've always feared the farm would one day become too difficult for them. For a moment I entertain the possibility that there won't be years between now and having to set about selling the farm, and the picture seems different, and I feel panic gathering in me. Things that are going to end some indefinite time in the future look very different from things that could end any day. I know as I sit by the bed how much of a betrayal it really is for me to be resolved against ever coming back here, against ever taking it on.

We spend perhaps an hour and a half together, trying to reassure Mum that she's going to be all right, trying to talk about ordinary things so she doesn't feel like the whole world's ended, telling each other stories about what we'll do when everything's all right, the family gatherings, the reunions. Amy disappears a couple of times to let Ivan out of the car and make sure he's all right. Then when the plate's been taken away again, Mum starts talking about going to the toilet, and Chris suggests that perhaps we should leave her now to rest. She's having to use a bedpan as she's too weak to move or stand at the moment, and doesn't want us around to watch.

I don't really want to leave. It feels like I've only just walked in, and I know once we get home there'll be five hours of driving between me and her, and getting to her bedside will become more difficult. I don't know how to say goodbye to her. What I want to do is open up, say how I'm feeling, talk about love and things that matter. But I hold back. I don't want to make a big deal of this leave-taking. If I say too much,

I worry it will seem as if I think she's going to die. So I kiss her on the forehead, as she must have kissed me on the forehead when she used to tuck me into bed as a child, and tell her I'll visit again as soon as I can, and we leave with Chris, and say goodbye to him in the car park of the hospital, and tell him we'll call him that evening once we're home, again not saying enough because I don't want to say the wrong thing.

Then we let the dog out for a minute, and get into the car, and turn for home. Neither of us speaks for the first mile of road. Neither of us knows what we ought to say.

'Look,' Amy says to me, eyes on the road. 'Don't go home to your place tonight. Actually, don't go back there again. You don't want to be on your own right now. Come and be with me. If you want, I mean. Why don't you come and be with me?'

The offer strikes me as almost impossibly romantic. I realise that she had hoped we'd have this conversation out on our holiday, too; she had also been wondering when we'd get round to mentioning that.

'I really want that,' I say. 'But I don't want you to feel you have to because my mum's not well. We should only do that if we would have done it anyway.'

'Would you have done it anyway?' Amy asks.

'Yeah,' I say. 'I would. I don't know when I'd have asked, but I wanted to ask you.'

'All right, then,' she says, 'let's do it. Because that's what I wanted as well.'

'It changed while you were away, didn't it?'

'Yeah. It was always going to, though. It was always going to end or get more serious. Being apart does that.'

'You're sure you're up for it?'

'If it's where you want to be too.'

I want to say to her: I would go anywhere you wanted. I would follow you anywhere, because you want me with you. And to know someone cares whether or not you're around is the heart of all meaning, the heart of belonging; that's what people search for all their lives. I would go anywhere if you wanted me to go with you. But I don't know how to say it without sounding like a greetings card.

'I'm up for it,' I say to her instead. And we drive on together. And just like that, the world is different. I glance at her. Something happens that's never happened before.

'I love you,' I tell her.

She smiles. 'Yeah, I think I might love you too actually, but right now I'm going to concentrate on driving.'

1952

Years before her husband killed himself, Mary was just a
young woman from Llandrindod Wells who wanted to
be happy, who met a man at a dance in Builth Wells who said
he was going to take over a farm near Erwood, and fell in love
with him, and fought with him sometimes because he had
black moods but always loved the making up together. Who
looked after her parents-in-law until they died. Mary was a
young woman who had a daughter with her husband, and
she loved the raising of that girl, her angel, her Angie. She was
a young woman who kept the house while Leo kept the farm.
As the years coursed through her, she gathered in the store of
her memory a trove of things which seemed to her to have the
gleam of love, and life became more and more about the act
of remembering for her with the passing of each year, as she
went on collecting up these things that gleamed like prayers,
one beautiful image after another that made her grateful to
have been alive. The day she found a shrew with all its babies
in the pantry of the house, and lifted one of the baby shrews
up on the palm of her hand and watched it groom itself; the
day she travelled with her parents to St David's, and for the
first time saw the sea; the first time she helped birth a lamb;

the feeling of biting into good beef bought from Builth market and carted the miles home for the family after Lent; the feeling of sitting at Evensong in church, looking up at the stained glass in the windows while the organ music seemed to speak to her, catching chords in her heart she'd never previously heard, lifting her up out of herself. Like the feeling she got when she climbed up mountains.

Her life on the farm was one of unremitting labour, but each of the thousands of tasks she carried out were essentially straightforward in what had to be done, the number and constancy of them being what really wore her down. If people ever asked her, she'd say she had a simple life, though each morning she woke before first light to put fires in the grates and open the shutters, let the chickens out and feed them grain, take the bread dough from where it had been proving under its cloth overnight and get water from the well and heat a kettle and make breakfast for her family, clean the house and keep the fires stoked and get her child out to school at the top of the hill in time, clean clothes in the big tub with the washboard in front of the fire, and wash herself, and change the sheets, and make her husband's lunch, and make bread and churn butter, and maybe go down into Erwood for provisions, and mend things, always patching or darning, and help Angie with her reading, and make the dinner, and get her child to bed and then help her husband clean up from the day, and a thousand other tasks besides this. Leo always knew this and was always appreciative, always grateful for the work she did keeping the house together while he was out on the hills with the lambs or mending fences or feeding the sheep, all the daily work of a farm. It was barbarism really, she thought sometimes, but that was life in that part of the world in that moment in time, and she accepted it. It wasn't as if there was anything else. Or rather, there might have been once, when she was young, and could have gone anywhere or fallen in love with anyone, but that never happened, and now was long gone. She was in her life and she decided she would love it. Years later, when Angie's marriage ended and she came home to the farm, Mary would sit with her grandchild Edward while Angie and the man she'd hired to run the farm were out doing Leo's old job on the backbreaking land, and tell stories about the lives she hadn't lived, the things that might once have been different.

'It's the pattern with the women in this family,' she'd tell Edward. 'They follow the men and that becomes their lives, for better or worse – that's been the pattern. I followed your grandfather back here and now I will die here, I suppose, and your grandfather's mother followed her husband the whole way across the world when he wanted to come home, from the place where she was born in India. And the cost it took on her, you wouldn't believe it, she was a very ill woman, but that's what happens in this family; we all come to the farm, the women following the men.' She shouldn't have, really. Probably sowing trouble like dragon's teeth. But that was the story as she understood it, and she liked to tell her stories to them; she thought love was storytelling, the sharing of a life the meaning of love.

All the time she told this story of herself, there was another life happening within her that she never knew how to share with people. These feelings, these vast feelings that she could not fit into language, would assail her every day as she reeled, dizzy sometimes, with how much she loved being alive for this span of time. The sunsets at the end of the valley, and the way the hawthorn foamed with flowers upon coming into bloom. The trees seeming to speak to her in the wind, the shelter of tall oaks, the shelter of beeches. It was all breathtaking to her, and she wished she could have found more ways to say it. Instead she satisfied herself with telling her family that she loved them, trusted that they saw the world the way she did, trusted that they would know what she meant when she spoke of love.

Leo took a lot of looking after. Sometimes he would sit and cry in the mornings before he went out for the day, and for many years she kept her distance from him, afraid he would become violent and strike out, but that never happened and as time passed she realised what he wanted was to be comforted, because there were things terribly wrong with him. It was the legacy of his mother, she supposed, the years when she had been mad but nothing had been done about it, when she used to sob and scream and try to throw herself from windows, the cost of that on this poor boy who should have been looked after by her, not the other way round. He had to do it all, right till her dying day, because his father didn't know what to do, and there was no one in the area who could have helped her. Really she should have been sent away, but asylums in those days were not places for anyone you loved, perhaps they still weren't, perhaps they never would be, so she stayed upstairs in her own private kingdom in the attic and looked out at the alien hills and the abandoned farmhouses falling down, and Leo would cook for her, wash her, keep her living, although Mary doubted that was what Phoebe herself really wanted. She would have rather been dead or gone home, but no one can ever go home, not really. That was what she thought Leo might have been doing the day he died, those many years later, when he fell from the roof. She remembered Phoebe's funeral in 1952, the two of them standing side by side in the churchyard in the village, holding her husband's hand. She was looking down into the grave as the coffin was being prepared to be lowered down into it, as the young men who had dug the grave started to take the weight of the straps wrapped round the box, and she glanced at Leo, worried he would be appalled by this, traumatised by the physicality of it, the huffing and heaving, and saw to her surprise that he wasn't looking at the coffin at all. He was looking at the tower of the church and the sky beyond.

'Are you all right?' she asked him, knowing she had asked a stupid question, because of course he wasn't, his mother had died, and just as difficult as the sorrow of this was the sheer relief, the knowing she wasn't in pain any more, and that all the work of keeping her alive had finally ended; the guilt of that relief would be as difficult as the sorrow.

'She used to love to look at the tower from her bedroom window,' Leo said to her.

'It's very beautiful.'

'It wasn't so much the tower itself. She liked to be up high. When she was high up, she could see further. I think she dreamed of one day getting so high she could see all the way home. Of course, she got it all wrong. She could see further from the farm, she could see for miles from the top field over the valley, and if she'd climbed the tower, she'd only have seen the valley from the bottom. But she loved to be up high, my mother, she loved a tower, loved a spire.'

Mary looked up at the little church tower, which seemed so pathetic when you thought of ever getting high enough off the ground to see all the way to India, but of course she knew home wasn't a place, it wasn't somewhere physical in the world you could return to. What Phoebe must have liked, she suspected, was the look of distance, the blue of distance falling over hills, which must seem beautiful from the top of the church tower in the estranging wind. A chance to see out to the edge of the vision, not to spy any particular place, but just to know the distance and take it in. She watched Leo watching the tower. She knew as the years rolled on, he might fall more and more in love with the look of distance too, a way to take in what had become of him, to remember his mother. And she was right. And then he fell. And then he was buried in the same graveyard where they had stood together in 1952, newly married, not yet parents, barely begun on the journey they'd share until he took it away from them, because the black moods became the whole of him, because no matter how hard he tried he couldn't outswim the current any more, which had been pulling at him ever since his mother left India, before he was even born. She had the strangest feeling later, after he had gone, that she had seen it all coming, as early as that day in that churchyard. It had all been contained in that moment when she watched him staring fixedly at the church tower while his mother was lowered into the ground. She remembered how she used to wait to meet him from the bus into Llandrindod when they were courting, standing on tiptoes to see in the windows of the bus as it arrived, to spot him looking out at her. She remembered the crackle of the air when he got off the bus, the joy in both of them, their faces lighting up with smiles and him shyly leaning down to kiss her on the cheek, and him taking her hand, and her heart in her chest as they walked into Llandrindod together, or out the other way into the fields to be alone together. The glory of taking a man's hand, and loving him, and knowing as you did that he loved you, that you wanted the same things, that one day you were going to be together. Couldn't life have been that? Might there not have been something she could have done to make things different?

2019

WE TRAVEL HOME. In English we don't have enough words for 'home', the precise nuances of what we mean are never spelled out clearly enough. The same word has to stand for this place I'm from that I'm leaving behind, and this place where I lie down to sleep each night. The traffic of London slows us down for the last hour. The city we live in rises to meet us, funnels us along its faceless roads flanked with dirt-caked houses and the walled-in soundproofed lives lived inside them, the people hiding. I feel the city climbing into my head, making room for itself, overturning one thing after another, setting everything spinning. The ceaseless noise, the light, the fear, the anger. In this place we cling to each other and try the best we can to survive the huge indifference of the metropolis all around us.

All cities are built like maps of a mind, and when you spend time in them they come to map your own, you can't help but fall into the rhythms offered up to you. As we return, I feel all my thoughts start to press together. This jealous city where no one looks anyone in the eye. We crawl through the leafy outskirts, then on to the concrete and empty shops that make up the place where we live, the part of the city where things are sent that people want to forget or ignore or cover over. This is us for now. We find what life and dignity we can in this place where voices are not heard, where memories are being obliterated.

We reach Amy's flat and I get Ivan out of the car while Amy brings the first of the bags inside. I look around the place with new eyes now, imagining moving the things I own into this space, becoming part of it, for however long we stay here. I try to imagine my books on the shelves.

It's growing dark and for the first time in a week I find I can't feel the weather. Behind this double glazing under the low growls of the road, under the flight path and disoriented as the orange lights turn on outside with the nightfall, I can't feel what's happening in the air in the evening. This is living in the city, desensitized and numb. I hadn't noticed how numb it made me feel.

So this will be us for a little while, then. Four rooms to go round, the big living room at the front, the bedroom, the kitchen and the bathroom. The flat was once the first floor of a house on the end of a terrace built at the end of the nineteenth century; all those houses were cut up into flats many years ago. Amy lives above a Spanish family with a three-year-old child, who I have learned loves nothing more than to run up and down the length of the house, screaming at the top of his voice. It seems to me sometimes when I stay here and listen to him as if there must be something emotionally wrong with him: the child seems to cry at the slightest provocation, and his parents, who are kind people, and can't be blamed for the noise their son makes, don't know how to calm him down. If we pass in the front hallway, we greet each other like friends, but in the back gardens, our garden being the one nearest the house and theirs being the scrap of lawn beyond it, we pretend not to see each other, and get on with our reading or sunbathing in silence. This is how I've come to characterise life in this city – impossibly close together, yet somehow miles apart.

Before Amy lived in this flat it was, I believe, a cannabis farm. Both the downstairs and upstairs flats had stood empty for some time, as this part of the city, though still undesirable now, was practically dangerous five or ten years ago, and flats could often be hard to rent out. At some point, someone must have noticed the flats were abandoned and found a way to break in. I've only been able to piece the story together by reading around online, but the pieces seem to fit. Our building, being on the end of the terrace, borders the playground of the neighbouring primary school, and I came across an article one day describing a police raid on a property next to the school that discovered a farm with a hundred plants growing in it. As all the refurbishment work done on this flat to make it habitable dates from about five months after that raid, and the only other property next to the school has been a family home for many years, it seems likely to me that the owners of this place, having been informed by the police of what had been going on, had decided to give the flats a lick of paint and persuade some more legitimate tenants to live in them. Very little sign of this chapter in the life of the flats remains to be seen today; only the front doors seem to give a hint of it. The outer door, which contains several glass panels, has two very different kinds of glass in it, the panels nearest the door handle being much newer and more recently installed. The inner door, meanwhile, is a cheap fire door installed very recently. These, I think, are the traces of the police raid that ended with Amy's flat being reclaimed for human habitation. The outer door was opened by breaking a couple of glass panes; the inner door had to be kicked in completely.

We eat a light supper, take Ivan for a last walk round the woods up the road, phone Chris and tell him we hope he's able to sleep tonight, and promise we'll call the ward for an update in the morning. Then we watch an hour of TV sitting side by side, take our books to bed together, and make love, then sleep.

For a little while after Amy has fallen asleep, I lie awake and watch her. I used to laugh at people who talked about watching someone sleeping. I didn't understand how it could be a tender moment. It was a moment, after all, when the person you were watching wasn't really there. It was just that I hadn't loved anyone back then. In these quiet moments of looking unselfconsciously at someone else, taking time to take them in, the mind unspools the life you have together, the things you've shared in the last hours and days, and you find out what they mean to you as the feeling creeps up and makes itself known in all its depth and complexity, the feeling swells because it's given its acre of silence to stretch out, like light falling lazily through the window of a kitchen, taking a whole day to roll across a table, loving slowly, tracing every knothole and lineament. I watch Amy while she sleeps and the feeling is almost like grief, that once I didn't know this woman, I missed so much of her life in the years before I knew her, and one day not so far from now our togetherness will end again, it is all of it ending every minute we live.

When I call the ward the next morning and ask to speak to the nurse in charge, then apologise for taking up his time and ask how Mum is feeling, I don't get the reassurance I hoped to hear. Strange, how in these times we always seem to expect the best. I had called up thinking whoever I spoke to would tell me that things had improved with the passage of time. People, given any reasonable inducement, will look away. The rubbernecking traffic that builds up on motorways is misleading, it's not really a marker of human behaviour at all; when the accident happens in their own lives, most people don't slow down to look at it if they don't have to. Most people will deny it's even happening.

'Your mother's been moved to intensive care; she's no longer here on this ward, I'm afraid. You'll need to redial and speak to them.'

'What's happened to her? Why was she moved?'

'In the night she needed a boost in oxygen, and she's continued to need that today. She can get that more easily on intensive care, so the decision was taken to move her.'

'But she's not getting worse?'

'She wasn't getting worse, no. It's just that she wasn't managing to get any better, so it was decided a stronger intervention would help her turn the corner.'

'All right. Thank you. I'll call intensive care now and see how she is.'

But I don't. I ring off, then decide to call up Chris instead, guessing he'll know all this already and just hasn't got round to calling me yet, guessing I'll learn as much from him as I could from the overworked nurses. It makes me uncomfortable calling the hospital; I feel like I'm taking people away from their work. I call him straight away without going to find Amy, because I'm looking for quick reassurance. The memory comes to me of the last days of my grandma's life, my father's mother, when the hospital kept sending her back to the nursing home and the nursing home would simply send her back to the hospital, because within an hour of getting there she'd need oxygen again, and they didn't have a ventilator. Three times it happened; there was nothing technically wrong with my grandma when she kept getting sent in, so the hospital would send her home, then six hours later she'd be back again. I was there for two of them, and watched her being wheeled along on her trolley bed, tiny and birdlike, looking suddenly fifty years younger without her glasses on, her face stripped of old age, perhaps because she had lost a lot of weight, and she looked so like my dad that it was frightening. In a corridor waiting to be given a ventilator room, she shifted and moaned, and I asked her where it hurt, and she roared out to me with all the strength left in her body in a voice that seemed to come from some supernatural depth the one word 'everywhere'. There was nothing I could say. I held her hand. I told her we were all so proud she was our grandmother, that she'd set us all a wonderful example. She looked very deeply into my eyes and nodded, and the pain seemed to clear while she thought of that. Then the pain came back again, and she lay on her back, and all life had shrunk down to focusing on her breathing, the whole world, which had once been hers to travel round and explore and visit on cruises, reduced down to breathing in and out. She died later that same day. I'd left the hospital, and wasn't with her when it happened, and I wish I had been, I wish I hadn't gone home that afternoon.

And remembering her always leads me back further to the death of my grandad, her husband. One memory always spurring the next. His death was even more horrifying to me, in part because it was the first; he died before Dad died and I had never gone through it before, I had never seen how hard it was to die till then and the knowledge shocked me, the knowledge made me far less certain than I had been that it was a fortunate thing to be born into the world, when there was so much pain waiting for us all in the leaving of it. And there was the fact that there was nothing really terminally wrong with him either; he seemed to just decide he couldn't go through with it all any more, so he stopped eating and drinking, and starved himself to death, and was overcome by waves of fear and panic in the last days when we sat with him and asked him to drink a little water, and begged the nurses to help him with the pain.

I think of them both, my beautiful grandparents, the kindest people in the world to me, who never deserved the way their stories ended, and I can't believe Mum could be next along the line to face all that. It's ludicrous to me, at her age, in her robust health, it's unimaginable. Although I realise, having seen her lying in the hospital bed, that it will happen one day; and I realise that now she's one of the people in my life who might be next, impossible as it is to really take that disturbing thought in. So I call Chris's number and he picks up, sounding a little out of breath. I can hear that he's outside, and I guess he's in the hospital car park again.

'I'm sorry I haven't called yet,' he says, once he's heard that I know she's been moved to the ICU. 'When they told me, I just got in the car and drove. I've just parked up.'

'Of course, don't worry. I'm guessing you don't know any more yet than I do?'

'Not really, no. I don't think your sister knows yet.'

'I can call her, don't worry.'

'Are you sure?'

'Of course. You just want to be with Mum, you don't want to do all that.'

'Thank you.' He's silent for a moment. 'I thought I'd be stronger, you know.'

I don't know what to say to that. I still don't know what conversation Chris wants to have, how much further he's thought than this moment, whether thinking past this crisis and getting Mum back home would just be an irrelevance to him. I want to ask him how long she's been ill, and whether he's cleaning the house for when she gets home, where she'll sleep while she recuperates, how his work's been affected, whether he's getting help in. All of this might just be chaff to him, could even make him angry while his wife's there in the hospital and that's all he wants to be thinking about.

'Why don't you go in and see her, see what's going on?'

'All right. Thank you. I'll call you in a while, then.'

He rings off, and I look out the window and don't know what to do. I can see the back of the allotment site beyond the gardens, a line of trees dividing the allotments from the gardens of the houses. I can see the light falling on the trees, and catching the high fences of the gardens, picking out the slats of the fences in stark dark and light. Amy is in the next room. I go through to her.

'I'm guessing you heard all that?' I say.

She nods.

'Do you want to go back?'

'I don't know what to do yet. It might just be she needed the extra support, and that will mean she turns the corner. I don't think we should do anything till he calls back.'

'All right.' She stands up and crosses the room to me, and we kiss. 'Are you all right?'

'Kind of.'

'Can I do anything?'

We smile at each other, because of course we both know she can't. Absurd as it is, there's nothing to be done. Even travelling to see her might be more for us than her, really. But what else are we supposed to say at times like these? What else can we offer? Is it better to stay silent and say nothing at all? The words are really just a form of kindness, just a way of telling someone you love them.

Ten anxious minutes pass, time I spend in the kitchen putting the washing-up away, then Chris calls again, and I answer. I'm slightly surprised he's called so quickly. When the phone rings my stomach drops, as if I already know it's going to be bad news.

He tells me he didn't stay long, because she's not conscious any more. He came back outside to tell me so I could call my sister and get in the car and start driving. She has sepsis, and for some reason he can't explain she's not conscious now. I hear the news through a dim, deep roaring, as if there's a waterfall crashing down to drown the air between Chris and me. It's the blood in my ears, I think, the panic, the urgent heartbeats. He hangs up. Amy has come to the kitchen doorway. I turn and we look at each other.

'I thought she was recovering,' I say.

'She might still be recovering. She might just need more help than she was getting.'

'But why is she unconscious? What does that mean?' I try, but I can't get my head round it. I didn't ask what he meant, whether she'd passed out or whether her unconsciousness had been somehow induced. Did he mean sleeping? Did he mean a coma? She's still a young woman, my mother, she's just turned sixty; it's going to be a long time before her health fails. There's going to be a long time yet for us to plan what to do when this kind of thing happens. We don't have to be thinking about days like these, not for a decade yet, not till she's older. What on earth is happening? How could this moment be real? I call my sister and she answers on the third ring.

'You OK?' she asks.

'I'm OK. But I think we need to head home.'

'What's happened?'

'I'm not completely sure, but Mum needed more oxygen so they moved her to intensive care. Your dad's there with her but I think we should go.' I finish the call, and ring off, and again I don't know what to do, I feel frozen by the significance of what might be happening even now, right now, even though the day outside the window looks unremarkable to me.

'Shall we go?' Amy asks.

'Is that OK?'

She smiles as if in exasperation. What passes unspoken between us is my apology for still behaving as if this might not be an emergency, still pretending we might have some say in what we do with the next few hours, when in fact we've fallen somehow into a crisis, and none of the normal rules are going to apply for a while. I'm still pretending a drive back to Wales might be putting her out, because if that were true, if there were still any say in the matter, maybe the situation wouldn't be as frightening as it suddenly seems.

We get the dog back in the car and drive, only stopping at a service station once the fuel light's come on. There's a text from Chris to tell us he's still with Mum. No more than that.

Rachel is my half-sister, though I've never used that term about her. She went through a phase of calling me her half-brother. I didn't understand why at the time. It was a long time before I realised she must have been upset when I left home, and relegating me to the status of half-sibling must have felt a bit like what I'd done to her when I went away. Because she was born after Mum and I came to the farm, the place is closer to being the whole of her life. I always find that strange to imagine, because in many ways we're extremely alike, and it's easy to imagine we think all the same thoughts, share our memories. But there's an essential difference between us. Her image of the world was never broken. She never lost the geography of her childhood, never experienced being uprooted and having to accept a new place as her own. Her first memories belong to the farm, so for her there's still one place she can call home, one centre. She's never even had to work out what it means to have divorced parents. I can't imagine what it would feel like to live her life. I suppose there are things I distrust that she can never have doubted. Because she doesn't have the same grounds I have for believing the world could suddenly end at a moment's notice. It occurs to me, thinking of this, that she might respond more calmly to this current situation than I have. It may be that I'm catastrophising, expecting the worst because I always look out for it.

Amy drives, worried I won't be able to concentrate on the road, and I sit in the passenger seat beside her and think of the past. I remember the first time I ever needed stitches, falling from a tree and impaling myself on the stump of a low branch Dad had sawn off at the base of the tree I was climbing. Mum and Dad rushed me in the car to the doctor's surgery, my lower half covered with only a towel because the cut above my coccyx was open and bleeding. While we waited, I sat on Dad's lap and Mum crouched down and put her face in front of mine so that I could see her smile, I could see she was calm and listen to the soothing words she was trying to say to me, persuading both of us at once that I was all right. They took me into the doctor's room and I lay on my front on a bed, and the doctor sewed up the cut. I screamed as the needle went in, but it was mostly for show because Mum was holding my hand and I knew that I was safe and that I'd be all right, and the local anaesthetic the doctor had applied, a cold gel I remember him rubbing on, meant that I couldn't really feel any pain. I remember falling on a walk, and my front tooth cutting right through my upper lip, and the screaming, the blood and the pain, my mashed lip, and Mum kneeling down to pick me up and carrying me away again, back to the doctor's. This was the rhythm once, falling and being picked up. I watched her do it with Rachel, when Rachel broke her arm so clean at the elbow that when she held it out to show us all, it swung the wrong way. We would fall and she'd pick us up. And then, ever so slowly, everything changes, and it's her turn to be falling, and all of us feel like the same person we used to be, we hardly realised any time had passed at all. But everything is different and we can't go back.

When we get to the hospital Mum's awake again, and I can't get a straight story from Chris about what he meant when he said she was unconscious, whether she was sleeping or delirious or something else. The tension he feels is written on his face now, the colour all fled from it, the lines gouged deeper than I've ever seen them. He looks decades older than he did the day before. Rachel is there with him, holding Mum's hand. Mum tries to smile, but seems afraid, and I worry the fear on all our faces must be making it worse for her. So I try and see the positives. The new breathing machine Mum's been hooked up to makes it easier for her to speak and drink and eat; because the tubes go into her nose now, there isn't a mask to cover her mouth, and this makes talking easier.

'It must be such a relief to be able to drink without having to take a mask off,' I say.

'What?' She speaks like someone who's been up for a week – which she has, more or less, the shortness of breath and the other patients previously lying alongside her in the hospital ward making sleep impossible.

'The tubes. These must be so much better.'

'Oh,' she says. 'Yes. That's right.'

'And it's calmer in here, isn't it?'

She has her own room now in the ICU, a window that looks out, comically, on to a brick wall about three feet beyond the glass, like something from a movie, a cliché of a hospital view. The walls of the room are painted in that blue that people call either duck egg or eggshell, I can never quite remember, and the nurses are in earshot beyond the swing doors, which are pinned open. Through the doors we hear the nurses speaking and the beeping of machines, but there's quiet around Mum, where before there were five other people in beds on the shared ward, visitors, the scraping of chairs, nurses fending off questions. Mum growls in the back of her throat at the memory of it.

'Fucking place.'

We laugh.

'Yeah. Was it really awful?' I ask her.

'This woman opposite. I don't know. Theresa. Seems to have had a difficult life, and fair enough. But my God. All night, she wouldn't stop.'

'Stop what?'

'There was this programme she was listening to. About jazz music in England. About jazz music after the Second World War. And it was all about the kinds of jazz and where people heard it, and the kind of venues there were and the record shops, that kind of thing. And Theresa listened to this whole programme, and the thing is that after the war there was a lot of motorbike manufacturing. People made a lot of motorbikes because they were cheap to produce and cheap to run and because they were popular as well. And Theresa thought there wasn't enough in the documentary about motorbike manufacturing. And she was calling up the station for hours and hours to complain.'

Rachel and Chris laugh uneasily. I lean towards her, try to catch her eye.

'So this was a programme on the radio, was it?'

'Yes, but she kept calling in.'

'She was trying to complain about a programme on the radio.'

'Yes, again and again and again.'

I try to look her in the eye, make out whether this really happened or if she had been delirious. She seems to doubt what she's saying herself, already what had seemed so clear a moment earlier becoming dim and cloudlike.

Chris leaves the room to go to the toilet, and Mum beckons to me and Rachel, drawing us closer, so we both lean in around her.

'You have to look after him,' she says.

'We are, Mum, don't worry,' Rachel tells her, taking her hand.

'But you have to make sure he's all right.' This time neither of us speaks, because it's clear she doesn't mean just for now; she doesn't mean till she gets better. It's shocking, to see her planning for life after she's left it. And neither of us knows enough, neither of us knows whether she's truly in danger or whether she's just frightened. 'He won't be able to look after himself on his own.'

'He won't need to, Mum, you'll be home with him,' I say.

'But if he couldn't look after the farm,' she carries on, determined, a little out of breath now from this speaking.

'We don't need to think about this.'

'If he couldn't look after the farm, would you help him?'

Rachel and I share a wild glance, and don't know what to say.

'Of course we would,' I say.

'He can't just leave it. It's his home. You'd have to help him keep it going.'

'We'd do whatever we could, Mum.'

'No, but I mean it. You can't let him leave. Couldn't you take it on? For me, couldn't you do that? He can't do all his cooking himself, you know.'

I lift up my head again and this time share a look with Amy, trapped at the edge of the room, not knowing how to help me. 'We'd do what was best for Chris, Mum, don't worry.'

'You'd live there with him?'

'We'd work out what was best. Sometimes when people get older it's better for them to move somewhere easier to man-age, it's not just a case of saying we'd help him stay. But all this is years away anyway, Mum, we can talk about all this another time.'

'You don't want it,' she says with sudden force.

'What do you mean, Mum?' Rachel says.

'We built it. We all built that life.' Her face seems to fall in on itself, with the sad sullen rage of a child. She has seen it for the first time. She's taken it in. And we should be changing our minds to reassure her. If I was a better man, I'd say what was needed. But I say nothing. None of us says anything for a moment, because I can see Rachel feels the same way I do; Rachel doesn't feel like the farm is her life, and neither of us wants to lie to Mum just to make her feel better. Perhaps we ought to, but we don't, and then Chris comes back into the room, and the moment passes.

After a while, the nurses tell us we have to leave. It's different here to the rules on the ward, where we were allowed to stay late and no one noticed. The ICU is full of people fighting for life. So we say goodbye to Mum, trying to keep it light, trying not to say too much and frighten her, and I leave with Amy and Rachel while Chris stays behind for one more minute. Mum seems frightened, under the surface of her saying goodbye, but she tries to be brave, she tries to hide it. We tell her we love her and she says the same. We kiss her on the forehead and then we leave. We go outside and see to Ivan while Rachel uses the loo.

'She's pretty scary,' Amy says.

'I know. The machine she's on seems better, though.'

There is a fear that's taking me over, and I don't know how it got so strong, or whether it's rational, and whether I should mention it. The feeling of having no more control over what's going to happen, the knowledge that even Mum can't make it on her own now, and needs the machines to help with her breathing, makes me feel suddenly very weak. I wonder how many times in my life I'll have to feel this. I wonder how often I'm going to have to cope with this feeling of weakness. I can't quite dismiss the thought that this, now, is the beginning of a long and drawn-out ending that will slowly build up till it encompasses everything, drowns out everything. In and out of hospital for one person or another, turning the years into a long goodbye. I could see it stretching ahead of us. The world going round in ever-decreasing circles for my parents as they grew older. One thing after another becoming impossible, the walks they used to take getting shorter, the back aching worse first thing in the morning. Before they knew it, they'd have bought their last overcoats.

'Do you want to stay?' Amy asks. I guess we've both assumed since the moment we left home that that was what we were going to do, for a while at least, though neither of us has mentioned it, though neither of us actually packed a bag.

'What do you think?'

'I think while things are scary, it would be the supportive thing to do, don't you?'

'Would you mind?'

'Of course not.'

'If we're welcome, of course.'

'Of course. But I think we will be.'

Rachel comes back out of the hospital. 'What are you two going to do, then?' she asks.

'We thought we'd see if we could stay for a few days. If we wouldn't be getting in the way.'

'I think that'll be good for Dad, yeah. He's not dealing with this very well, is he?'

'Understandably.'

'Told me he spent all of last evening online looking at houses in town.'

'Did he?'

'He said it was a useful distraction.'

'Really?'

'He's worried the farm will be too hard for Mum.'

'Jesus.' I don't know what to say to this – I ought to feel glad we're thinking along the same lines, but in fact a kind of panic sets in.

'We'd been talking about that,' Amy says. 'You can't know with these things, can you, but we wondered whether the lifestyle could have been what made her ill.'

'It's so fucking hard there, in the winters,' I add. 'I don't know whether now's the time, because there might be too much else to deal with, but it's interesting that that's what Chris's doing.'

Then Chris comes along the hall from the ICU and joins us by the front door. We smile at him, tentative, and he smiles in return.

'Shall we have a cup of coffee?' he asks. So we go to the hospital café and I order drinks, and we sit down.

'We were actually wondering whether we might stay with you for a night or two?' I ask once we're all seated. 'If you didn't mind.'

'No, of course. I'd be really grateful,' he says. 'I know your mum would be too. That's really kind, thank you.'

'All right. That's great. Thank you.'

We finish our coffees.

'Did she seem OK when you left her just now?' Rachel asks.

Chris shrugs. 'I think so. I hope so. I think maybe she had a wobble this morning, but things are levelling out. This is going to be a long road,' he says.

'Yeah.'

'The doctor tells me maybe six months, before she's properly well again. And while she's recovering, there won't be that much she can do.'

'We could make up a bed for her downstairs, so she doesn't have to go up and down too much.'

'That could be good.'

None of us speaks for a second then. I have a feeling that all of us are holding back. All of us scared, and imagining different futures. But none of us wants to be the first to say these terrifying things out loud. Eventually my stepdad looks up and smiles.

'I spent the whole of last evening on Zoopla, you know. Looking at cottages in town. Silly, I know, wrong time to think about it, but it was where my mind went. Seeing if there were easier places for us to live while your mum recovers. God knows how we'd ever sell the farm, though, selling it would take years. I was only distracting myself.'

We walk to the cars, putting Ivan back into the back seat, and Amy and I are alone together once the doors close and the silence closes round us. While we travel, a buzzard flies low over the road, and seems to stare in through the windscreen at us both. The sun catches its wings as it passes, so it looks like it's burning, and I feel as if the world's trying to speak to me. Perhaps that's just the ghost of religious faith making me read significance into a bird in the air, and light on its wings. Sometimes I can almost hear God singing through these landscapes, though I don't believe in that story any more. But it's hard to start life in a place like this and not believe the world has secret currents, because of the cold, heart-stopping sunlight on the grass. After forty minutes we come to the road that leads to the farm, and drive through the village, slow and easy, then on up the lane till we come to the left turn, and bump over the last few yards of unmade track till we come to the gate.

I half expect the house to be a mess when we walk in, but Chris has been cleaning up to keep himself busy, and the house actually looks better than I can remember it in a long time. Mum and Chris's dogs are overjoyed to see Ivan, and they race out into the garden together, chasing each other, inscribing circles in the grass and the quiet air and the afternoon. I make tea, and we take it out to the garden and sit by the vegetable beds, the three of us together.

When we first came back here, I think Mum saw the farm's history as a challenge, a story she could try to rewrite. For a long time she managed to pull off that trick – we all did it together, made the place where we lived fill up with noise and life and the clatter of living. That had lasted a long time. I don't think I'd ever noticed till now how long we'd held all that life in the air. A quarter of a century is a long time to make anything work. Was it going to end now, I wondered? Was this what it felt like to enter a new phase of the life of your family, for everything to change? People don't seem to age at all till they get ill one day, and suddenly they realise they're getting old, and then they can never get back to before. Would the farm reassert its true self now, its real face, and cast a shadow across us again?

'We could go back later today, I think, but I'm not sure that we ought to,' Chris says. 'Not unless they tell us we need to. I worry that what your mum needs most is rest rather than visitors.'

'We can leave it for today and go tomorrow. What can we be doing for you for the rest of today?' I ask.

He smiles weakly. 'You don't have to do anything. It's just great having you here.' He drinks his tea, and no one speaks for a minute. I watch a red admiral fluttering past us to settle on the flowers of the pea plants in the bed beyond. There are other butterflies feeding there already, blues and coppers and a swallowtail. 'The thing I need to start thinking about is what your mum will need when she gets home,' Chris says.

'Shall we set up a bed downstairs?' Rachel suggests.

'That would be good.'

'And if you wanted us to really go over the house and hoover all of it, I don't know whether that might help her breathing.'

'It's made me wonder whether we're getting old.'

Amy glances quickly at me, then looks away again. 'I don't think you're getting old,' she says to Chris. 'But it must make you realise how hard the life is.'

'That's it,' he says. 'Even a couple of days, when it's just me on my own, it's too much really. All the time you're out in the fields there's nothing happening at home. There's no way of keeping up. It makes you think.'

'We could come and help a bit more,' I say.

'You're kind. But it's not a solution, is it? You can't be always making that drive.'

The swallowtail catches my eye as it leaves the pea shoots and takes flight.

'It makes me wonder whether perhaps we might be coming to the end of this story.' He throws his arms wide then, and looks around him, to indicate that it's the place he means, the farm he's spent his life on. 'We've talked about it before, the two of us.'

'In a few months she might well be fine.'

He shrugs. 'Maybe.'

We finish our tea then, and talk of other things, work and our plans for our house move, unimportant stories, ways to distract us from talking about the thing that makes us all afraid. Even the talk of selling the farm is no more than that really, no more than a way of steering clear of the thought of Mum in the hospital, fighting the infection that wants to kill her. We all feel useless, because in the end we all are. We have all realised there isn't really anything we can do, and that shames us.

As the day passes and the shadows lengthen, we convert the sitting room into a bedroom in the hope that before too long Mum will be able to come home. Chris hopes it won't be too long, and talks about hospitals being dangerous places, where one infection might follow another. Then we spend a couple of hours in the garden, fixing the wooden frames on some of the raised beds and trimming a hedge, and mending a fallen section of dry-stone wall. It's good to find work to do with our hands, and in a small way all of it feels useful. Everything that makes Mum's home an easier place to live might help with her recovery. Chris calls the hospital to check what's happening, and the news is neither positive nor negative, in that it seems nothing has changed. He asks if we ought to be going back in, and the nurse in charge tells him Mum's stable, she's OK. We start preparing dinner when the evening comes, and don't need to light a fire because it's been a hot day and stayed dry, for the first day in weeks, Chris says, so we all work together on a chestnut casserole. When it's cooked, Chris starts serving the casserole on to plates while we lay the table, and that's when the call comes.

He goes to the phone with the ladle still in one hand, and answers, and asks who was speaking. These are the last moments. I try to remember what they looked like, the end of that world. Dust in the air and the cobwebs shadowing the roofbeams, logs piled up in the baskets by the hearth. The lights bouncing off the wood of the dining table, the wicker chair catching at Amy's top as she leans forward to fill a glass with water, a single candle flame on the table the centre of the scene. The phone is just round the corner from the kitchen, just out of sight, and none of us stop talking to listen in, none of us suspect. Then Chris comes back into the room, and we see his face, and stop talking, because we all know suddenly that Mum has died.

1964

A NGELA WALKED OUT into the wood beyond the home fields on her birthday, dreaming of knights in armour, dreaming of learning to fly. She threaded her way through the trees past the camp where the old soldier had slept last summer, past the old stones where the barn once stood, and watched the leaves weaving over her head in all their autumn glory. She saw how, when the clouds passed over, the colours of the wood hid themselves all away, and the place became damp leaf mould, deep shadow, shivers up her arms, so she hugged her cardigan tightly round herself and wondered, irrationally, if someone was watching. And then she saw how, when the clouds cleared once again, the colours of the wood flamed out once more, as if there was some wild light hidden in the trees, and the sun brought it out of them.

A thought struck her for the first time in her life that day that would haunt her for all the years that came after. A thought that would always remind her of this birthday, this moment in the wood when the clouds cleared, just before she heard her mother's voice calling her home for cake and presents. It occurred to her, watching the trees wake into beauty once again, that perhaps the same wild light might be hidden in everything, only waiting for the sun to bring it out. Years later, she would think that must be what people talked about when they talked about God, and why people went to church and bowed their heads, to feel close to moments in their own lives just like the moment Angela experienced in the wood. Years later, she would take comfort in the memory of that day when hard things happened to her or the ones she loved, and remember that sometimes in the world you did glimpse divinity, you did glimpse peace, and perhaps the passage of time was all a falling away from those moments, but that didn't mean such moments never happened.

She stood in the wood and drank in the reds and yellows of the autumn, watched the leaves twist and twirl in the air. A year later, at school, she wrote her very first poem about that moment, and felt a rhyme happen in her head for the first time, the way the words seemed to dovetail like a knitted stitch. 'Autumn leaves are falling down, whirling whirling to the ground.' Nothing so special about that, really. But the words seemed to go together because they echoed each other, and Angela felt very deeply, years before she had the learning to understand it, that words, when you strung them together, were like a map of the world, and the rhyme, the act of rhyming two sounds, was just what it had felt like to stand in that wood. As if the world wasn't just one thing after another. As if there was a shape to her different days when you looked at them together.

'Angie!' She heard her mother's voice filtering distantly through the trees, and turned to look for her, through the shade of the autumn wood to the light beyond and the home fields and the cottage. She saw her mother waving from the other side of the fence, leaning on the fence in a blue dress like a smock, as if she was living in a painting. And she thought nothing of it. She was just a little girl, five years old today, and wandering through this world that had been given to her to make the most of. Her mother was there, and she loved her. Inside the house her father might be washing his face, or perhaps he was still working and would get home soon. It didn't matter. They were together. And their lives were a dance like the leaves that fell through the endless blue air all around her. Back at the cottage there was poppyseed cake, and five candles for her to blow out when her father was with her. She started to walk back through the woods towards home. Years later, she would remember that walk towards the light, towards her mother, and wonder if that was the journey that she had been making ever since.

2019

H ARD TO REMEMBER the following few hours. The moment we knew Mum had died was filled with agony the first time I lived it, but I've lived it so many times since then that I seem to have drained all the blood from the memory, so it hardly feels like my life at all, more like a story I've told too many times. What happened to me next seems to exist now on the other side of a glass separating my past from my present self, and I can't get back to it. It was a moment when my life changed, I suppose, when I became a different person; so perhaps it's natural I can't think my way back into the body of the man I was when that happened. This must be why people who've been through pain will sometimes talk about it so much they seem proud it happened to them; they've relived it so many times the shock of the story has died. And they go back into the story just to check there's no way of crossing back into the past and recovering the person they were before.

Rachel lets out a cry that seems to last a long time as she crosses the room to Chris, and they hold each other, tears in their eyes. I look at Amy, and then we seem to get up as one and go to Chris and Rachel, who part as we approach them and hold out their hands, so I take my stepdad's hand in one of mine and Amy's in the other and for a moment, almost absurdly, we all stand holding hands in a kind of ring, and everyone is talking; perhaps I might have spoken too, but I don't know what I said, and no one else's words go in. Again, the rush of blood is roaring in my ears, and I hear nothing of the outside world. I stand in the dark stone room instead with my left hand in Amy's hand and my right hand holding Chris's left, and feel very close in that moment to all of the darkest days of my life. They all come rushing in, because they all felt like this, it always felt like this; when trouble came, it always hurt me in the same way, so that new tragedy always had the strangest way of feeling simultaneously like a retreat into old pain.

I remember the blood spattered over the floor in the rented farmhouse where Amy hit her head, the blood on the floor and the shock in her eyes and her fast, shallow breathing, and listen to her breathing now and hear the same sound, all of us drawn back into the same pain body by this grief, it seems, and then absurdly I find myself thinking of Tolstoy, who said all happy families were alike and all unhappy ones were different, and how wrong he was, because happiness had always seemed so infinite and various to me, whereas pain always seems to gather life back into the same narrow darkness. Each of us knows exactly what the others are going through, right down to our secret fear that it won't affect us as much as we think it properly should, each of us caught in the tide of sudden mourning that sweeps over everything and then retreats, emptying us all and leaving only a hollowness, leaving only a silence behind. Radiohead country. It was the same when Dad died. I'd worried for so long that, when it happened, I'd feel only relief. Then the day came, and I walked home in shock from the hospital along narrow pavements by myself, down quiet shabby backstreets linking the hospital to the estate where I lived, and went through the house and found the bottles he'd hidden, and emptied them into the toilet, then sat alone in the dark on the sofa where he'd slept till he went into hospital, and wished I could have my dad back again, and felt like a child, felt so small in the world, and wished I was young, wished that none of this had ever happened, because in that moment all life felt like an unravelling, a long litany of things gone wrong.

'We just saw her, though,' Rachel says. 'We only just saw her.'

'Oh my God.'

'She was fine, she was talking to me.'

'My God.'

'Jesus fucking Christ.'

'I don't understand.'

'What are we going to do, Dad? What are we going to do?'

'Should we go? Are we meant to go there?'

'They said that we shouldn't.'

'Jesus Christ.'

'They said that it's late; we should go in the morning.'

'This isn't possible.'

'What did they say happened?'

'I don't know, I don't know.'

'Fuck.'

'Oh fuck.'

'Oh Jesus Christ.'

I sink back into my chair and stare at my hands, and think of the time when Mum and I weren't speaking, while Dad was dying, the things we didn't say and the things we hadn't mended, and I feel my lips peel back in a rictus snarl as something takes me over and pulls back the muscles of my face till I bare my pain and show it glinting in the bright, broken snarl of my mouth. I feel welling up inside me a need to do violence, some desperate violence, to kick out and reject what I've just heard.

And there are no words for it. Language stops short here.

The nurses hadn't seen it coming, we learned; if they had, they would have told us to stay, or called us and asked us to make our way back. It was her heart that failed, they said. That was why they didn't see she was going to go downhill; if her breathing had deteriorated, they would have had more warning. Her heart had been under strain for several days, and all of a sudden it gave out and stopped. They attempted to revive her but didn't succeed. It seems almost impossible, in this day and age, that a whole hospital can muster its resources to try and jumpstart someone whose heart has stopped working, and somehow not manage it. But that's how it goes, I suppose, every time someone loses a loved one. It seems impossible that it could have ever happened. I was angry when we first knew what had happened. It seemed outrageous to me that, all the time they were trying to save her life, no one called us and urged us to get back there. They waited till the death had been pronounced before they called. But of course, there was no one free to make the phone call. And we'd never have got there in time. And perhaps we'd have died trying, killed by some blind bend, killed trying to overtake and running into another vehicle while driving on the wrong side of the road. Heart trouble ran in her side of the family, they'd seen on her notes. A couple of relatives who'd gone that way. As if that made it normal. They told us that because she had turned sixty, she didn't even count as having died young. Just a fatal heart attack in someone with a family history of cardiovascular weakness whose age made them vulnerable to the same fate befalling them. They made it sound so normal, when it wasn't, when it felt like whole continents had been hacked away from us, as if all of our memories had been torn out.

I had learned already what it felt like to lose a parent. The loss of a father had left me thinking of the future, the world I would have to live in without him in it, the man I might become as a result, the way his story ended and the way I wanted my story to be different. The loss of a mother was something else. Somehow it drew me in the other direction, back into the past, into memory. She was the shell I had sheltered in whenever things went wrong. She had always been the place of safety. Now there was no safe harbour to turn to, only the life I would have to make for myself, and I thought with sudden grief of all the ordinary afternoons we'd spent with one another, all the small acts of connection that would never come again. The loss of a mother was like all the lights going out on the shore, and I was left alone on the waves, turning back in the hope of receiving some encouragement, seeing only the dark instead.

We stay at the farm for the next seven days. A neighbour agrees to keep an eye on Amy's flat, and Amy and I stay with Chris. There are a lot of phone calls and paperwork that need to be done and that we'll try and help with. Chris goes to the hospital and sees Mum the next morning. The doctor warns him he might not want to, but he goes all the same. We don't travel with him; he comes home, and says nothing, and needs to be alone for the rest of that day. I try not to think of what he must have seen, but of course I think of her, and the way bodies look in the movies, and the room he must have seen her in, and the corridor he must have walked down to reach her, and then had to walk back the length of it to get back out into the light. I can't stop seeing it the rest of that week, and I almost wish I'd gone with him. Perhaps that would have broken the spell, I don't know. Numbness. Like paralysis creeping through me, turning me into a statue, killing me cell by cell. Shock, someone tells me. It's OK not to be able to cry. I try to tell them I have been crying, I've done nothing but crying, but then I realise I don't know what I've been doing, because of the shock, because I'm living in a kind of fog. Rachel stays for a few days, then says she has to travel back to the city. I think of asking her why she isn't taking the week off work, but she seems determined to leave, so we say no more about it.

The injustice of it all makes me speechlessly angry. That she just got ill, and was taken in, and never got the chance to go back home. Never got to climb the hill above the farm for one last time, and see the view, and fix the place where she had lived her life in the mind's eye for a last time, for ever. Never got to sleep out in the cold beneath the stars one final night, or go to the bluebell woods in May and lie down among them, the river of their scent and colour, dousing her senses in the world she had loved before she left it. She would have deserved that. Anyone would. A deliberate goodbye to what they were leaving, all they had loved and lived among, everything that had shaped them.

It feels like we spend a week on the phone, then just as the first wave of work is almost finished, the funeral date is set and we have to do it all over again, sending out cards to people to let them know, preparing an order of service for the funeral directors. It's relentless, remorseless. It's shocking to me, the way that time goes on, and the world seems to be speeding away from what's happened without our having had time to stop and examine and understand it, so that already, before I've even taken this moment in, it seems to be turning into part of the past. I can't believe how quickly the moment is moving away from me. Chris spends most of his time in the garden, staring at nothing, trying to write a speech. He was determined from the moment we started planning that he wanted to deliver one. Rachel and I will stay silent, letting him speak for all of us, that's the plan; and a colleague of Mum's will say something, and a childhood friend. I don't envy any of them. When I go to funeral services, the speeches people make just sound like rain. I wish the whole thing could happen in silence, because all anyone wants to do is sit with the feeling of being there, surely?

'You don't mind if I say something, do you?' Chris had asked me, and we had looked at each other, and the moment had seemed absurd.

'Of course not. What do you mean? If you say something at the funeral?'

'I just mean you kids won't mind if I speak.'

'Of course not.'

Every second has become an unravelling, a shredding of the narrative order of our lives, the sense that we knew who we were to each other, the sense that we knew what to do. But now none of us knows, it seems, who's supposed to be in charge here. Rachel and Amy and I had assumed it was Chris, but something had been holding him back too, preventing him from feeling that he could take whatever decision he liked.

'I don't want to say a lot.'

'You don't have to. You should just do whatever you need.'

'Whatever your mum would want.'

'Yes. Of course.'

Day by day we navigate around each other, leaving space for one another's silences. Then after a week, Chris suggests Amy and I should go back to the city till we have to come together again to face the funeral. Again, I feel the world beneath my feet spinning madly, barrelling on.

'You've done so much,' he says, 'and I'm so grateful. But you shouldn't have to stay here with me for ever. I'll be all right for a week. I'll be all right.'

'We don't want to leave you on your own if there are things you still need help with.'

He looks into his tea and I realise he might have reached a point where he doesn't want people round him; he might want to spend the next week alone with the ghost of his wife before he has to say goodbye to her for the last time. The strange, in-between weeks after a death and before the funeral, when nothing seems final, nothing seems certain, everything seems to need to be done. Life at its most provisional, life as survival.

'I know. And you're kind. But I'll have to be on my own at some point, won't I? So will you both.'

I worry, once we've agreed we'll leave the next morning,

that we've somehow ended up outstaying our welcome; that Chris has grown tired of our voices and wants above all to be on his own. When we heard the news, it seemed the only thing we could possibly have done was to stay and do whatever we could, and I didn't want to leave and head home. Perhaps we should have left when Rachel did; perhaps Chris has been wishing we'd leave ever since. Amy does her best to reassure me.

'He's trying to do something to help us,' she says. 'He can see as well as I can that you're not processing this, you're not taking this in, and you need to get home and try to work out what's happened. And maybe he does want to be on his own as well, but why does that matter? We were always going to have to go at some point.'

'What do you mean I'm not processing it?'

'I just mean you're in shock. You know you are.'

'Do I?'

'OK, maybe I'm wrong. I just mean what's happened is a lot to take in.'

'Do you think I'm not doing that?'

'I think it will take you a long time to do that.'

So we leave, promising to come back for the last few days before the funeral. Chris hugs me when we go. I hug him back. We get in the car and I feel as if it's gone so fast, that week, it can't really have happened. Perhaps I won't believe in it till the day of the funeral comes; perhaps I should have gone to see the body after all, because the time since Mum died has all seemed like a dream, and I don't know what's going to shock me out of it. It is so brief, this thing we're in, so fragile, and its disappearance is so sudden, so impossible to bear. We drive away from the farm and I look back once, see Chris still waving at us from the gate. Next to him stand the dogs, who have no idea yet about what's happened, who will take a long time to accept they won't see Mum again, who will be months still rushing to the gate when they hear a car passing, always hoping it might be her. The lane leading down from the house is rutted and uneven. I look at the farm standing behind Chris, and it seems to me that it's become like all the other empty barns around it; one more vanished life disappearing back into the waters, as time closes over, as time moves on.

A week passes. Another week in the city, feeling like life lost, life half lived. The heat of the city in these days of apocalypse, the shirt clinging to your back, the news screaming murder, and no bugs to clean from the windscreen, no water running in the brooks that ran year-round through my childhood. In this heat it's difficult to think. My skin is tight over my face from being out in the burning sun. Mosquitoes rule the park and the wood at the end of the road where we walk Ivan morning and evening, and bats raid the air when night comes. In the dark of the trees, chicken of the woods stands out, luminous among the fallen tree trunks, the wild garlic has died and disappeared in the heat, and the other dog walkers loom up out of shadows, slapping at their legs where the mosquitoes bite. I work as best I can and stay out of the centre of London, walking Ivan and catching up with emails, plugged in, trackable. I feel the weight of this working life like an anchor.

Chris says there's no more to do for the funeral, so I move

all my things into Amy's flat instead. Anything to distract me, any way of turning my mind elsewhere, because I find I can't talk, I can't let out what I'm feeling. I lose hours rereading Marcel Pagnol. I make a pile of all my old CDs. I haven't listened to any of them for years now; no point keeping what we don't use any more. Moving house a lot in my early twenties taught me only to keep what I couldn't bear to lose. In the end it turns out that's not ever so much.

Moving house will reveal things you'd lost and hadn't noticed. As I move my things from the converted garage into Amy's flat, I go over what I'm going to keep and what I'll give to charity. The grandfather clock my grandfather made in 1976, the hottest summer. The bookshelves he made for my dad. The coffee table he made in 1988, the year after I was born. His harmonium, which I can never play now I'm at Amy's because the first time I try I find Ivan barks at it, thinking it's another animal. The guitar he made, which never comes out of its case because I can't play it. The carpet I stole from the theatre I worked in, a beautiful old rug they were keeping in a store room no one ever looked in and which I claimed for my own when I left. The armchair my father gave me because I never got out of it and he said it didn't suit him, which I think he only really gave me because he knew I was in love with it. All these were days once, now they're the memory of those days. I lug the things across London, sweat in my eyes, and hope they won't overcrowd the flat, hope that they'll go with everything else Amy has gathered around her already.

When thoughts of what's happened begin to overwhelm me, I go out into Amy's little scrap of garden, and sit there quietly, and stare at the sky. This is the one small space I've found in my day-to-day where something like peace is sometimes possible. In the garden I can still hear the planes overhead, the ice-cream van at weekends, boy racers, the football ground nearby on match days, drills and electric saws from the home improvers, the traffic noise underlying everything. But all I see is stillness around me, and that's something, that's precious. Sun on the back of my neck, the fence shifting in the winds, oak leaves whispering, blackbirds and wagtails calling to each other, crickets in the grass, the bees coming and going from an apiary somewhere nearby. There are hedgehogs living along this row of back gardens that crawl under the fences at night, there are admirals and whites, jays and green woodpeckers coming and going. There is life going on here under the radar of the big world and it comforts me.

Rachel texts me and asks if I want to go for a drink. I read her message, and think for a while. The truth is I'm not sure I do. Since we've got back from the farm, the best way I've found of coping is not to talk any more than I have to. Going to see Rachel will just mean having to talk about it all over again. And there's a part of me that resents Rachel for having left so quickly, when I know she could have got the time off work and stayed at the farm a little longer if she'd decided that it was the right thing to do. I resent her because we stayed, and she didn't, and I resent her because we were wrong to stay as long as we did, I feel sure of it now; we ended up being a burden on Chris when he needed to be on his own, saying nothing, seeing no one for a few days, and Rachel saw that coming and left when we should have done too. I resent her because when Dad was dying he came to me and I had to help him, and Rachel never had to deal with all that, because he was nothing to do with her, he wasn't her father; it was me who had to watch my dad die, I faced that alone. Rachel kept a distance then as well, knowing when not to be around, because really Dad's death was nothing to do with her, but it felt like she was taking sides, avoiding the flat I lived in for as long as my dad was in it out of some kind of loyalty to Mum. I didn't mind at the time: I would have liked to have nothing to do with all that vomit and shaking, either; I would have enjoyed the privilege of being able to remember Dad as he had been when I had lived with him originally, when I was very young, and not how he was in the end. But he came to me and I took him in, and I did that on my own, and Rachel was no part of it, because, really, it was nothing to do with her. But now Mum had died, I found I resented her for that. It seemed to me now that, during that year, she had become closer to Mum than I was, because I was living with Mum's ex-husband while he died. So Rachel ended up in league with Mum, while I looked after Dad. They had shared things that I hadn't. Now Mum was gone, and I'd never catch up with Rachel on that missed time. That was that. I had thought there would be longer, and there wasn't, and that wasn't Rachel's fault, but I felt angry nonetheless, and in the moment of getting her text, I focused that anger on her.

'Rachel's asking if I want to go for a drink,' I say.

'You should,' says Amy.

'I'm not sure.'

'Why not?'

'I don't know whether I want to go through it all. Talk about it all right now.'

'It'll be easier to talk now than it will be when you get to the funeral. There'll be too much happening then to think. And you should be there for her if she needs it. If she's asking to see you, it's because she needs it. You're her big brother. You should help.'

'I think it's easy to say that if you don't have siblings,' I say, and instantly regret it. Amy gives me a look. A lot of the time this last week, she's found herself needing to be patient with me while I say the wrong thing.

'How do you mean?' she asks.

'Well, I can see that you're right,' I say. 'In black and white, that's what I should do. But it's not black and white with your sister. Because there's so much between a brother and sister. We're still furious at each other over things that happened fifteen years ago, or hurt by something the other one said that no one else ever heard, that no one else would ever think was important. That's how it works between siblings, isn't it? All these things that seem so small, except to the people involved. Things we couldn't even remember any more if someone asked us, which make everything political.'

'But not so political you'd refuse to have a drink with her when your mum's died and she needs someone to talk to?'

I shrug. I know I'm wrong. Whenever I start to feel angry I know that I'm wrong, and I know that the person I'm feeling anger towards is actually myself. So I swallow my unhappiness, and text Rachel back, and we agree to meet in a pub halfway between our flats the next evening before dinner. I don't want to see her, because I know things will be different now. The world has given way to something new, and I can't take it in, I don't want to. Not least because I worry that, spoken out loud, it would all seem small, it would prove inexpressible. A break-up for me; the loss of a parent for both of us. These are things that everyone goes through. But they seem like the whole world for now. It's the same stake as Lear's, except for the scale of it, except that we have to fit the worlds inside us into these stories, these lives.

Rachel is the eternal student, working on her doctorate, still living on beans. She tops up the funding she got to finish her studies with teaching work at the university, and lives in one room in a shared flat in the far-flung south of the city, on the fifth floor of an old block of flats overlooking the train station that connects her to the centre of the capital. One day the work will have been worthwhile, but it takes a long time to make your way in academia, and I can't really say I envy her the years spent waiting. Too much of your life is spent waiting to start. I get to the pub first and sit outside in the afternoon sun, and see her approaching, the bob of her walk.

'How are you?' Rachel asks, as we embrace.

'You know. Want a pint?'

'Thanks.'

I go inside and get the first round, then bring it back out, and we sit down together at a pub bench in the sun.

'How long did you stay for in the end?' she asks.

'Till the end of the week.'

'Was that OK?'

'You know. I think we stayed too long.'

'I just felt like I couldn't be there any more.'

'You didn't feel like you were closer to her there?'

'I can't be closer to her anywhere. That's the point.'

'What have you been doing since?'

'Nothing, really. I try and work. I've been teaching. Then when I get home I stare at the wall. You sleeping?'

'No.'

'I've been angry with myself,' she says. 'That's part of why I wanted to see you, really. I can't talk about it with Dad, but I can say it to you.'

'Go on.'

'I've been thinking that I should be doing more.'

'I don't know about that.'

'No, but I should. I should be doing more. But I've found there's a limit I can't get past. There's a point where I have to stop. Because I can't support you or Dad or anyone. Because I have to look after myself.'

'I know. It's the same for everyone. It's all right.'

'It doesn't feel all right.'

'No. But it's the same for everyone, all over the world.'

She tilts her head back and drains her glass. 'There should be a way for us all to be together now, though, don't you think? A thing like this should mean that just for a little while, for as long as it takes to come to terms with this, we become one unit, like we've never been before, or not since we were young. And I don't know why that isn't possible, why it feels like we're just as far apart as we were. I want it to have changed more than it has. Because otherwise it's just loss.'

'But that's what it is, Rach. There might be no positives to it. It might just be loss.'

'Yeah. But I hate that. Another?'

'I don't want to get drunk.'

'No, but you'll have another.'

'All right.'

212

She stands up.

'Want me to get it?' I ask.

'Fuck off,' she says, and disappears inside. When she comes back out with the drinks she's silent for a moment, looking at her pint. 'Is it true that in Japan they pull down a house when someone's died in it?'

'I don't know. I think they pull down houses because it's humid and they rot.'

'I think we should do more of that. I'd like it if everything was got rid of, and nothing left behind after you'd gone. Every time I go back home, I feel this guilt that I wasn't a better kid to Mum and Dad, and I wasn't kinder, and I didn't say thank you more often, and I wasn't nicer to them. I feel this shame that I didn't get it right, that's what the place reminds me of. And I feel this sadness because when I go home, it's not like it was. It just never can be. Even when Mum was still there, it never could be. The times I've spent there since I moved away always remind me of those shadows of people that get left on walls after nuclear bombs, you know what I mean? Those ghost people. I'd never feel all that if the place wasn't there any more.'

'Is that really what you want?'

'Maybe. I don't know. Did you like going back there? Before Mum, I mean, when they were both there and you went home. To the land of lost content.'

'It's too complicated to say yes or no.'

We finish our drinks, and in the end we agree not to have a third, and we say goodbye to each other, and go our separate ways. I walk away thinking how cruel I was being, to think I shouldn't see my sister. How cruel of me to think we should keep apart at this moment. Why could I not see straight away that that was just what I should have been doing? Why could I not have known instinctively that the best way for each of us to break our own silence would be to start sharing one another's? The selfishness of grief, maybe. Or maybe more evidence I'm sleepwalking through life.

2000

E D HAD MADE the treehouse with Chris's help the previous summer. That meant it wasn't particularly well made, because Ed had only been twelve back then, but he'd hammered nails in as best he could, Chris finishing off the job after he'd done his bit, and tied string round things, and got a platform together. It had stubbornly refused to cohere into a whole, remaining instead like several planks of old wood that were up in the tree, and that he could sit on, not a coherent house at all, but Ed was still proud of it because it was his. There were many sheds and outhouses in the farmhouse garden that he played in and out of. They included Chris's workshop where all the tools were kept, which Chris had started talking about padlocking this year, because he was worried the tools might be stolen, and because Ian from down in the village had taken to sleeping there on nights home from the pub if he couldn't face the whole walk back to his farm. Mum had first mentioned it six months earlier, her suspicion that someone was sleeping in the workshop some Saturday nights. She'd find things disturbed, and the dogs would bark. Eventually Chris woke early enough to see Ian slipping back out of it to finish his long walk home, and then they knew what had been happening. Ian was a drinker, especially on nights off, so in order that he could have his preferred skinful he'd walk from his farm to the nearest pub on Saturday, a walk of about three miles down to the river at the bottom of the valley. This meant that at the end of the night he had to walk three miles all the way back up, usually with a dozen pints in him. Ed's home was just off the road he walked back up, on a little lane that split off invitingly just before the steep hill up to the school and the Buddhist retreat centre and Ian's farm. Clearly, on some nights, Ian gave in to temptation and found temporary shelter among the tools. Chris and Mum didn't mind this at all, it seemed, and would have been happy to let Ian sleep on the sofa, as long as he wasn't sick, they said; but it had got Chris thinking about security, about whether tools were even insured if you left them in an unlocked building, because maybe there needed to be a padlock for the insurance to kick in. It was one of those jobs he said he always meant to get around to doing, which never quite got to the top of his list.

Next to the workshop there was the shed inside the chicken wire, which contained nothing but grain for the chickens and a huge old chest freezer Chris had run a cable up to under the ground, where the family kept bags and bags of frozen lamb they'd set aside for themselves to eat. This wasn't a shed Ed particularly liked to go into – rats got in to eat the grain, and had to be dealt with by the farm cat because you couldn't leave rat poison in with the chicken feed. The shed was damp and starting to rot away, and he thought it was spooky, though he didn't know why any ghost would go in there.

Above the workshop, further up the hill, there was another shed, very like the grain shed in the chicken wire, where Chris kept the lawnmower and tubs of varnish and paint and twine and manure and bamboo poles and forks and things for the garden, except this one wasn't rotting away because he'd put a cement floor in, and then at the bottom of the hillside, right by the house, was the woodstore, which was open on one side, covered only with a tarpaulin. Here, the family stored everything they could burn, because fire was life and they needed a lot of wood. This varied in character, from old junk, old furniture, to trees they'd chopped down on the farm and some firewood they ordered in to make sure they had enough in the winters. Chris didn't like ordering firewood in, but the fact was that theirs was a sheep farm, and all their land was grass, so they just couldn't get by on the trees they could grow. And the man who brought the firewood was the doctor's nephew anyway, and Mum liked to say it was a good thing to send some business the way of the doctor's family, because then they'd look after you when it was needed. Ed didn't know why the doctor wouldn't look after you anyway.

All of these could be the sites of various games that Ed would play, whether that be simple hide and seek or gangsters or World War Two, they all had their uses, and were tolerably full of interesting things, but Ed was also aware that none of them were his. He could be turfed out of each of them at any minute, and wasn't really allowed to change anything, and he wanted a place of his own, high up above everything, where he could look down on the farm and feel as if he was sailing away into the distance far from this place, someone on a spaceship, someone on a plane. He'd been on a plane once, flying to Guernsey, a little yellow plane called Joey that Mum had bought him a book about at the Guernsey airport, and it had been the most thrilling experience. Far better to be up in the air and strapped into one of the rattling seats looking down at the miracle world below than enduring the drive to Cornwall, the catamaran to France. Guernsey itself had been so-so – the most memorable event of the holiday had been Ed cycling downhill into a wall and sending himself flying over his handlebars, barking both his knees and his chin and his elbows as he fell – but he had been very in love with the plane, and that was in his mind when he asked for his treehouse. A way to be up high above everything. He asked if he could build one, and Chris picked out the sturdiest tree, and they worked together to get a platform up there. Ed had initially imagined walls and a roof, a little window to look out of, but Chris was always busy with the farm and could only help in little bursts in the evenings, and in the end Ed decided just sitting up there on dry days was enough for him. He could tell he hadn't made the platform very well, and had plans to ask Chris to make him a better one the next summer, when Rachel would be old enough to play up there as well, and the treehouse would have to carry more weight.

Rachel had been furious to be banned from the treehouse in its first year, of course, but Mum was determined that it was too dangerous and she couldn't go up there in case she fell. But this year, Rachel had been given permission, news that she had initially met with joy. Once she was up on the platform, though, she found the whole thing less impressive.

'There's nothing to do here,' she said. 'There's no walls on.'

Chris said that perhaps one weekend later this summer, they could all work together to improve the treehouse, which Ed and Rachel agreed to readily. So Chris said they'd spend a day on it next weekend, and make a really good one with walls and a roof and a door and a ladder. It would be easy for him to do, Ed knew; he'd held back the year before because Ed had been in charge, and Chris hadn't wanted to take the job off him. He felt a little embarrassed now he was older that his efforts had come up so short, but it was understandable; he'd only been twelve at the time, and would be better placed to help Chris make a really good treehouse now he was a year older.

In the meantime, he tried to encourage Rachel to enjoy the one they had. It was difficult; she had noticed straight away that Ed felt responsible for the treehouse's shortcomings, so poking fun at them was a way of poking fun at him, and she pursued this mercilessly. But he showed her there were games that could be played. You could, of course, be a pirate in the lookout post on a pirate ship; or you could be a fighter pilot in a plane; or you could be a panther, stalking puny humans, looking down from the trees to jump on them. Rachel attempted all these games, but enjoyed making fun of Ed much more, so their attempts to play up in the treehouse didn't get far. The third day Ed tried to play pilots in the treehouse with Rachel, and she refused to be a rear gunner and protect their tail, preferring instead to pick bits of splinter off one of the platform planks, he lost his temper and climbed back down to the ground.

'You're stupid,' he shouted up at her, not really knowing what stupid thing she'd done.

'You're the one who's stupid; you can't build a treehouse – how am I meant to play up here?' Rachel shouted after him as he stormed inside. Ed didn't look back, but went into the kitchen instead and poured himself a glass of milk. He took the biscuit tin down from the high shelf he could reach now, and got himself a biscuit, and took that and the milk through to the sitting room where his Mum was typing at the work table on her old typewriter with the radio on. Ed sat by the bookcase and thought about taking down something to read, but he was too angry to concentrate, so he just ate his biscuit instead. A bite of biscuit, then a sip of milk, then mixing them together was his favourite thing, the best meal in the world, the meal he'd ask for if he was on death row. He'd tried McDonald's at a birthday party in Hereford, and it wasn't anywhere near as good. Biscuits and milk was the best meal imaginable.

'Everything all right, darling?'

Ed looked up at his mum. 'Fine.'

'Where's Rachel?'

'In the treehouse.'

'You're not fighting, are you?'

'She says it's no good.'

'But next weekend you'll make a better one.'

'I suppose so.'

'Why only "suppose so"?'

'I don't want to play in it if she's up there.'

It was at this point that Rachel came into the room, and it was immediately clear that something was very wrong. She was deathly pale and her breathing was fast and shallow, as if she was trying not to cry. Ed watched, stomach lurching, as his mum stopped what she was doing and turned round and then stood up.

'Are you all right, darling? What's happened?'

'Mum,' Rachel said, and then couldn't say more. She held out her arm instead, and Ed recoiled as her arm from the elbow down fell back the wrong way, as if it wanted to stay by her side, snapped at the elbow and hanging loose from the rest of her. Rachel saw what had happened and screamed, and then Mum became a sudden whirlwind of action, bundling Rachel out of the room, grabbing her car keys, thinking of the hospital. She turned once to Ed before she left.

'Will you go and tell your stepdad what's happened? And he can take you with him to the hospital.'

'Where is he?' asked Ed.

'He's out in the fields.'

Then Mum and Rachel were gone. Ed drained his milk as he stood up from the chair by the bookcase. He looked around, shocked by the sudden quiet, queasy because of what he'd just seen. He shouldn't have drunk the rest of the milk really, but it was automatic, he hadn't been thinking. He put the glass down on the table by the typewriter and went outside to the garden. He wondered whether he should lock the front door, but he had no key, so he didn't know how to. He could get the spare one from under the flowerpot, but maybe Chris would want to get things before they left.

Halfway up the garden, he could see the treehouse. He stopped and looked at it for a moment. He knew already what must have happened. Rachel, on her own up there, had decided she was bored, and started to climb down, or otherwise she'd tried to test her bravery by leaning over the edge.

Either way, she'd overbalanced somehow, fallen to the ground, and landed on her arm and snapped it badly. He looked at the treehouse, tried to spot some malevolence in it. He was very afraid this was all his fault; that he had wished this on her somehow, when he left her alone. Had the tree-house hurt her because he was angry? Or was she just too young to be up there? Either way, he shouldn't have left her alone. He realised he should have looked out for his sister, and his heart sank at the thought of the telling-off he'd prob-ably get later. He decided then and there that he wouldn't go up in the treehouse again, and he wouldn't say any more about Chris building a new one. He turned his back on the abandoned island he had hoped to make his own, and went to look for his stepdad.

2019

A DAY COMES WHEN I'm supposed to go into the office for work, the first time they've asked me to go in for a few weeks. I walk the mile to the nearest train station, and find it's closed, the area cordoned off for half a mile around. On the roof of the flats looming ten floors over the station a woman is standing on the concrete edge, her back to the police negotiator trying to talk her down, doing little practice jumps, visible to all the crowded street below, her eyes fixed straight ahead of her. People throng the streets to watch. I turn around and go back home. She wears a blue cardigan over a T-shirt, and looks cold up there in the wind keening over the city, which must blow stronger and more frightening up there above the buildings. I can't watch the fragility of the woman, desperate to be noticed, desperate not to be invisible any more, but powerless to end her silence any way other than threatening to throw herself down that endless drop. Why do people watch these atrocities? Does it make us feel better that we're not her? Or is she really a part of all of us, acting out something we've all thought of doing?

I get back home and call the office and tell them I can't make it because there's a jumper above my train station so all the lines are closed. They commiserate with me, and I say I'll go in tomorrow, and then I put down the phone. A whole conversation come and gone as if what I had seen was something normal, as if it happened all the time and it was just one of the many reasons meetings are rescheduled every day. Because where we live, it is. I remember a woman who had stood next a jumper saying to me once on a station platform, 'They always put their bags down on the platform before they get on the track. What I don't understand is why they bring their bags at all if that's what they're going to be doing. She wasn't even dead after it hit her. She was screaming and the bottom half of her was gone. She wouldn't have made it. Poor woman. I wish she hadn't done it, though.' In a place like this, sometimes the only way people can think of breaking out of their silence is to do something so terrible no one can look away. Among these atrocities we make our lives.

I pick up the car keys and leave the flat again.

As I try to go forwards through the story of my life, the feeling takes hold that somehow I am going in the wrong direction, that really what I want to be doing is going back, not flicking through the picture book towards its ending. I can't find it, the secret of myself, the person I'm supposed to be; the key is lost, and I feel it must lie deeper, I must have lost it earlier, it must be buried longer ago. What I am trying to fight against is a sense that I regret having lived my life, that I would almost rather my life had never happened than for so much of it to be lost and unrecoverable. I don't want to feel like that. I want to feel like I'm glad about where I'm going.

The drive south feels like travelling back in time. Money has preserved these places more or less as they must have looked in the nineteenth century. The green south of this island, repository of the most extraordinary wealth ever collected by people almost anywhere. The vast estates sprawl out, the beautiful cottages, tree-lined roads. I listen to Bill Evans as I drive, thinking he'll keep me calm, but it's been a long time since I heard *Undercurrent* and the rhythms surprise and mislead; I find myself listening uneasily, not knowing what's coming next. The music is a journey back into memory as well, songs I listened to as a student, songs Dad introduced me to as a child. An hour's drive and I pass the village where I first went to school. It is still the place I knew, and yet entirely different. New buildings have sprung up around the old schoolhouse. Past the school is the village green where we used to go in November to see the Guy burned, the bonfire stacked up on the grass and the mannequin sitting at the top. He tried to burn us down once, so now each year we burn the memory of him. I've seen his signature on display in the Tower of London, the shaking, ruined hand of a man stretched and broken on the rack. I used to stand hand in hand with my parents, watching the flames lick their way to the sky till he was consumed once more. How many years till he's burned for the last time, I wonder? Or will people still burn his image after no one remembers who he was? I drive on through villages I called home a life ago, but there's no sense of belonging to any of these places, no point of connection between them and myself. It unnerves me to see the buildings that have changed. For decades I left this place behind, and never revisited, and the buildings seemed only to live inside me. Their independence from the way I imagined them is a reminder of the smallness and hubris of my life. I come to a wood and leave the road, changing down into first to bump along a rutted dirt track through shadows that darken the middle of the day and beckon me back into childhood. An avenue, dark, nameless, without end. I turn off the music, watch the silent woods on either side of the track till the sky opens up again ahead of me and I see the lodges waiting.

We were here for a few years, living in one of the two hunting lodges at the edge of this wood. There are photographs and home videos of my family together in this place, the only place we were together, on a bright day in summer. Is that why I've thought of this place today, and felt compelled to return for the first time, because this seems like the closest we ever came, where the idea of family and the idea of home once almost cohered into some clear meaning? I drive up to the gate between the two lodges and turn the engine off, and there is the view I remember from childhood, the silence of the birchwood, empty fields stretching away, grass in the sun and the hum of crickets. I walk through the gate and there is the house where we once tried to be a family. Empty now, panes missing from two upstairs windows. I walk around the building, looking in through the windows and the glass in the doors to the bare living room with its red-tiled floor, the bedroom where I used to sleep just visible to me on the first floor through its quarter-moon window that we curtained off with spaceman curtains, and the stairway curling round three sides of the hall as it descends, the cupboard under the stairs where Mum hid Christmas presents, and the little porch over the front door and the white Formica kitchen. I stare through the kitchen window for a long time, because the fittings haven't been replaced since we left, and I am transfixed by their dim familiarity. I turn away and stare into the garden. At the end of the lawn I'm standing on, two apple trees, a russet and a James Grieve, with fruit already ripening. I walk towards them, take them in. I take a russet from the tree and bite down, the dryness of the skin and the acidity of the flesh sharpening the day as if it's being etched into me.

I turn back to the house, walk towards it again. A pane of glass in the kitchen window catches the light when it shouldn't, and I realise the window is slightly ajar. I walk back to it, open the window all the way, stick my head through. There is a sound sensor plugged into one of the power sockets on the kitchen wall. I reach across and turn it off, then clamber up on to the window ledge and into the kitchen, my feet in the sink, before lowering myself down to the linoleum floor. I walk out of the kitchen and into the hall, take in the living-room fireplace of rough brick, turn to the staircase and begin to climb. At the top of the stairs I walk through the first doorway on the landing and stand in the room that used to be mine. Let the stillness settle for a moment. No one speaks, nothing happens. No one is waiting for me. I bend down to look through the quarter-moon window. I look at the empty field falling away towards the blue of distance. The colour we can never know or ever put our hand on, the light that never reaches us, which spends itself on what is far away instead.

I am cast down in the flood of remembrance.

I could have been telling her all this time that I was grateful, and that I loved her, and that I was glad I'd come into this world, and been her child, and lived this life and no other. I could have been telling her that all along, and driving to see her, it wasn't so far really; a hundred years ago the distance would have been insurmountable but I have a car, it wasn't all that far to travel. I could have stayed closer to her, or at least called more often, or at least forced us to set aside whatever silence sprang up between us while Dad was dying, and find our way back to each other, find our way back to being a family again. Because she was my mother. Had she not been, I would have been someone unimaginably different. And so how could I not have loved her all along, if I had any time for my own self? How could there have been a day when we let each other doubt that, when I didn't go back, when I didn't call, when I let that silence linger on between us? I used to think it was because of the divorce. Because my parents ended up apart, there were gaps in our family, there were hairline fractures. But it was me who chose them. Me who let them last. I could have left them all behind, and now she was dead, and I realised I'd always imagined that there'd be more time. Of course I had. Who doesn't? There would be time to fix things and create togethernesses we'd never known while she was living. Except there wouldn't. Except there hadn't been.

After a minute I straighten up and walk away from the window and down the stairs and climb back out of the house. Push the window closed behind me. Take another russet from the tree and walk a little way into the birchwood. I feel like someone's watching me, but there is no sound, no sign of anyone. Only an avenue, dark, nameless, without end. As I walk further in among the trees, here and there I pass oak and holly, the ghost of an older forest that grew here long ago. Someone has crammed a sheep's skull in among the branches of an oak, its empty eye watching as if it knew I was going to come back. Two hundred yards down the track, a fox breaks cover from the green bracken, stops and sees me, then disappears into the wood once more. I turn around and look behind me, and for a moment I'm convinced I'm going to see Mum walking towards me.

I drive back to the flat and drink alone, and then Amy comes home and sees the gin bottle out on the kitchen table, and sits down next to me, and puts her head on my shoulder.

'You all right?' she asks.

'There was a woman on the roof of the flats above the station,' I tell her.

'I know, it was on the news.'

'I watched her. She was doing little jumps up and down like she was trying to psych herself up to something. And the policeman was leaning out of the window trying to talk her back in. And everyone was watching and recording on their phones.'

'She's done it before, they said. They shouldn't let her have that flat.'

'I suddenly felt as if I was her. I felt like I was up there on that roof and looking down and only feeling alive because of the drop waiting for me. And I felt that if I had been up there, I'd have jumped. I'd have jumped for sure, much better than the embarrassment of going back in.'

'OK.' She takes my hand and closes both of hers around it. I know I'm drunk and talking nonsense now. I know that I should go to bed and sleep.

'I didn't go into the office in the end. I drove south instead.

I went back to the place where I used to live with Dad and Mum, and they weren't there, and it was totally empty. No one living there or anything. I actually broke in and looked around, there was a window open. And I felt so awful once I was inside. Because I don't know why this got into my head, but I think I genuinely thought I'd find them waiting. But they're not. They're dead.'

Amy rubs her thumb across the back of my hand. The thought occurs to me that skin on skin is love. It speaks more eloquently than anything else, and any other language is too finely nuanced to be really understood. At the start of the summer, this girl beside me might have died, I might have lost her when she hit her head and her blood was scattered over that strange room where we were staying. Now it's the rest of the world that seems to have gone, and she's still mine.

'We have to get out of here,' I say. 'I can't be here any more, in this city. This isn't my life. I don't know where it is, but it's not here, and I have to get out – I'm sorry.'

'It's all right,' Amy says. 'Don't worry. We'll leave, then.'

For a moment I can almost see the course of this year laid out around me, like a view from the top of a hill. From the vantage of this moment, I'm astonished by the strange unmooring that's taken place, one thing after another cut away. It seems as if I've been carried very far from where I used to be, and I wonder when that started and where it will end. Not here, that's all I know right now; this is not my place. Time to move on and look for my real life. Because I didn't find it living with Juliet, and I never did find it back home at the farm. And I'm not going to find it here in the city, or lost in the past, or anywhere like that. My real life is waiting in some place I haven't found yet.

The day of the funeral breaks over us, heavy and inevitable, a wave scattering sandcastles, and we change into our mourning clothes and travel back to the farm to be with Chris again, and drink together again, and then we get into our cars and make the long journey to the crematorium. I remember the mourners at Dad's funeral, which was small, with only half his relatives and a few friends in attendance. Drink had cut him off from the world. This is different. A crowd of people are thronging outside the crematorium when we get there. We file in first and they all follow after. We were offered the chance to carry her in, but Chris didn't want to, he said it felt religious, and Mum had wanted a secular cremation. So we follow the coffin in, and I feel the old familiar sense of drowning, which is how grief always feels to me. When we get to the front row I want to sit down, but we stand and wait till everyone's come in. Some people around us seem to be trying not to cry, but I let it happen, and the tears run down my face, and the ceremony happens, and we listen to the music, and we listen to the readings, none of the words anyone says going in, till the moment I've been fearing comes, and an electrically operated curtain is drawn across the plinth where the coffin's resting, and I know I'll never see my mum again. Amy holds my hand.

I am thinking of the will she left behind. That she called to talk me through just a year ago. That she wrote in the knowledge neither Rachel nor I would be carrying on the life she had built up, that once she and Chris had both gone we'd sell the farm. I'm thinking of how easy it was then to reject that idea, and how important it seemed to me to maintain independence for myself. Maintain individuality. And how unimportant it seems to me now that Mum should have known that that wasn't what we wanted. We never needed to tell her at all. We could have let her go through life believing that things would carry on after she'd gone, and she might have been happier. We could have made our decisions now. And I am sure they would have been the same ones, but there would have been no need for her to know about them. We could have been kinder and said nothing at all. Then in the last year we might have been together, we might have been a family in the old-fashioned way. If any family is still that any more. The ceremony ends, the music plays. We file back out of the room in the knowledge that right now, as we shuffle together, as we hold each other, she has gone into the fire, she has gone for good.

'They don't do it while we're still here, do they?' asks Rachel, tears smudging the make-up on her face.

'I don't know,' I say. I watch Rachel as she presses the heels of her palms to her eyes, her body shaking as she cries, and I wish I could say something that would help. We get into the car and drive to the wake, and stand in silence, in awkward groups, as people come up to us to offer condolences and then step gently away again. I want to smile and thank them all for coming, but I find I can't, I don't have the energy. When everyone's gone, we go back to the farm, Amy driving with me in the passenger seat, Chris and Rachel getting a lift in another car. I look out of the window and think of nothing, head heavy, sleep tugging at the corners of my vision; I feel so tired now, I just want to sleep. This is the land of lost content, and I have wondered in the time since she died whether I was wrong, whether I want to be here, but I can't stir the feeling. I know I don't belong. I have to reject this inheritance, be a citizen of nowhere, even though it means in the years to come there will be less and less left of the life my mum lived. Chris will leave this place in time as well; one way or another our family will leave here, and then there'll be memories, a few sticks of furniture, and the furniture will mostly break with time, and the memories won't all be passed down. The way my grandchildren tell our stories will grow shorter and shorter, just a few sentences to say what became of us will one day very soon be enough. We see the house as we end the journey. I remember I never asked Mum if it was our family who built it. There's no one to answer that question now. Perhaps it will be somewhere in some old parish record. But that's beside the point; it's not the fact I'm after, it's the story. It's the tales I left it too late to ask her for that I'm thinking of as I let myself into this childhood home, the old rooms that hide their secrets just under the surface, burying memory, saying nothing.

Once we sat and read about Narnia here. And about Middle Earth, and the Faraway Tree, all the escapes from this world we lived in, while out on the hills the lambs grew up, apart from the ones who sickened and died and had to be disposed of. Shepherding taught you strange things about love. You couldn't devote too much attention to the lambs, for fear of infecting them with something that might kill them. People could be carrying all kinds of viruses that might be fatal to a lamb if it caught them. It was important to keep a safe distance. And you couldn't let yourself see what city people saw in lambs either, because you had to witness so many of them dying. The ones who keeled over and rotted in the fields, that needed to be burned or buried; the ones that went away to the butcher. I had gone to the livestock market in Hereford often enough, ever since I was young; I knew what became of them. You couldn't feel too much for the lambs you raised or you'd get your heart broken. I had been amazed when Mum and Chris started keeping dogs as pets, really, because it seemed like a softening that might hurt them. But it wasn't the whole story that shepherding taught you to close your heart up. When I was younger, I had bottle-fed lambs whose mothers had died; I had worked with Chris and Mum to put ropes round a sheep that had fallen into a ravine to lift it out again to safety. The truth was that you worked to stop yourself getting too attached to the animals in your care, but it meant nothing. Everything was still felt just as deeply. You just learned to turn your face away from what you were feeling. Pretend your heart was different from everyone else's, when really your heart beat just the same.

After we've drunk ourselves into a stupor, after we've staggered upstairs to bed, after we've slept through half the next morning then come downstairs to find Chris has been up for hours and all of the washing-up's already done, and he's out in the fields, and we've missed the chance to help him, we start to pack our bags and get ready to leave, then sit around drinking coffee till Chris comes back for his lunch. When he comes in he sees us and smiles, but a veil seems to have come down on what's left of this family, shrouding our sadness, preventing us from sharing our feelings with each other, or not knowing how. We eat some toast together, and not knowing what to say, we speak mostly of the weather.

'I'll understand if you need to come here a little less now,' Chris says all of a sudden. We look at him, not quite knowing what he means.

'Why?' I ask.

'Now your mother's not here. I'll understand it.'

'Don't be silly, Dad,' Rachel says.

'Maybe not you, sure,' Chris ploughs on. 'But Ed, if it feels strange. I'd understand it.'

'Is that what you want?' I ask. I don't want to sound confrontational, but I simply don't understand what he's saying.

'God, no,' Chris says. 'I just wanted you to know.'

Amy steps in and rescues me, because she sees I'm on the brink of crying.

'We'll still be here,' she says. 'You're still here, aren't you?'

Chris smiles, and seems relieved, eyes suddenly bright. 'That's good,' he says. 'This is still your home.'

'Yes,' Rachel says, and for a moment none of us look at each other.

'You'll be glad to have me out here,' Chris says, getting up from the table to clear away the plates. 'People need to get away from things sometimes. You'll be glad to have this place to escape to.'

I say to myself that I must make sure he's proved right about that; I must ensure the rhythms of my life don't change, and I keep coming back here. It will be harder now, it will be a stranger journey, but my stepfather still needs us to visit just the same. I look round the farm. The Welsh have a word for this feeling, *hiraeth*, but there's no word in English. And that's strange, really, when you think about it. Because what country could be more haunted, more crowded by the remnants and the echoes of lost worlds than rain-soaked England? How could a feeling be more English than this one? It is a failure of our language, a failure of our culture, not to know how to speak of the things left behind.

We come back to the city and I start to feel that the place is making me sick. The feeling of having been unmoored in the midst of life gets steadily worse, and I observe the process of one day turning into another with a growing bafflement, because nothing seems to have changed at all, though the landscape inside me feels unrecognisable.

We start to look for somewhere we can move to, spend the evenings on Zoopla and Rightmove, searching for ways of escaping the city. I find it's the only sure way of taking my mind away from what's happened, a kind of dream therapy. Project yourself into the lives in these photos, the bright colours, impossibly tidy kitchens; imagine that's you, not this life, not this feeling of dislocation. And not the life behind you either, the farm, the things that are gone, the people who died and the places where their lives happened, but the future, the unwritten, where you might step outside of where you come from and find out who you really are. We book some viewings. Strange to search for a new place in the midst of grief, and feeling distracted while trying to make what ought to be one of the most important decisions, and completely unable to focus. But this is how life always seems to happen to me. The future can never just be created on its own. The ebb of one part of life turning into the past is what always seems to give birth to the future, so that every decision ends up being a reaction to something, not a thing in itself; every new choice is born of a kind of grief.

We travel out into the home counties looking at flats and houses, till a day comes when we see one we can afford, and call up the estate agent, and plan our escape. Then once we know the place is ours, I worry we've rushed, that we've done the wrong thing. The flat we're leaving doesn't mean a great deal to me, it's something Amy and I are sharing while we wait to begin, but it is one more stage in this casting adrift that has overtaken me in the course of this year, so I worry about what I'm losing now as the day of our leaving approaches.

After you leave them behind, I've found that for a time some places become impossible to revisit. After I finished school, that was what happened to me. It disturbed me to walk down the street past my school as it filled me with thoughts of things that had ended. I stopped going back. When I visited Mum and Chris I'd just drive straight to them, and stay on the farm. I didn't go anywhere else, because everywhere else was a lost world, and the indifference of those places to the memories I kept of them unsettled me. But it wasn't like that for ever. I walked back down the street past my school a year or so ago, going round old places while visiting the farm, and though I felt some apprehension on the way there, wondering what dragons' teeth I had sown when I left, I found when I walked along that street that somehow the ghosts had faded, and the place wasn't haunted any more. Time has a curvature like the earth has curvature, and over time things pass out of sight.

I start to pack the flat up into boxes. Everything we own tucked away into boxes and turned into bulk, into ballast. I look at it all and feel it weighing me down. A few days later I have to go into town, and I'm waiting for a train on an Underground platform when I see Juliet looking at me through the crowd. She's waiting for the same train as I am, and she's seen me standing by the yellow line, and held back, I suppose, in case I wouldn't want to speak to her. I smile when our eyes meet, walk through the crowd, and we embrace awkwardly, like distant relations.

'Hi,' she says.

'Hello.'

'How are you?'

'You know.'

'I'm so sorry. I was so upset when I heard. How are your family?'

'Yeah, you know.' I wonder what people are supposed to say in these situations. 'How are you, though? Are you doing OK?'

'Oh, I'm fine. Carrying on.'

'Yeah.' We're both wondering now, I guess, whether we should ask each other about our partners, about Amy and whoever has moved into Juliet's flat.

'Where are you living at the moment?' she asks instead.

'Actually, we're moving house quite soon.'

'Oh, right? Where are you moving to?'

'Out to freedom, actually, out of the city.'

'Really?' She seems surprised by this. 'You don't need to be here for work?'

'I don't know,' I say. 'I guess we'll find out.'

She smiles at this, and shrugs. 'I guess so. I hope we'll still bump into each other now and then when you come to town.'

'Yeah, that would be good.'

'It would be nice to stay friends.'

'We ought to go for a drink sometime.'

'Wouldn't she mind that?'

'Who?'

'Your girlfriend. Is her name Amy?'

'That's it. No, I don't think she'd mind.'

Juliet seems uneasy now. 'OK. Well, maybe we should, then. I'd better get this train.'

'Me too.'

'Will you give my love to all your family?'

'I will. Thank you.'

'And are you going to be all right?'

I find this question difficult to answer. What does she mean? Not in the long run I won't be, no; in the long run, I'm going to end up dead, as we all are. But what does all right amount to in the meantime?

'I'll be fine,' I say. Then the train pulls in, and we get on at different doors, and I guess unless we meet by chance at some mutual friend's wedding sometime, we'll probably not see each other again. Strange how quickly life can change.

I go to my meeting and my boss says he could move me to the company that owns his business, and I could do the same work I already do for them, and make a bit more money. There's a vacancy opened up there, and he knows a lot is changing in my life, and the work might suit me, and could be done remotely most of the time. He could take on a kid to do what I've done, and he'd be doing his boss a favour because he'd be sending them someone good. It's one of those strange, kind-hearted interactions that happen now and then, when you're reminded that the people around you are watching how you're doing, and do want to help you, and do want to make sure you're OK. I always find such concern for my well-being slightly disquieting, but I tell him I'll take the job, and thank him for it. I ask him what I'll have to do there, and he's not certain. More advertorial, certainly. But they sell a lot more stuff than us, he says, they own a lot of different companies. So it'll be all sorts of things, but it's all the same work really. And perhaps I should run a mile from that. But if you can earn enough to live, and leave your work behind at the end of the day, that's not so bad, is it? I head home feeling calm about the future, because I know quite soon there'll be more money coming in.

Amy is on the sofa, watching TV. 'How was it?' she asks me.

'They offered me some work. Good work,' I say.

'That's good. Well done.'

'I saw Juliet on the Underground.'

'Oh really?' Amy shifts on the sofa, turns her body to face me. 'Was that OK?'

'It was fine. I'd felt bad for not getting in touch with her, actually. She got on well with my mum. She sent me a text when Mum died, but I didn't get back to her. I thought she might be upset by it all; I probably should have called.'

'Why didn't you?'

'I don't know. It all felt like the past.'

Amy turns the TV down.

'Did it feel strange to see her?'

'No, it was fine. There's nothing to talk about, it's fine.'

'You sure?' She looks at me. She always knows when I haven't finished talking. Usually better than I do. There is something very finely tuned between us, so we can hear each other when we need to speak.

'I've been feeling bad about the way all that ended,' I say.

'Why?'

'Because I thought it was something to do with her. And it wasn't her, really. I just wasn't happy.'

'And how are you feeling now?' she asks.

'Strange.'

'Why strange?'

'Because I shouldn't be happy, should I? I ought to be grieving. But everything that's happening now is my life. Everything that happened to me before this year, I feel like it was someone else's.'

Amy doesn't say anything to that. She smiles at me, as if she knows better than I do that there's something else I meant to say, and that wasn't quite it, I haven't quite said it. I look at her. I feel as if I'm waking from a dream. It was something else, something to do with love. Whatever that means. That was at the heart of it.

'I was thinking we should try and book a holiday this winter,' she says.

'Yeah?'

'Somewhere hot.' It feels impossible, so soon after getting back from the funeral and as we plan our stepping out of London, to be thinking about going away somewhere again. But Amy has learned to look further ahead than I have.

'Where do you want to go?' I say.

'I don't mind really. Just anywhere hot.'

'I'd like to see Turkey. Turkey and Greece have the best food.'

She checks the weather app on her phone. 'Not hot enough. Sixteen degrees on average in November. What about Bali?'

'I'd rather not fly that far.'

'Where, then?'

I try and remember the advertising I've been subjected to in the last year, seeking to dredge up a place, a name. 'The Azores, maybe? They're off Portugal, I think.'

She checks. 'Still too cold. But what about the Canary Islands?'

We look them up, read about them, look at pictures. All hotels look the same online. The same empty chairs, anonymous spaces. Why are there never any pictures of people? Who wants to stay in an empty hotel? Still, we look them all up.

'I don't know whether we'll be able to afford it,' I say after a while, not wanting to burst the bubble but knowing it has to be said. 'With the house move.'

'I know,' she says. 'I just thought it might be nice to look it all up and see what we'd need. Let's just save the pages maybe,' she continues, 'and come back to this in another month, and see how we're feeling then about money.'

And I say yes, though I know we're not going to find the money we'd need in the next month. But I say yes, because it's good to dream about something.

When I was twenty or twenty-one, I had this feeling that I was swimming in the shallows of the world, and there was a current pulling at me that would carry me into the way the world worked before long, into holidays and tax bills and weekends off and mortgages and pension funds and planning for decrepitude, and that for a moment I had an opportunity not to be caught in that tide, if I just had the intelligence to see some different direction, some different way of living, and strike out on my own into new water, and live clear of the current that took hold of most people's lives and wore them down. But somehow I never found a way. I dreamed of living away from this ordinary world, but the current caught me, and now here we are, and we make do, we fit our vast dreams into these circumscribed rhythms, and we look up holidays online, and make sure we have things to look forward to. But I can still remember the feeling that there must be other ways. There must have been different directions, if only I'd had the wit to see them in time before the current caught me.

Two months pass after the funeral before the call comes. I'm drinking coffee when it happens, staring out the window and thinking about going to the shops for milk because I've just used up the last of what was in the fridge, when I feel the vibration in my pocket, take out my phone to see Chris's name on the screen, and answer, and hear what I'd wondered might be coming.

'Ed, hi.'

'How are you, Chris?'

'I'm fine.'

'You sure? You don't have to be.'

'No, I'm fine. I wanted to talk to you about something, though. You and Rachel, maybe.'

'OK.'

'I won't be too mysterious. I think that I should sell.'

'OK.'

'It's not mine, is it? I just lived here. And keeping it going for you doesn't make sense. You and Rachel aren't going to want it.' He pauses here, lets a silence open up. Even now, at the very last moment, even now he wants to be wrong.

'No, I'm afraid we're not,' I say.

'I thought not. I think you're probably right about that. But it leaves me with a bit of a puzzle.' He pauses again, sounding a little emotional now. 'Of course I could keep it on for your mother. In memory of her. But it seems a little perverse somehow. And I'm knocking seventy, and I don't want to work this hard for ever.'

'No.'

'I could sell it, and take my pension, and buy a place that was easy to keep up, and that would be just fine with me, as long as you two didn't feel let down.'

'Why would we feel let down by that?'

'If you thought it was letting down your mother.'

'Of course not. Of course we wouldn't think that, Chris. We'd want you to be happy.'

'Sure.' Again, he stops speaking. 'Very modern idea, that. Very unhealthy.'

'Happiness?'

'Always running after it. I don't know why people do that, really. It will come and go. It seems a bit perverse to go in search of happiness this year, you know?'

'Of course. I'm sorry.'

'No, sorry; it's coming out wrong. And I appreciate the sentiment. I just don't know whether I understand it.'

'No.'

'Whenever anyone asks me whether I'm happy, I want to cry, really. I don't know how it would ever be possible just to say yes. Which is not to say that I'm an unusually unhappy person.'

'No, you're not.'

'I actually think that I'm quite a happy person. But I also have nights when – well, you know the kind.'

'Yes,' I say, 'I do.'

'But I do appreciate the sentiment; I'm sorry. I don't know why I'm responding so strangely.'

'Should Rachel and I come over sometime soon, so we can all talk about it?'

'I thought that might be good, don't you? Then we could have a dinner and have a few drinks. Tell old stories. You should bring Amy.'

'That would be nice.'

'All right, then. When would work for you?'

'Can I check diaries with Amy and text you?'

'Of course. I'll call Rachel in the meantime.'

Then he said goodbye and rang off, and I sat thinking of him, staring out the window. Thinking how barbaric it was that we had left him alone in that place, how like a cage it must have been for him, what it must have been like there over these last two months for him to have come to this decision so quickly. We should have stayed while he reached this point, at least. I feel ashamed at the thought of him sleeping there alone on that hill where you hear nothing, where the buzzards circle overhead, on that hill where everything is always slowly rotting away. I open my phone again, and text Rachel.

Chris called you?

There's a moment's wait, and then the ellipses of her reply

are pulsing on the screen, and I think of her on the other side of town, sitting like me, staring at her phone like I am.

Yeah. When can you go?
I can probably do this weekend?
OK.
If that works for you?
That's fine for me.

So we go. Amy accompanies me, and Rachel travels with us in the car this time, sitting next to Ivan in the back, a journey we haven't made together in a long while. The sat nav takes us out over Hammersmith flyover, and as we crest the road and start to descend out of the city and into the wide world, the sun strikes all three of us, lighting us up. For a moment the fantasy takes hold in me that this might be a launching-off point into anywhere, into memory, other worlds, into the past. Then the road glides down to ground level again, and we're motoring, the speed limit gradually releasing us, a leash getting longer as we go. We drive for most of Saturday morning, and get to the farm, and Chris has made lunch for us. Just bread rolls and tins of tomato soup. He never did much of the cooking. He stands in the doorway as we get out of the car, and I see that he's burst into tears, and find that I've started crying as well. This man who has been there virtually all of my life. This man who has shaped me as much as anyone else has. Alone now out here, with no one to help him. I wouldn't wish this on him. Wouldn't wish it on anyone. He holds out his hand to me. I give him a hug. We all go inside and Rachel goes straight to the kitchen without asking, makes a pot of tea, and we all see the soup waiting for us in a pan on the hob and imagine the night that Chris must have had, knowing we were coming, wondering what to do. The place looks clean, and I guess that he's hoovered. I guess he's worked all morning so that we can sit down in this place with it feeling uncluttered, and work out what we're going to do with it.

'Thank you so much for coming,' he says, tears still on his face. He wipes at his eyes and seems frustrated. I suppose he didn't want to cry.

'We're really glad to be here,' I say.

Rachel brings the tea through, and we talk about nothing for a little while, Amy doing most of the talking, because she can see that none of us knows what to say. Mum's not here now. She won't be again. We have to work out how to connect with each other now she is missing. And we will work that out, because we have to, for Chris's sake, and for our own, but we don't know yet, so Amy talks about photography, tutoring, the government, anything she can say to fill the air, and I feel grateful, and I guess that we all do, as we smile and nod and feel sheltered for a moment. Then once the pot's emptied and all the tea drunk, Chris leans forward and changes the subject, and it's like opening a door into the night and stepping out into a hailstorm.

'So I think we ought to put this place on the market.'

'OK,' Rachel says. 'I think that's a good plan.'

'But I don't want to sell it if that's not what you want.'

'No,' she says, 'don't think like that. What we want can come later. Right now we want this to be about you. If you don't want to be here any more, we want to sell it.'

'But it will be gone for ever then. You won't get it back.'

'No,' she says, 'we know that. And we won't want it later. We don't think you're selling it from under us.'

'I'm sorry if we made it feel unwelcoming to you.'

'You never made us feel unwelcome. It's just not who we are, Dad, that's all, OK?'

After lunch we look at estate agents' websites together. There's one place that sells most of the houses round this way, so it makes sense just to call them and ask them to come round. Chris speaks to a young woman who arranges for someone to visit on Monday, make a valuation, offer some feedback. Then we call another agent and book them for the same day, so that Chris can have a second opinion.

'I was thinking it would make sense for you to have whatever money we get for it that I don't need,' Chris says.

'Don't be silly,' I say, 'we don't need it now. You should be keeping it for now.'

'But you having it now could help with inheritance tax, and you could buy a home,' Chris carries on.

'And you having it now would mean that you were all right, and we didn't have to worry about you and money.'

Once the estate agents are booked, Chris starts walking round the house, going into the kitchen then the living room to take them in, breathing deeply, clearly emotional. We follow him, not speaking. Rachel takes his hand. I suppose he's been building up to this for some time. I remember he said almost the first instinct he had when Mum first got ill was to go on Zoopla. This place was always going to be too difficult to manage once their strength had gone. And there, in the back yard, the place where my grandfather landed when he fell, the weeds that grow up differently round the flagstones.

This place was always going to be too deep in memory for one person to weather it all on their own. There must be a sense of release to having started, I guess, as I watch Chris watching the garden. It must feel like shrugging off a heavy weight.

'You two ought to think about what you'd like to keep, maybe.' I look around the room at the things that were once the carapace of my childhood.

'Really?'

'I won't need somewhere as big as this. If there are things you want, you should pick them out.'

It's like a fresh grief, to think of taking things back with me. A new breaking up of the world I used to know. But at the same time, I can see that it's inevitable. He is right that we should let some of this go. I stand and stare at all of it. It's just such a big thought, it's hard to take in. There is an old chest by me that Mum used to say had once come from India, carrying my great-grandparents' luggage with them when they travelled to England at the outbreak of the First World War. There is a plate my family have kept fresh fruit on for as long as I've been alive, that came to this house from the woods in West Sussex with us, a decorative ceramic plate, dark and heavy, patterned with broad strokes of rich colour, reds and browns. There is a tall bookcase of old pine where Mum's cookbooks are still stored, all the favourite cookbooks falling apart. Delia Smith. *The Complete Vegetarian*. All of this was part of her once, part of me, part of my becoming someone. How much of it should I be carrying with me into the future? I look around me. I can't take it in.

'Perhaps that's something to work out later,' I say in the end. 'It'll be a while before you sell the farm, I think.'

Chris laughs. 'You've got that right. Farms can take years. It might be years before I can leave here.'

'If it's hard to be here, you could always rent it out to some-one till it's sold, and live somewhere else?'

'No, it's all right. I think that would be stranger.' He turns around to look at us. 'There was something else I wanted to talk about with you while you were all here.' I nod, though my stom-ach drops, because it seems suddenly obvious. I feel certain I know what's coming. 'We ought to talk about scattering her ashes.' It's what I thought he was going to say. I can see Rachel flinching as the thought hits her. I fight the urge to turn away.

'Of course,' I say. 'Do you want to scatter them here?'

'I think that's what she'd have liked, don't you?'

'Unless you wanted to take them with you.'

Chris shakes his head. 'I'm not likely to forget her, am I? But this was her home, this is where she ought to end up. It's just slightly difficult, because once she goes—'

'It'll get harder to come visit her,' Rachel says. Chris nods, saying nothing.

'Not really, though,' I say. 'Not really.'

'Why not?'

'Because it's this valley, isn't it? This whole valley was what she loved. We can just come here, and that would be enough. We don't need to go traipsing through the garden.'

Chris nods at this, and almost seems to be smiling. 'Yes,' he says, 'I guess that's right.'

'Where are they now – they're here now, are they?' Rachel asks, seeming suddenly agitated. I suppose the thought of Mum actually being in the house with us in some way is freaking her out.

'Yes, over there.' Chris points into the corner, and there on the table where Mum used to do her sewing is a little urn I hadn't noticed until now. It's not conspicuous, half in shadow by the sewing machine, in front of the curtain by the French window. The world seems to stop for a moment while we look at it. None of us seem able to breathe.

'Fuck,' says Rachel. We keep on staring.

'Not today, though,' Chris says, 'not just yet. We don't need to scatter them till we go.'

'Sure,' I say.

'Unless you want to.'

'I don't think we'll ever want to. We should do it when we go.'

'Can we go outside for a bit?' Rachel says. 'I feel like I'm going to fall over or something.'

We go outside. I look up at the house. I think of the generations that it's been home to. Mum and Chris, who were happy here. My grandparents, to whom it was a place of grief. Up there on the roof, my grandfather climbed one day and must have looked at the view, which must be very beautiful from so high up, then ended his life and fell back down again. Because he had not had a proper life. Because his mother had been an invalid here, mad and bedbound, in need of constant nursing. And that was what became of him. A parent to his mother. Who had been nursed before that by her mother-in-law. Who had lived here all her life long, raised her child, passed the place on to him. All those lives poured into this one place. All that continuity about to be broken.

Let it break. It seems to me like good news after all that hardship. Let it all go. This place isn't who I am. It's somewhere I came from. I stand staring at it, and Amy takes my hand. She hasn't spoken for a long time. She looks at me now.

'You OK?' she asks me.

'Yes,' I say. 'I'm fine.' And we stand together in the garden.

All of us eat together that night, cooking together with music on loud, George Michael and Sting and Rickie Lee Jones because that's what Mum used to like to listen to. We play their music from Mum's old CDs, not on our phones, a way of having her here with us. None of us speaks about the urn in the sitting room, because after the shock of seeing it for the first time, I don't think any of us thinks of it as her. Mum was always a storyteller, and home always seemed to me to be in the stories, not in this house, not in the world at all, really. So it might be in the stories that we'll find her, if she's anywhere to be found. I remember when I was very young Mum used to say when I was falling asleep, 'I'll meet you in your dreams by the trees in the top field. Walk up to the top field and I'll be there.' Perhaps it's in those stories that she's still waiting.

All of us go to bed too late, then wake hungover the next morning. Chris looks tired, but there is a calm to him that I didn't see when we got here the day before. As if he's breathed out, let go of something.

'Thank you,' he says to us.

'Are you going to be all right?'

'I'll be all right,' he tells us. And I almost believe him. And I hope in time it will be true. After breakfast we pack the car, and then get ready to drive away. The next time I see the farm, I guess there will be a 'For Sale' sign in the driveway. I try to imagine what that will feel like. I suppose it will feel neither good nor bad, but just like letting go. Chris embraces each of us before we get in the car.

'Drive safe, won't you?'

'We'll call when we get home,' I say.

Then we get in the car and drive away.

Amy and I pack boxes, book a removal van, order a sofa for the new house online that's due to arrive in time for Christmas. Then comes moving day. The bell rings in the flat and I go to the door and the van's outside, waiting for our life to be loaded into it, everything we own wrapped up and muffled and sealed inside boxes, ready to disappear into the exhaust fumes and speed of the motorway, bliss of speed like forgetting that sidles along motorways. Three men tramp up and down the stairs to our flat all morning, and slowly the place clears, stripped of personality, of memory, and I realise that for as long as these things are in boxes, the rubble we've used to shore ourselves up in this little eyrie at the edge of the indifferent city, we have no home at all, nowhere and nothing to belong to. Because it's not quite in places. That's not the heart of belonging. It's not in things either, but they are part of it somehow; take away everything you have gathered and called your own and you're left unmoored and damaged staring at the empty living room, the filthy carpet. On my hands and knees I clean black mould from the walls that must have been giving us fever dreams all the time we've been here. I pour bleach straight on to the walls and scrub, and my head aches, and I daren't think of what I'm breathing in and what the mould and bleach are doing to my lungs. Then the back of the van is closed and all the objects we love enough to take with us to the next place are packed away and out of sight and don't give off any meaning any more. They're only a stacked van, shut up and leaving, driving away from us into the future. It dawns on me that every removal van you see is loaded with the same dense and potent meaning I can see in the retreating form of our van, what I think of as our van because our lives are crammed inside it – every one of them is always filled up with the lives of people, all the hopes of people, all the dreams they have that aren't going to come true.

After the van has gone we hoover the rooms and check the flat one last time, and the place feels haunted and absent, as if it has already forgotten us. Perhaps it's us that have been haunting the place all along. We load the house plants and Ivan last of all into the car and then head west, through the grim streets and industrial units, past the scaffolders and run-down pubs, through the angry traffic and over the tram lines till we get to the open roads and accelerate, away from the nightmare of our youth spent trapped in this place, away from the cramped compromise of living in the city, towards a future we haven't yet written.

We get to the new house after an hour's drive and find the removal men waiting in a layby, eating fish and chips from the shop across the way. We open up the house and they start to take the boxes of our life inside and stack them in the rooms. I join in, carrying the boxes through the front door while Amy takes Ivan out into the garden. It should feel like a beginning, these boxes filling up the house, but there's a sense of loss to it as well, I find. To love is to want to keep everything, not to miss anything, to live in grief at the thought of someday saying goodbye, until everything, every action, becomes a farewell. After the van has been emptied and the three men who got us to this new place have gone, we spend two days unboxing our possessions.

The house has seven rooms. The first when you come in through the small hallway is the living room, which faces north. There is a wood-burning stove in the hearth and bookcases built into the alcoves on either side of the chimney. Through a door at the back of the room you enter the dining room, and beyond that is the kitchen and the bathroom and the garden. The front of the house was built in 1880, but the bathroom is an extension, added only thirty or forty years ago. The garden is a bare vegetable patch where I won't grow anything because the dog would only dig it up again. I will sow grass seed and plant apple trees there instead, a russet and a James Grieve, and have an orchard of my own.

In the dining room, the staircase to the first floor is boxed off by wooden panels that date from the time of the house's construction. Climb them, twisting once as you go, and you will find three more rooms: the main bedroom at the front of the house where the traffic whispers past; the spare bedroom at the back of the house; and then another, strange room that narrows towards the back window like the prow of a ship and which I will turn into a study. From that window there is a view of hills stretching fifteen, twenty miles away, into the blue of distance. An olive tree in the next garden rising up above the vines that shelter the neighbours' patio. Telegraph wires looping away from view to join up the dots of the world. It is a far cry from the place we've left, the living room, one bedroom, kitchen and bathroom and the back stairs down to the garden and the garden shed. By coming to this place, changing the landscape around me, I feel almost as if I will become a different person.

After the removal van has gone, and the house is secure, and the dog's fed and watered, Amy gets back in the car with me. I've told her about my superstition, about always going back one last time to check the house we've left. We strap Ivan into the back of the car and drive back into the city, into the suburb where we used to live, up the road that's already forgotten us. I get out of the car and take the house key from my pocket, and Amy and I walk up to the front door that used to be ours. I start to put the key in the lock to open the door, and then check myself. Take the key back out. Turn back to Amy.

'We didn't leave anything, did we?'

'No,' she says. 'We didn't.'

'I might just post the key, then,' I say. She looks at me quizzically, wondering why I've changed my mind.

'Yeah?'

'We don't need to go back in, do we? We could just go home instead.'

So I post the key through the letterbox, and we walk away, because people are made out of stories, the ones that led to them and the ones they tell, and I don't have to live looking over my shoulder. I could try and tell a story about what happens next, see what that changes.

Next morning we wake up in the new house, everything beautiful and strange, everything a chaos of unpacked boxes, and we eat breakfast, then walk Ivan in the big park that separates our new village from the nearest town. We walk down gravel roads away from our house, past the church and the village hall and the working men's club, then over the cricket green till we come to the mouth of the park. My mum's not here in the world any more. But we're still here for a little while longer. Ivan runs away from us into the oak woods, and we follow him, down holloways that have carried people for almost a thousand years through this place to their squatters' homes or to work at the gravel pits that used to be beyond our cottage, that have now been built over by the council and turned into flats. Magpies chatter in an alder tree; two rooks are trying to get at their young. We come to the first of the streams that tiger-stripe the park, and cross the footbridge, the water running under. As we pass out of the tree cover into an open field, a deer bolts, sudden and startling, from the hedgerows, dashing past us towards the next stand of oak. Ivan hares after her before we can stop him, pitched headlong in a race he'll never win, vanishing away from us as we both call his name. We hurry after him along the path that bisects the field, two more visitors drawn through this place, caught in currents that will become our lives.

Acknowledgements

I would like to thank Suzanne Bridson, Kate Parker, Kirsty Dunseath, Kate Samano, Bobby Mostyn-Owen and everyone at Transworld who supported this work; Caroline Michel and the team at Peters, Fraser and Dunlop; my family, who I have borrowed from to tell this story; Lamorna Ash, George Duncan-Jones, Aidan Grounds, Beth Lawson, George Spender, Jonathan Webb, Laura Williams and her colleagues at Greene and Heaton, Lydia Wilson, and Charlie Young.

I wish the dedicatee of this novel, Sophie Christopher, was here to read it. Her death in 2019 was a huge blow to everyone whose life was made richer and happier by knowing her. She was the most brilliant colleague I have had the privilege of working with, and the most steadfast friend through an extraordinarily difficult period in my life. I count myself incredibly fortunate that books afforded me the opportunity to meet her. I choose to remember her by the unbelievably characteristic last thing she tweeted:

'Joy!'

Barney Norris has been the recipient of the International Theatre Institute's Award for Excellence, the Critics' Circle Award for Most Promising Playwright, a South Bank Sky Arts Times Breakthrough Award, an *Evening Standard* Progress 1000 Award, a Betty Trask Award and the Northern Ireland One Book Award. His work has been translated into eight languages. He is a Fellow of the Royal Society of Literature, teaches Creative Writing at the University of Oxford, where he is the Martin Esslin Playwright in Residence at Keble College, and regularly reviews fiction for the *Guardian*.